Handbook of Vitreoretinal Surgery

Vitreoretinal (VR) surgery has steadily evolved over the years and this handbook provides a comprehensive overview about its past, present and future. It covers a wide array of topics ranging from its fascinating origins to recent technological advances, from surface anatomy to their clinical relevance, from anaesthesia to building and maintenance of operation theatre, from major surgical steps to sub-steps, from preventing to managing complications, and from routine surgeries to rare surgeries. Included in addition is a section on futuristic surgeries and another on important studies in relation to vitreoretinal surgery. Hence, **Handbook of Vitreoretinal Surgery** serves as a ready reference for both fledgling and experienced VR surgeons.

KEY FEATURES

- Includes recent developments like 3D surgery, telescopic IOL, bionic implants, and robotic surgery.
- Highlights the importance of surface anatomy and provides a deeper view into the working of vitreous machines, microscopes, and other surgical components.
- Text is supported with videos of rare surgeries like endoillumination-assisted scleral buckling surgery, placement of retisert intravitreal implant, suprachoroidal drug injection, intralesional injection into a subretinal abscess, and endoillumination-assisted biopsy of intraocular mass lesions.

Handbook of Vitreoretinal Surgery

Pradeep Venkatesh MD, DNB
Professor of Ophthalmology,
All India Institute of Medical Sciences [AIIMS],
New Delhi, India

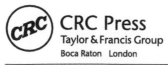

CRC Press
Taylor & Francis Group
Boca Raton   London

CRC Press is an imprint of the
Taylor & Francis Group, an **informa** business

First edition published 2023
by CRC Press
6000 Broken Sound Parkway NW, Suite 300, Boca Raton, FL 33487–2742

and by CRC Press
4 Park Square, Milton Park, Abingdon, Oxon, OX14 4RN

CRC Press is an imprint of Taylor & Francis Group, LLC

© 2023 Pradeep Venkatesh

Library of Congress Cataloging-in-Publication Data
Names: Venkatesh, Pradeep, author.
Title: Handbook of vitreoretinal surgery / by Pradeep Venkatesh.
Description: First edition. | Boca Raton, FL : CRC Press, 2022. | Includes bibliographical references and index. | Summary: "Vitreo-retinal (VR) surgery has steadily evolved over the years and this handbook provides a concise and focused approach to its past, present and future. It discusses the setting up of a VR operating theatre, viewing systems and highlights the utility of a particular surgical step/ misstep"—Provided by publisher.
Identifiers: LCCN 2022015565 (print) | LCCN 2022015566 (ebook) | ISBN 9781032016191 (paperback) | ISBN 9781032016221 (hardback) | ISBN 9781003179320 (ebook)
Subjects: MESH: Vitreoretinal Surgery | Retinal Diseases—surgery | Retina—surgery | Vitreous Body—surgery
Classification: LCC RE551 (print) | LCC RE551 (ebook) | NLM WW 270 | DDC 617.7/35059—dc23/eng/20220412
LC record available at https://lccn.loc.gov/2022015565
LC ebook record available at https://lccn.loc.gov/2022015566

ISBN: 978-1-032-01622-1 (hbk)
ISBN: 978-1-032-01619-1 (pbk)
ISBN: 978-1-003-17932-0 (ebk)

DOI: 10.1201/9781003179320

Typeset in Times
by Apex CoVantage, LLC

Access the Support Material: www.routledge.com/9781032016191

To
HKT [my beloved teacher]
&
Ron J. Michels [an inspiration]

Contents

Videos and Legends

Foreword

Vitreo retinal surgery is an ever-changing speciality that is heavily dependent on technology in addition to the skill of the surgeon. While it is one's own experience ultimately that stands in one's good stead, textbooks serve an important role in the formative years of a vitreo retinal surgeon as well as for the more experienced surgeon. With the ready access to the internet and the plethora of publications available, it is easy to discount the role of textbooks. However, one should realise that the textbooks contain distilled information from the diverse material that is available. The author carefully weighs the evidence and includes selected information that in the opinion of the author is the most acceptable and useful. Hence the experience of the author is intricately woven into the textbook.

Prof Pradeep Venkatesh is a widely respected vitreo retinal surgeon from a premier institute in the country and has years of immense experience in all facets of vitreo retinal practice- medical and surgical. He has used his enormous experience to bring out a 'Handbook of vitreo retinal surgery' for the benefit of the vitreo retinal fraternity.

Handbook - as the very term indicates - is like quick reference. It should not be too verbose but should contain all the relevant information in a very condensed format - a no mean task for the author. Prof. Pradeep should be congratulated for the excellent effort he put into making this handbook extremely readable and informative. It is well structured. The introductory chapter pays obeisance to the masters who are responsible for the creation and propagation of this specialty. This is followed by a thoughtful chapter on training in vitreo retinal surgery with discussion on the role of surgical simulators. Very rightfully, Prof Pradeep dwells significantly on the preoperative evaluation, anaesthesia, operation theatre design, surgical anatomy and instrumentation. As was alluded to earlier, technology is very important in the practice of vitreo retinal surgery. Understanding the mechanics of the vitrectomy machine and various other accessories is very vital for the smooth conduct of vitreo retinal surgeries. Prof Pradeep devotes a significant number of pages on this important area introducing us to the latest in the technology.

The surgery itself is well illustrated and lucid in the presentation. After describing in general the various steps of vitreo retinal surgery, the subsequent chapters elaborate the techniques specific to important conditions for which vitreo retinal surgery is commonly performed. These again are well illustrated. There is detailed description of the nuances of membrane surgery in diabetic retinopathy, PVR etc. Most important conditions including macular disorders, endophthalmitis, paediatric retinal detachments etc have been covered. Relatively rare indications for vitreous surgery have also been covered in a separate chapter. The last few chapters deal with important studies that guided the present day vitreo retinal practice and a prediction of how the future of vitreous surgery is likely to be.

Prof Pradeep has packed a lot of information in this handbook to make it an excellent handbook. While it benefits the budding vitreo retinal surgeon most, it has enough material for use by even experienced surgeons.

I deem it a great honour to have been asked to write this foreword for an important contribution to ophthalmic literature in the field of vitreo retinal surgery.

Best regards,
Dr Lingam Gopal MS, DNBE, FRCS, MSc (epidemiology), FAMS
Senior consultant, Medical Research Foundation, Sankara Nethralaya, Chennai, India
Senior consultant, National University Hospital, Singapore
Associate professor, National University of Singapore, Singapore

Preface

Vitreoretinal surgery has steadily evolved over the past three decades. Unlike in recent times, support from advanced technology to perform a surgical procedure was rarely available to surgeons. Despite this, satisfactory visual outcomes were achieved. This was made possible by adhering diligently and patiently to every guideline and recommendation made by pioneers in the field of surgical retina such as Dr. Charles Schepens, Dr. Ernst Custodis, Dr. Harvey Lincoff, Dr. Paul Cibis, Dr. Robert Machemer, Dr. Steve Charles, Dr. Ron Michels, and many more. The advantages, disadvantages, limitations, and outcomes of surgery for retinal disorders like simple and complex retinal detachment, diabetic vitreous surgery, and macular hole surgery were evaluated through unbiased, randomized studies. These provided guiding principles and a benchmark for most retinal surgeons. Currently, improvements in technology have enhanced the overall safety and ease of carrying out some surgical steps. However, the foundations, components, and principles of managing a patient with vitreoretinal pathology remain the same. Also, the future belongs to the young residents in training today, a future wherein procedures like robotic surgery, bionic eye surgery, Argus-like implants, precision surgery, retinal vascular surgery, gene therapy, and molecular therapy would be carried out as routine procedures. It is useful to keep abreast on these developments, so a brief overview on these approaches has also been highlighted.

In *Handbook of Vitreoretinal Surgery*, an effort has been made to incorporate varied approaches that have been reported and to highlight their advantages and limitations. An effort has also been made to subdivide each surgical approach into multiple smaller steps, with a detailed description of each step. Repetition of the surgical steps during the description of specific surgeries has been avoided when it is not very different from the standard approach. It is, however, emphasized that repetition enables better understanding, decision making, and implementation of surgical steps, and so the reader must refer to these steps in specific sections, as and when necessary. Reproducibility of well-established guiding principles and attention to small details hold the key to achieving maximal success and with minimal iatrogenic complications. It is hoped that this book will help readers achieve this objective in all their surgical endeavours. Being concise and up to date on the past, present, and future of vitreoretinal surgery, this book is expected to serve as a tabletop assistant to both fledgling and experienced surgeons in the field of vitreoretina.

In this compilation, an attempt has been made to amalgamate my experience of performing more than 5000 surgeries in over two and a half decades, assisting and observing many more thousands of surgeries, reading a dozen outstanding books on vitreoretina and hundreds of related manuscripts, and the opportunity, as co-investigator, to undertake procedures such as Retisert implantation, Iluvien implantation, and suprachoroidal drug delivery. This experience includes being a witness to the evolution from limbal ring localization and removal of retained intraocular foreign body [RIOFB] using giant electromagnets, use of 20G surgery with cut rates of just 1000/minute to 2500/minute to the current standard, 25G surgery with cut rates from 5000 to 10,000 cuts/minute, using the most advanced visualization platforms such as Ngenuity and vitrectomy systems [e.g., the Constellation and EVA]. The figures and animations are amateurish because they have been created by the author, and for this I hope to be excused. Readers are requested to kindly provide a feedback on any possible errors that may be evident and also suggestions that could be incorporated into future editions.

Acknowledgements

I would like to express my immense gratitude to my teachers Prof. VK Dada, Prof S. Ghose, Dr. Vajpayee RB, and Dr. Ramanjit Sihota, who provided me with the initial impetus, motivation, support and opportunities and to my mentors in the field of vitreoretinal surgery, Dr. Lalit Verma, Dr. Atul Kumar, Prof. Satpal Garg, Dr. Dinesh Talwar and Prof. Yograj Sharma.

I would be non-existential without the love, care and freedom given to me by my parents, L and V; and the shield provided by Pras and Praps. To Ng, I shall always remain indebted and to Chinnu, I shall always look up for sunshine.

I would also like to thank Shivangi Pramanik and Himani Dwivedi at CRC Press for their guidance, assistance, and patience throughout the course of creating this handbook. Without their support and gentle prodding, it would have been difficult to take the book to completion.

I would like to acknowledge the efforts made by March Hecht at Taylor and Francis, and Ganesh Pawan Kumar Agoor, at Apex CoVantage, towards the overall production of this book.

About the Author

Dr. Pradeep Venkatesh MD, DNB is Professor of Ophthalmology at the All India Institute of Medical Sciences [AIIMS], New Delhi. He has been practising medical and surgical management of retinal disorders for the past 25 years and has performed about 5000 surgeries over this period. His areas of expertise include management of retinal detachment and advanced diabetic retinopathy. He has been a co-investigator in several multicentric trials, including those involving sustained drug delivery systems such as Retisert, Iluvien, Posurdex, and suprachoroidal injections. His PubMed indexed publications are over 250 and include those on endoillumination- [chandelier-] assisted scleral buckling surgery, endoillumination-assisted biopsy of intraocular mass lesions, posterior vitreous wick syndrome, the role of ultrasound biomicroscopy to detect status of peripheral retina in opaque silicone filled eyes, small-gauge endoresection of choroidal melanoma, concept for inflatable drug delivery device and a simple means of harvesting peeled internal limiting membrane for laboratory studies. In the past, he has edited/authored books on fluorescein angiography, optical coherence tomography, retinal imaging, and the eye in systemic disorders.

Introduction

Life is all about learning, and vitreoretinal surgery is no different. The objectives of the two are also no different — to do the little good you can in improving the quality of living for someone in need. Learning is in itself very fascinating as there is no end to it, and there is always something to explore and to understand. Learning has many phases and forms: learning that occurs as a natural instinct, as seen during our early years of growth, learning from curiosity and sense of wonder, learning that is formal and aimed at providing us with the basic foundations on which to build further, learning that is driven by challenge and competition, learning that comes from simply spending time with elders and mentors with years of experience, and learning that results from reading the masterly work of pioneers. The strongest form of learning, however, results from self-motivation and a sense of restlessness to understand better and do things better than yesterday.

The tools or sources for learning in life or in vitreoretinal surgery also share a common thread and include stories from the past, reading and watching classics created by masters in their field, daily happenings in the present, a keen sense of observation, arduous efforts, infinite hours of practice, and experimentation [with new approaches, based on current understanding and situation]. It is hoped that the 12 sections in this book will complement the desire of vitreoretinal surgeons to keep abreast and achieve the best for their patients.

Being aware of the pioneers who made this journey possible, from a situation of not being able to provide any solution to one wherein surgical intervention enables restoration or maintenance of vision, is in itself a stupendous learning experience, and this is covered in the first chapter. Some useful resources, including a simulator, that can make a significant contribution to further the growth of fellows training in vitreoretinal surgery is covered in the next chapter. Investigations, when chosen and applied well, could have a major impact on the decision-making process, surgical plan, prognostication, patient counselling, and postoperative secondary interventions, and this aspect is discussed in Chapter 3. This is followed by a discussion on anaesthesia, which is critical to increasing the safety and efficiency of the surgery. Within a hospital, the operation theatre is the most sacred region for both the surgeon and the patient. Maintaining the sanctity of this zone is crucial for the translation of our endeavors into successful restoration of human function, and this is covered in Chapter 5.

It is necessary for vitreoretinal surgeons to be aware of certain recognized surface landmarks, anatomical dimensions, distances, and so on, to implement the surgical steps accurately. These are covered in the section on surgical anatomy. Although the microcircuitry of advanced vitreous machines is complex and difficult to comprehend, it is necessary for surgeons to become familiar with their various modes of operation and their advantages and limitations. This is covered in Chapter 7. It is imperative for the ocular volume to be replaced with biologically compatible substances, either liquids or gases, after vitreous humor has been removed at surgery. The choice of vitreous substitute depends on the preoperative pathology, intraoperative considerations, and the intended purpose and duration of action, and this aspect in discussed in the following chapter in addition to the use of specific dyes to enhance tissue visualization at surgery. The subsequent chapters [9–12] provide a description of the surgical approaches, surgical steps, common and rare surgeries performed, and the complications that could occur. A summary of randomized studies, systematic reviews, and metanalyses relevant to vitreoretinal surgery is provided in the next chapter. The last chapter is dedicated to surgical approaches that vitreoretinal surgeons are likely to perform frequently in the years to come.

DOI: 10.1201/9781003179320-1

1 Milestones and Pioneers

The first step towards tackling retinal problems through surgery, in a logical and systematic manner, was taken by **Jules Gonin** [Figure 1.1]. He was the first to propound that retinal detachment was caused by a tear in the neurosensory retina and that surgical closure of these would result in successful reattachment of the retina. His approach of search a break, seek a break, and seal a break [3S] still remains the cornerstone of retinal detachment surgery. It is ironic that it took more than a decade for his views to become widely accepted. It soon became established that retinal detachment could be successfully repaired by accurate localization of the retinal tear, external drainage of accumulated subretinal fluid, induction of sterile inflammation around the region of the tear, and then supporting the tear externally by an encircling element. Some of the methods used to achieve sterile inflammation were ignipuncture and chemical cautery. The first description of using an external support was made by **Jess** [1937] in Germany [a gauze pad was used as a temporary indent]. Scleral buckling using an episcleral implant was first conducted by **Custodis** [1949]. He was also instrumental in introducing Polyviol as an explant material [1953] and later for the concept of non-drainage retinal detachment surgery.

However, a major limitation for the concept to gain traction was the inability to visualize the peripheral retina and locate the retinal tear(s), owing to the narrow field of view provided by available ophthalmoscopes. The problem of difficulty in visualization of the retinal periphery, wherein most retinal breaks are located, was solved with the pioneering work of **Charles Schepens**, who introduced the binocular indirect ophthalmoscope [1947] and propagated the application of contact fundus biomicroscopy. In addition, it was realized that materials such as Polyviol, used for indenting the sclera, were not optimal and were themselves causing tissue damage. So, Schepens initially used polyethylene tubing [1957] as a material for providing external support. Initially, the support was only to the region of the tear and for a clock hour on either side. The barricade with polyethylene was called a *scleral buckle*. But failures were observed because of leak across anterior part of the tear. To overcome this anterior leak, the buckle was extended to 180 degrees and thereafter to 360 degrees, thereby introducing the concept of encirclage [1957]. When this failed to reduce the leakage, it was decided to increase the width of the scleral buckle. However, the concept of encirclage has remained because it may retain the height and position of the buckle and counter tractional forces from the anterior vitreous. To anchor the external plombage, partial-thickness tunnels were made in the sclera. A year later, **Arruga** [1958] reported using Supramid, Mersilene, and nylon sutures instead of polyethylene tubing. Silicone was first used by **Girard** [1959] for scleral indentation [as a rod made of silicone rubber]. It was again Schepens and his team who first reported the use of solid silicone as buckling material [1960]. They developed several designs of buckle, some of which are still being used. **Lincoff Harvey** [1965] and his team used silicone sponge to treat large breaks, and these were in use until the late 1990s. With advances in vitreoretinal surgery, large tears and radial tears are now better managed with an internal approach, so silicone sponges have lost their importance. Major disadvantages of silicone sponge were the high risk of infection because of the air pockets and extrusion. Hydrogel buckle [1972] and expandable silicone [1973] were described by **Grignolo** and **Banuelos**, respectively. Two types of balloon implants have been used in the past: permanent and temporary. The first permanent [sutured] balloon implant to support the macula was reported by **Hoepping** as early as 1969. Currently, macular buckling seems to be regaining attention for management of macular pathologies in patients with high myopia. Use of a temporary [sutureless] balloon buckle was tried by Lincoff in 1979.

Methods to induce sterile inflammation around the retinal tear have included thermal cautery [ignipuncture, Gonin, 1930], chemical cautery using potassium hydroxide sticks [**Guist**, 1931;

DOI: 10.1201/9781003179320-2

RD Surgery: Time-line

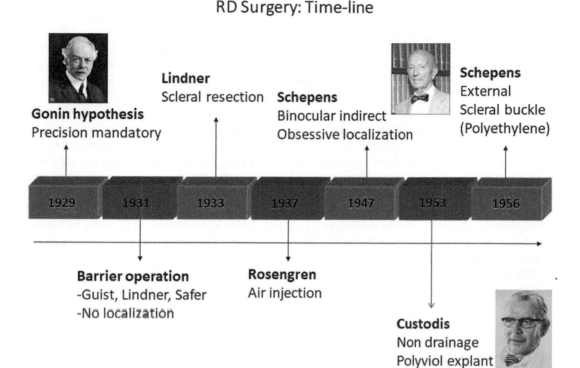

FIGURE 1.1 Timeline in the evolution of retinal detachment surgery.

Lindner, 1931], electro-diathermy [**Safar,** 1931], and diathermy electrode. Multiple diathermy burns were applied to the bed of a partial-thickness scleral flap created over the location of the tear. After a series of explant related infections, Lincoff undertook some experimental studies, which revealed that the cause of infections was not directly related to the silicone sponge but to diathermy. He established that diathermy had a tissue-destroying effect and often caused scleral necrosis with its associated complications. Subsequently, curious about the carbon dioxide probe being used by his dermatologist, Lincoff introduced **cryotherapy** [see section on cryotherapy] as a method for inducing sterile inflammation during retinal detachment surgery. However, CO_2 was not conducive for use within the orbital spaces. So, Lincoff and **Mclean** modified a nitrous oxide cryoprobe being used by neurosurgeons and applied it to retinal detachment procedures [1964]. Very soon cryopexy replaced diathermy and became the method of choice to induce retinopexy. Unlike diathermy, cryotherapy had no damaging effect on the scleral fibres and could also be safely applied across an extraocular muscle, with no lasting complication. Lincoff also introduced silicone buckle as a better alternative to Polyviol. These landmark contributions significantly reduced the complications of retinal detachment surgery. Lincoff was also instrumental in throwing light on the pioneering work of Custodis, in successfully treating retinal detachment without external drainage of subretinal fluid [non-drainage surgery]. Having spent time with Custodis in his clinic and noticing the successful outcomes, Lincoff introduced non-drainage surgery into his own practice in New York. Until then, external drainage of subretinal fluid through a scleral cutdown was routinely practiced despite some serious adverse effects that could result. In the course of analyzing the first 1000 cases of retinal detachment treated using silicone buckle and cryopexy, Lincoff and **Gieser** provided guidelines for preoperative localization of the retinal break based on configuration of the retinal detachment [**Lincoff's rule,** 1971].

Despite high success rates [90%] with this procedure, failures were noted at a higher rate in patients with large tears. It was observed by **Norton** [1973] that the reason for this was leakage through radial folds that developed along the posterior margin of large tears following surgery with a segmental buckle. To counter the radial folds, he suggested injection of air into the vitreous cavity, thus reviving an approach that was first reported by **Rosengren** [1938] several decades earlier. The short half-life of air within the vitreous cavity was a limitation, so efforts were made to seek inert and biologically compatible gases with longer duration of action. The half-life of a gas within the eye was identified to be related to their solubility. This led to evaluation with short-chain perfluorocarbon gases on the suggestion of a chemical engineer, **Andrew Lincoff** [1984]. In the next few years, after the introduction of perfluorocarbon gases to salvage some failures following scleral buckle, **Hilton and Grizzard** [1986] described a new approach for primary management of simple retinal detachments. This technique, termed *pneumatic retinopexy* by the authors, continues to polarize retina surgeons about its utility, even to this day. The concept of using iso-expansile mixture of perfluorocarbon gases as vitreous substitutes at the end of surgery was introduced by **Gary Abrams**. Evaluation with long-chain perfluorocarbons [which are liquids] began soon after the work on perfluorocarbon gases. Heavy liquids were, however, approved only later for use as an intraoperative adjunct to achieve temporary tamponade following evaluation of its utility by **Chang Stanley,** Lincoff, and colleagues [1989]. **Haidt** had, however, used perfluorocarbon liquid with vitreous surgery much earlier in 1982.

While these approaches to managing retinal detachment from an external route were in progress, some other pioneers were working on solving severe visual problems resulting from conditions such as non-resolving vitreous haemorrhage. Until about half a century ago, it was firmly believed that the vitreous contributes to the structural integrity of the eye, and its removal would result in permanent damage. Owing to serendipity, however, **David Kasner** [1969], while conducting experimental work on cadaver eyes in his garage, noted that vitreous could be removed using forceps and scissors. He soon applied this technique to the removal of vitreous that prolapsed out of the posterior chamber during intracapsular cataract surgery [calling it *radical anterior vitrectomy*]. He then realized that vitreous removal may also be helpful in patients with significant opacities in the vitreous, so he went on to undertake this procedure in two patients, one with vitreous amyloidosis and the other with vitreous haemorrhage. This approach, which he called *open sky vitrectomy*, involved making a 300-degree limbal section and flipping over the cornea before dissecting the vitreous. Significant improvement was noted in patients following open sky vitrectomy. David Kasner taught cataract surgery to residents at the Bascom Palmer Eye Institute and lectured about his research findings, including the outcomes on patients with vitreous opacification. During one such meeting, **Robert Machemer** [1971], a faculty member at the same institute, was intrigued by the ability of the eye to tolerate significant removal of the vitreous without resulting in serious damage. Following a few visits to Kasner's garage to observe his research work on vitreous removal, Machemer conceptualized the idea of removing the vitreous through a closed approach using a rotatory, motorized cutter. Then, Machemer along with his colleague, Buettner, and an instrument design expert, Parel, developed multiple prototypes of a motorized vitreous cutter. Initial experiments were conducted on eggs and involved removing the white without damaging the yolk or shell, using the innovative device introduced through a hole in the shell. The final version of this came to be known as VISC [vitreous infusion suction cutter] because it performed multiple functions of infusing fluid into the vitreous cavity, cutting of the vitreous fibrils and aspirating the fragments out of the eye [Figure 1.2]. This probe had an external diameter of 2.3 mm and a single 17G port [1.5 mm] and hence needed a large scleral incision [Video 1.1]. Infusion of fluid was driven by gravity, and suction was provided by manual aspiration through a syringe; only the cutting was motorized. The initial vitrector was prone to cause winding of the vitreous fibrils and was soon replaced by an oscillatory vitrector [Roto Extractor]. **Parel**, a colleague of Machemer, was not only involved in the designing of VISC but also introduced fiberoptic endoillumination. Unknown to Machemer, **Anton Banko** is said to have patented a vitreous cutter prior to the VISC. In the very subsequent years, **O'Malley** and **Heintz** [1975] demonstrated the concept and superiority of vitrectomy using divided function 20G [0.9-mm] instrumentation, with separate pars plana opening for infusion, vitreous cutter [with aspiration], and endoillumination. They also introduced the first pneumatically driven vitreous cutter

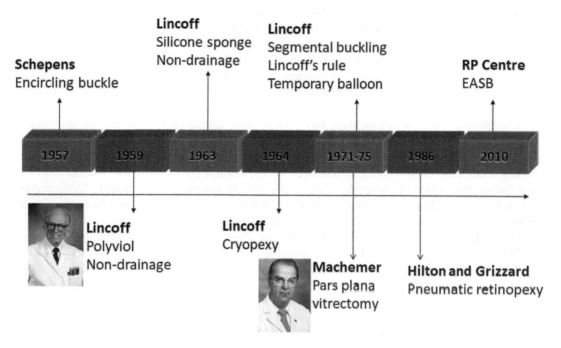

RD Surgery: Time-line

Lincoff
Silicone sponge
Non-drainage

Lincoff
Segmental buckling
Lincoff's rule
Temporary balloon

Schepens
Encircling buckle

RP Centre
EASB

1957 1959 1963 1964 1971-75 1986 2010

Lincoff
Polyviol
Non-drainage

Lincoff
Cryopexy

Machemer
Pars plana
vitrectomy

Hilton and Grizzard
Pneumatic retinopexy

FIGURE 1.2 Timeline in the evolution of retinal detachment surgery. EASB, endoillumination-assisted scleral buckling.

and active extrusion [by aspiration] through a foot pedal–controlled console system [Ocutome 800]. The first electric solenoid driven axial [guillotine] vitreous cutter was developed by **Gholam Peyman**. It is necessary to indicate here that both open sky vitrectomy and vitrectomy using a vitrector seem to have been reported a few years earlier in the **Japanese literature**. Ever since these developments, three port pars plana approach has become the accepted norm for vitreoretinal surgery.

A major shift in the drainage of subretinal fluid, from an external, transscleral route to an internal, transretinal route [by simultaneous air-fluid exchange] was introduced by **Steve Charles**, who went on to make several other immense contributions to vitreoretinal surgery, including endophotocoagulation, flute needle, power silicone injector, end-grasping forceps, diamond-coated membrane-peeling forceps, scissors segmentation, proportional or linear foot pedal control, xenon light source, servo-controlled intraocular pressure, proportional diathermy, the concept of system integration of all functions of the vitrectomy machine, no spring-dual actuation vitreous cutter, and so on. **McEwen** introduced the automated air pump to facilitate air-fluid exchange in a controlled manner [replacing the previous syringe-based method]. Retinectomy and submacular surgery were pioneered independently by both Machemer and Charles. For peeling of epiretinal membranes, Machemer used a bent pick, while O'Malley used a membrane pick [blunt margins], and Charles used end-grasping forceps. **Yasuo Tano** introduced the diamond-dusted membrane scraper. Chang, other than introducing perfluorocarbon liquid, also developed the dual-function, end-aspirating laser probe. Charles, along with **Carl Yang**, introduced the first 20G disposable, pneumatic guillotine cutter.

Further developments have revolved around adopting advancements in technology and material sciences to refine the functioning, precision, and control of vitreous machines as well as intravitreal instruments. Some of these developments include the introduction of first 25G [0.5 mm] by **Eugene de Juan** [1990] and colleagues, 23G surgery by **Hilton** [2002] and **Klaus Eckhardt** [2005], and 27G surgery by **Oshima** et al [2007]. The initial 25G system introduced by de Juan and **Hickinbotham** [first to describe a trocar cannula system] needed to be sutured. In 2002, **Fujii** and de Juan developed the first transconjunctival sutureless vitrectomy [TSV25] system. With the introduction of micro-incisional or small-gauge vitreous surgery, patient comfort and safety have significantly improved, and surgical time has substantially reduced, so much so that 20G vitreous surgeries have become rapidly relegated to the past. Improvements in the field of view of visualization lenses, including noncontact binocular indirect ophthalmic microscope by **Manfred Spitznas** and contact system [Advanced Visual Instruments] with stereo inverter by Stanley Chang, have also contributed to making vitreoretinal surgery safer by providing a panoramic view of the surgical field.

In addition to these advances, there has been a steady endeavor by vitreoretinal surgeons to extend the scope of retinal diseases in which surgery may be helpful. These conditions include conventional macular hole surgery by **Kelly and Wendal** [1991], macular hole surgery with internal limiting membrane [ILM] peeling by **Yooh** [1996] and Eckardt [1997], modified macular hole surgery [large, chronic] by **Michalewska** [2010], optic disc pit maculopathy by **Bakri** [2004], myopic foveoschisis by **Benhamou** [2002] and **Kishi** [2003], vitreomacular traction, resection of intraocular tumours, and so on. Some others have contributed by describing approaches that improve the safety of a procedure [e.g., use of triamcinolone, by Gholam Peyman and colleagues to improve visualization of the vitreous, indocyanine green staining for ILM peeling by **Burk** (2000) and **Kodononsono** (2000), and Trypan blue staining by **Perrier** (2003)]. More recent advances such as intraoperative optical coherence tomography and heads-up vitrectomy, have added a new dimension to vitreous surgery, one that may enable surgeons to perform procedures such as submacular delivery of therapeutic agents and endovascular injections with precision and safety. Heads-up vitrectomy was first pioneered by **Riemann** et al, and the first clinical publication using TrueVision visualization technology, was by Eckardt and Paulo in 2016.

But, what about the history of silicone oil? Industrial silicone oil had been available for long, much before vitreous surgery was described, and animal studies had shown that it was relatively well tolerated in the vitreous cavity as early as the 1950s. **Paul Cibis** [1962], considered as a gifted surgeon, was drawn to these reports, and following his own studies on animal eyes, began using silicone oil injection [while operating using an indirect ophthalmoscope] in patients with vitreous retraction [currently termed *proliferative vitreoretinopathy*] and giant tears [institutional approval was not mandatory during those times]. So, silicone oil was used almost 10 years before the advent of vitrectomy. Although silicone oil was ideal as long-term tamponade after vitrectomy, it went into disrepute owing to multiple reasons [including the untimely demise of Cibis]. Silicone oil injection after pars plana vitrectomy was first performed by **Jean Haut**. It was revived and is currently accepted as a standard vitreous substitute following surgery for complicated retinal detachment because of the quiet persistence of his colleague **Okun** in the United States and later by **John Scott** at Moorfield's in the United Kingdom.

SUGGESTED READING

1. Lincoff H, Kreissig I [2000]. Changing patterns in the surgery for retinal detachment: 1929 to 2000. *Klin Monbl Augenheilkd.* 216(6): 352–359.
2. Machemer R [1995]. The development of pars plana vitrectomy: A personal account. *Graefes Arch Clin Exp Ophthalmol.* 233(8): 453–468.
3. O'Malley C, Heintz R [1975]. Vitrectomy with an alternative instrument system. *Ann Ophthalmol.* 7(4): 585–594.
4. Mimura T, Nakashizuka T, Mori M [2011]. Recent advances and history of vitreous surgery. *J Healthcare Eng.* 2(4): 447–458.
5. Jess A [1937]. Temporaere Skleraleindellung als Hilfsmittel bei der Operation der Netzhautabloesung. *Klin Monatsbl Augenheilkd.* 99: 318–319.

2 Training in Vitreoretinal Surgery

Like most other surgical specialties, vitreoretinal surgery requires abundant preoperative analysis and planning, intraoperative focus, precision and patience, and an ability to introspect and learn from not only one's own past errors and errors of their colleagues but also from those reported in literature and presented at meetings. Terms like *good surgeon* and *perfect surgery* are only relative. Each surgery is different, and sometimes even a straight-forward case can go terribly awry because of a multitude of reasons [e.g., the surgeon may be faced with endophthalmitis following an intravitreal injection, haemorrhagic choroidal detachment during pars plana vitrectomy, lens touch and cataract in a young patient]. In brief, it is important to emphasize that there is no zero-risk vitreoretinal intervention. At the same time, it is also important for the surgeon to take all measures, both during the training period as well as later professional journey, to work towards making his or her interventions one of the safest. One way of learning steps of vitreous surgery during the training period emphasized currently is to practice several tens of hours using simulators based on virtual reality. Animal eyes and cadaver eyes have a limited role in that they allow for practice of only a few steps such as passage of scleral sutures, and for obvious reasons, they cannot be used routinely to practice intraocular steps such as posterior vitreous detachment induction, membrane peeling, internal limiting membrane [ILM] peeling, and so on. Another option is participation in focused wet labs, but these are infrequent and usually allow limited participation. In the absence of simulators, the fledgling surgeon must identify one or more mentors and spend hundreds of hours meticulously assisting, observing, noting, reading, and discussing each step in detail. This would help build not only confidence in understanding and decision making but also inculcate useful traits such as focus, systematic approach, patience, and making rational decisions in the face of unanticipated events. Once these traits steadily become evident to the mentor, hands-on opportunities, one step at a time, would show up and help one evolve into a meticulous and responsible surgeon.

A few of the simulators available commercially include Eyesi/VRmagic, MicroVisTouch, and PixEye. The Eyesi system remains the most widely used and evaluated simulator. These have been predominantly used for training in cataract surgery, and most studies have shown that simulator training improves the efficiency and quality of cataract surgery while reducing complication rates. Unlike cataract surgery, simulator-based vitreoretinal surgery lags significantly owing to lack of widespread availability, limited uptake by trainees, lack of standardization, and absence of robust comparative studies. Eyesi/ Vrmagic [Haag Strait Simulation] is based on virtual reality simulation of a surgical microscope, intraocular instruments, and vitreous cavity [Figures 2.1 and 2.2]. The microscope focus and zoom can be controlled using a foot pedal. Simulation for intravitreal instruments is provided through three real handpieces that when inserted [into two openings in the model eye located on the head of a vitreoretinal mannequin] assume the function of multiple instruments such as forceps, scissors, laser, and so on, in a virtual manner, based on the type of task chosen. In addition to modules for vitrectomy, endolaser, ILM peeling, and epiretinal membrane, it also has an anti-tremor and navigation module [Figure 2.3]. Experience of widefield surgery is made possible because the simulator is integrated with a binocular indirect ophthalmic microscope system. The training module allows the user to choose the level of difficulty in performing a particular surgical step. No special googles are needed to use the simulator. A step-by-step guide to the performance of a procedure, for example, ILM peeling, is provided along with performance scores of each task on a scale of 0–100. Positive points are allocated for the amount of task that was successfully accomplished, and then points are deducted from this for every error made, complication created, or surgical

DOI: 10.1201/9781003179320-3

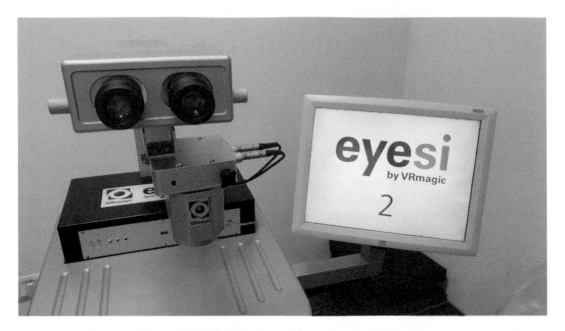

FIGURE 2.1 Eyesi VRmagic set-up: microscope, console, and display monitor.

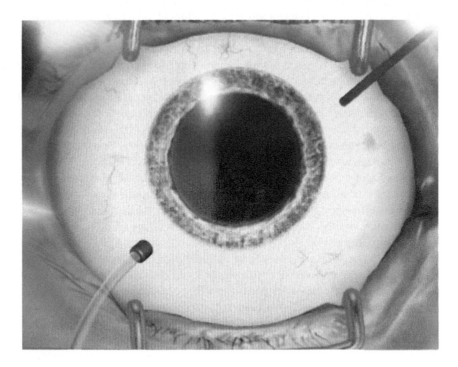

FIGURE 2.2 Mannequin eyeball with virtual vitreous cavity. Note the infusion line and one superior port.

time prolonged. There is a variable period of familiarization required for the beginner trainee. Disadvantages of virtual reality simulators include the inability to visualize elements of the real world such as grasp and orientation of the intraocular instrument, position of the surgeon's hand, and so on. Although technologically well crafted and having useful step-by-step instructions, the

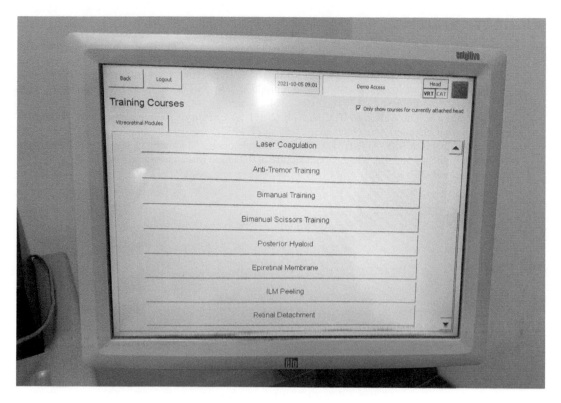

FIGURE 2.3 Surgical step modules on which training can be acquired.

simulator fails to provide a feel of the tissue. Also, the proprioception, while holding the tools meant for intraocular manipulation, feels different from that of performing the task [author's observation] at surgery. A major advantage of the simulator is that it provides microsurgical spatial awareness. Compared with cataract surgery, currently there is less validation on transfer of skills from simulation-based training to real vitreoretinal surgery. Despite this observation, if an opportunity exists, trainees and those wanting to remedy their skills should avail online training opportunity at the VRmNet portal.

Young trainees in vitreoretinal surgery should also prime themselves by going through standard textbooks written by pioneers in the field [e.g., Steve Charles, Charles Schepens, Ron Michaels, Paul Cibis, Gholam Peyman, AH Chignell, Ferenc Kuhn, Zivojnovic, John D. Scott, Ingrid Kreissig, William Benson, Heinrich Heimann, Stanislao Rizzo, Andrew Packer, and Paul Sullivan]. In addition, one must acquaint themselves with basic principles of ophthalmic surgery from classic textbooks such as ones by Stallard, George Spaeth, and Roger Steinert. In the current digital era, an ocean of edited surgical videos, with new approaches and modifications growing each day, is posted on several platforms such as Eyetube.net [registration is free] and YouTube [in the public domain] and several vitreoretinal societies such as ASRS, Euretina, and the European Vitreoretinal Society [all paid memberships]. That videos could substitute for a thousand words is only true if it accompanied by precise description of the technique and there is an expert review on the advantages and disadvantages of the surgical approach. However, a critique of surgical videos posted is very rare to come by. In this backdrop, it is emphasized that the books mentioned in this chapter carry an invaluable, immeasurable, and irreplaceable amount of clarity, emanating from years of expertise and experience of the authors, so they must be proactively read by all fellows in the field of vitreoretinal surgery.

SUGGESTED READING

1. Saleh GM, Lamparter J, Sullivan PM et al [2013]. The international forum of ophthalmic simulation: Developing a virtual reality training curriculum for ophthalmology. *Br J Ophthalmol.* 97(6): 789–792.
2. Saleh GM, Theodoraki K, Gillan S et al [2013]. The development of a virtual reality training programme for ophthalmology: repeatability and reproducibility (part of the international forum for ophthalmic simulation studies). *Eye* 27(11): 1269–1274.
3. Cissé C, Angioi K, Luc A, Berrod JP, Conart JB [2019]. EYESI surgical simulator: validity evidence of the vitreoretinal modules. *Acta Ophthalmol.* 97(2): e277–e282.
4. La Cour M, Thomsen ASS, Alberti M et al [2019]. Simulators in the training of surgeons: is it worth the investment in money and time? Jules Gonin lecture of the retina research foundation. *Graefes Arch Clin Exp Ophthalmol.* 257: 877–881.

3 Peri-operative Investigations

3.1 ULTRASONOGRAPHY AND ULTRASOUND BIOMICROSCOPY

When the ocular media does not permit detailed evaluation of the retina because of dense cataract, vitreous haemorrhage, amyloidosis, or capsular opacification, it is mandatory to undertake pre-operative ultrasonography [USG]. Relatively recent onset [fresh] and dispersed vitreous haemorrhage appears as bright dots on the B scan within the vitreous cavity, with corresponding low to medium reflectivity spikes along the A scan vector. When the haemorrhage is minimal [yet obscuring fundus visualization], one may have to increase the gain setting above tissue sensitivity to identify the haemorrhage on USG [however, beware of increased 'reflectivity' caused by increase in background noise]. This may be particularly necessary when trying to detect the presence of dispersed haemorrhage in a vitrectomized eye because blood remains in a liquefied state and is widely dispersed. As the haemorrhage becomes older, dehemoglobinized, and organized, the reflectivity becomes more easily evident. Sometimes vitreous haemorrhage that gets layered inferiorly over a detached hyaloid acquires the features of high reflectivity and can hence be mistaken for retinal detachment. To avoid this error, one must take other attributes of the membrane on USG into consideration before making a final diagnosis. Dot-like vitreous haemorrhage is often associated with membranous echoes, which could be indicative of the hyaloid posterior vitreous detachment [PVD] or detached retina. Dynamic ultrasound examination is very important in making a distinction between these membranes. As a general rule, if a PVD is absent, a retinal tear or rhegmatogenous retinal detachment [RD] is unlikely. If PVD is present, retinal tear [Figure 3.1] or RD should always be ruled out carefully before ascribing the haemorrhage to some other cause. Asteroid hyalosis too manifests as dot-like opacities within the vitreous cavity, but these are larger in size, and there is a distinct clear zone from the retinal surface.

PVD, when complete, appears as a membranous structure that is always tethered anteriorly [at the vitreous base], has low to moderate reflectivity, and has good after-movements. When incomplete, it may also be tethered posteriorly to one margin of the optic disc [never both, which is typical of retinal detachment] or one or more points on the retinal surface [usually to proliferative tissue or scars]. Unlike PVD, RD is tethered anteriorly at the ora serrata and posteriorly at the optic disc margin. Hence, the after-movements on dynamic evaluation are limited and sometimes appear like a whiplash movement. The reflectivity is also moderate to high in view of the higher thickness and multiple layers of the neurosensory retina. One could encounter a situation wherein the membrane is attached both anteriorly and posteriorly at the optic disc. In this situation, it is useful to study the posterior attachment to the disc more carefully; whereas a point-like attachment is suggestive of a PVD, a two-point attachment with a narrow separation is suggestive of retinal detachment. Also, a membrane may have features of high reflectively posteriorly and hence may warrant a diagnosis of RD instead of incomplete PVD. In this situation, it would be useful to determine the reflectivity along the anterior extent of the membrane, too. If the membrane is an RD, reflectivity tends to be high all along its surface; with PVD, it falls along its anterior extent. In addition, a tear may be picked up on USG in the presence of a retinal detachment. It is understandable from the mention earlier that it is very important to take scans through the optic nerve to make a precise diagnosis of a membranous structure. The configuration and mobility of rhegmatogenous RD are influenced by the severity and location of associated proliferative vitreoretinopathy. Accordingly, it has been characterized as an open- or closed-funnel configuration. Some long-standing retinal detachments may undergo cystic changes within the layers [intraretinal]. These cysts could be solitary or multiple and of variable size. They are generally without any echoes within the cyst, and the

DOI: 10.1201/9781003179320-4

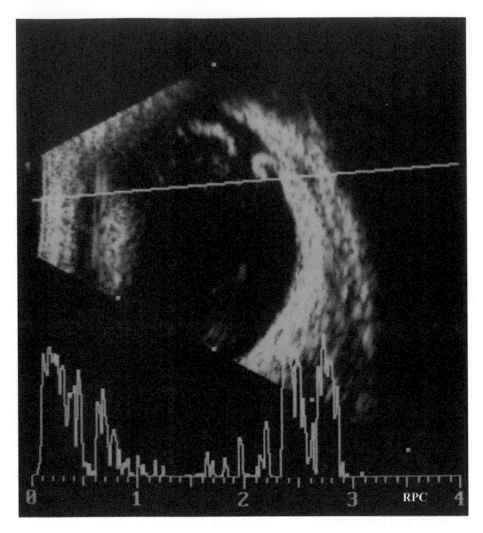

FIGURE 3.1   USG in the presence of vitreous haemorrhage reveals the presence of a retinal tear.

presence of such echoes should prompt the consideration of a haemorrhagic cyst, a transformation that is very rare. It may be challenging to differentiate a peripheral localized RD in the paediatric age group from congenital peripheral retinoschisis with vitreous veils and vitreous haemorrhage. Examination of the fellow eye and screening of other family members may be useful in this situation. A similar situation could arise in some adult patients with opaque media and senile retinoschisis. On USG, membranous structure caused by retinoschisis has a low to moderate reflectivity, is localized and dome shaped, and has no after-movements. In addition, senile retinoschisis is also frequently bilateral.

Dome-shaped elevation with limited after-movement on USG is also noted in patients with choroidal detachment. In this situation, history would be most important because most cases are secondary to an open globe injury, surgical complication, excessive retinal laser, or a serious systemic disorder with deranged body hemodynamics [e.g., malignant hypertension, hemodialysis, leukemia]. They could be limited in extent or massive, with retino-retinal apposition ['kissing' choroidals]. While serous choroidal detachment is echolucent, haemorrhagic detachments have variable internal reflectivity [that decreases as the blood liquifies with time].

Tractional retinal detachments are relatively easy to identify owing to their posterior and relatively confined location, multiple points of attachment, and absence of after-movements. Tractional detachments often have to be differentiated from vitreoschisis. Exudative RD has surface reflectivity features of rhegmatogenous RD, but the overall configuration is more uniform and smoother. In addition, dot-like echoes would be evident below the membrane because of collection of exudative material within the subretinal fluid. The shifting nature of the subretinal fluid could also be documented by undertaking the scan in different positions [sitting, lateral, supine]. The presence of a subretinal mass on USG is almost pathognomonic. When the suspicion of exudative detachment is high and no mass is discernible on a thorough scan, it would be useful to assess sclerochoroidal thickness, re-evaluate for signs of inflammation, and determine the refractive error and axial length of the fellow eye [for nanophthalmos]. Another source of dot and membranous opacities in the vitreous cavity is endophthalmitis. In this condition, the membranes are pseudo-membranes, aggregates of inflammatory cells and exudates that develop as an inflammatory response within the vitreous cavity. Inflammatory membranes may sometimes be accompanied by a cystic lesion with a dense focal opacity, pathognomonic of intraocular cysticercosis.

Ultrasound biomicroscopy [UBM] allows real-time microscopic visualization of living tissue using ultrasound waves at high frequencies [40–100 MHz]. UBM is a non-specific imaging technique that can be used for any ocular pathology that falls within its reach and penetration limits. UBM imaging has been very helpful in determining the wound-healing characteristics of scleral port using various gauges of trocar-cannula or microvitreoretinal blade, identifying status of the peripheral retinal in silicone filled eyes, and locating foreign bodies and tumours in the ciliary zone and peripheral retina and in the study of structural integrity of the ciliary body and ciliary processes. The pars plana sclerotomy site for vitreoretinal surgery has been the subject of considerable interest because of its implication in the causation of many postoperative complications and more recently to study differences in wound architecture and healing process of small-gauge surgery and conventional 20G surgery. Incarceration of the vitreous and growth of fibrovascular tissue at these sites has been noted in various histopathological studies. Vitreous incarceration is possibly also a major risk factor for anterior hyaloidal fibrovascular proliferation occurring in patients with diabetes, which is suspected to be responsible for rebleeds after surgery. Such proliferation has also been suggested as a risk factor for chronic hypotony, secondary to ciliary body traction, and for endophthalmitis [posterior vitreous wick syndrome]. Gape at the inner lip of the sclerotomy sites appears as an echolucent area, and we have graded this from 1 to 3 [Figure 3.2]. Grade 1 indicates no visible gape and grade 3 indicates the widest gape. Similarly, vitreous incarceration, denoted by echodense strands converging towards the sclerotomy site, has also been graded [Figure 3.3]. When early and late post-operative images are compared, there was a natural tendency towards reducing wound gape and increasing vitreous incarceration. Rhegmatogenous RD almost always reaches up to the ora serrata, and the ability of the UBM to scan this zone efficiently makes it a potential tool to predict status of the peripheral retina in silicone-filled eyes with media opacity [Figure 3.4].

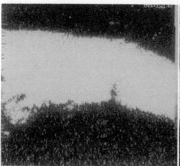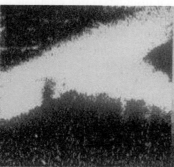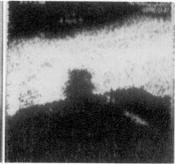

FIGURE 3.2   Grades of wound gape following 20G pars plana vitrectomy.

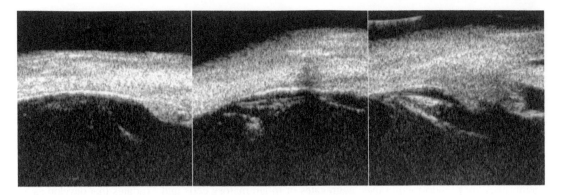

FIGURE 3.3   Grades of vitreous incarceration after 20G pars plana vitrectomy.

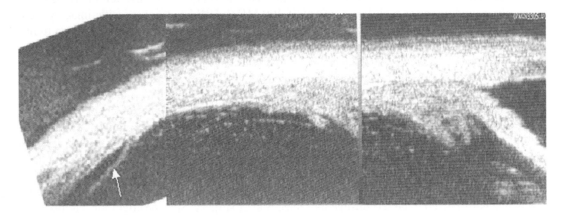

FIGURE 3.4   Montage of ultrasound biomicroscopy in silicone-filled eye showing detachment of the peripheral retina [marked by white arrow]. Note the aphakia and anterior migration of silicone oil.

3.2   OPTICAL COHERENCE TOMOGRAPHY AND OPTICAL COHERENCE TOMOGRAPHY ANGIOGRAPHY

Optical coherence tomography (OCT) has been a game changer in the management of a multitude of retinal disorders. It has provided objectivity to the treatment response, enabled better understanding of macular pathologies, and improved the ease and safety of follow-up. While the role of OCT in the medical management of macular disorders is well established, the same cannot be said of its role in the surgical management of macular disorders. Discussion on the importance of OCT to surgical decision making revolves largely around its ability to confirm a diagnosis [e.g., lamellar hole from full thickness macular hole, myopic foveoschisis, vitreomacular traction]. However, preoperative OCT has a strong potential to enable several micro-surgical steps to be carried out with greater precision, safety, and surety.

OCT images can be obtained in the enhanced vitreous view to identify the amount of vitreous and hyaloid attached to the optic disc margin. If none is found, then it suggests the possibility of complete PVD, so PVD may not have to be induced surgically. If hyaloid and vitreous is found adherent to the margin of the disc at only some regions, then the site of PVD induction can be chosen accordingly. In a similar manner, the relationship of the posterior hyaloid to the macular area and posterior retina can also be studied in detail. The amount and type of attachment to the fovea [broad or focal], the height of separation of the hyaloid from the retinal surface, and the presence

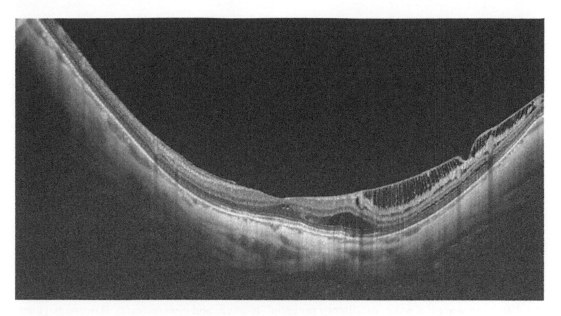

FIGURE 3.5 Schisis of the retinal layers on swept source [SS] optical coherence tomography in a patient with pathological myopia and clinical suspicion of macular hole.

or absence of the premacular bursa can all act as useful aids while surgery is being performed. In the presence of tractional retinal detachment, OCT again has the ability to provide vivid details of the tissue relationship, such as height of separation from the retina, multilayer separation, and so on [Figure 3.5].

3.3 FLUORESCEIN ANGIOGRAPHY

Fluorescein angiography, although invasive and associated with certain side effects, remains a useful and affordable investigation to assess the integrity of the retinal vascular bed. In the situation of non-availability of OCT angiography, it is useful for the surgeon to assess the status of the foveal avascular zone by fluorescein angiography. The presence of foveal ischemia is a poor prognostic indicator for the recovery of satisfactory vision following surgery for complications of diabetic retinopathy. This must be explained to the patient before obtaining consent for surgical intervention. In addition, fluorescein angiography may also reveal significant ischemia of the retina in other regions too, even in the absence of neovascularization. In this situation, it may be safer to first undertake retinal photocoagulation [if media permits] at least 4–6 weeks before planned surgery. This is likely to reduce the risk of postoperative complications such as severe fibrinoid reaction and anterior hyaloidal fibrovascular proliferation. Postoperatively too, it is useful to undertake fluorescein angiography within the first 4–6 weeks following surgery for complications of either diabetic retinopathy or retinal vasculitis. This would allow the detection of missed or subclinical neovascularization, and if present, prompt laser augmentation can avert recurrence of severe vision loss due to rebleed.

3.4 ELECTROPHYSIOLOGICAL TESTS

All living cells belonging to the neurosensory apparatus, when stimulated, undergo a change in the electrical gradient across their cell membrane, resulting from changes in the ionic equilibrium between the intracellular and extracellular space around the cell (sodium-potassium-calcium ions). The change in ionic charges results in an action potential. Action potentials may get transmitted to specialized centres to produce sensations of vision, noise, taste, pain, and so on or it may result in direct activity such as contraction of a muscle. Electrophysiological tests enable detection, characterization, and measurement of the action potential generated in response to an external stimulus. In retinal practice, the most important electrophysiological tests are electroretinogram [ERG], electrooculogram, and visual evoked response [VER]. Recent developments useful in the diagnosis and prognostication of retinal diseases include multifocal ERG [MfERG] and microperimetry [MP]. All these tests have three essentials: a characteristic stimulus pattern, electrodes to detect the action potential, and computer software that enables analysis of the emerging action potential. The stimulus is ideally presented within a Ganzfeld bowl (provides uniform background illumination). Electrode positions vary based on the test. ERG represents the collective action potential generated by all the cellular elements in the retina in response to light stimulus. Based on the type of stimulus used, several forms of ERG are categorized: single-flash ERG, flicker fusion ERG, pattern-evoked ERG, red-flash ERG, blue-flash ERG, and white-flash ERG. Based on the background illumination, ERG is categorized as scotopic (dark adapted), mesopic, or photopic (light adapted). Based on the area of retina stimulated by the stimulus, two forms of ERG are described: full-field or Ganzfeld ERG and focal ERG. ERG is a mass response of the rods and cones, so focal diseases do not alter the ERG. Scotopic ERG has the following waves: a-wave, oscillatory potential, b-wave, and c-wave (rare). A-wave is generated by the photoreceptors, b-wave by the bipolar and Mueller cells, oscillatory potential by the amacrine cells, and c-wave by the retinal pigment epithelium. Data must be interpreted with knowledge of normal values established for the testing lab and in comparison with the fellow eye. a-wave is the most negative and b-wave the most positive point on the waveform. Amplitude is the micro-volt measurement from the most negative (a-wave) to the most positive (b-wave) point. Implicit time is the time in milliseconds from the onset of stimulus to the development of the most positive (b-wave) point. Abnormal ERG waveforms that have been described are a very small to absent b-wave, making the wave look like a very deep V shape [negative ERG]; smaller than 2 standard deviations [SDs] below the normal mean A and/or B-wave [subnormal ERG]; more than 2 SDs above the normal mean B wave or both the A and B wave [supranormal ERG]; scotopic response less than 100 μV or a photopic response below 50 μV [minimal ERG]; and waveforms so small that they cannot be distinguished from the background noise, such as RD and siderosis bulbi [extinguished ERG]. In siderosis bulbi, ERG undergoes sequential changes [first described by Karpe] in three stages: negative-positive, negative-negative, and extinguished. It is believed that removal of a retained iron metallic foreign body when the ERG amplitude is less than 50% of normal [or fellow eye] may not help in arresting the progression of siderosis bulbi. This prognostic factor must be discussed with the patient before surgery.

Multifocal ERG [MfERG], as the name suggests, is a special form of ERG in which the retina is stimulated at multiple points in a unique pattern and the electrical response is recorded. Unlike conventional ERG, in which the recording obtained indicates the response of the entire retina, in MfERG, the response obtained indicates a combination of the response solely from the stimulated retina. Three waves are noted in an MfERG recording, N1, P1, and N2, and these are generated by the photoreceptors, Mueller cells, and inner retina, respectively. Preoperative MfERG may be useful in predicting visual outcome following surgery for conditions such as vitreomacular traction, myopic foveoschisis, and resistant diabetic macular edema. **Microperimetry** is a psychophysical test that allows testing of retinal sensitivity at some prespecified points on the retina. It is also designated as fundus-guided perimetry. Because the fixation pattern [stable, relatively unstable, and unstable] can be documented and the testing points can also be customized in newer versions, microperimetry may be a useful investigation to prognosticate the visual recovery following surgery for conditions such as macular hole, resistant diabetic macular edema, choroidal coloboma, and optic disc pit maculopathy.

SUGGESTED READING

1. Keshavamurthy R, Venkatesh P, Garg SP [2006]. Ultrasound biomicroscopy findings of 25 G trans-conjunctival sutureless (TSV) and conventional (20G) pars plana sclerotomy in the same patient. *BMC Ophthalmol.* 2: 6–7.
2. Venkatesh P, Verghese M, Garg SP, Tewari HK [2012]. Ultrasound biomicroscopy in silicone oil filled eyes. *Retinal Physician.* 9: 48–51.
3. Joshi D, Venkatesh P, Tewari HK [2005]. Ultrasound biomicroscopy of sclerotomy sites after pars plana vitreoretinal surgery. *The EVRS Edu J.* 4: 16–22.
4. Gupta S, Midha N, Gogia V, Sahay P, Pandey V, Venkatesh P [2015]. Sensitivity of multifocal electro-retinography (mfERG) in detecting siderosis. *Can J Ophthalmol.* Dec. 50(6): 485–490.
5. Kumawat D, Sahay P, Mahalingam K et al [2019]. Multifocal electroretinogram in eyes with intravitreal silicone oil and changes following silicone oil removal. *Doc Ophthalmol.* 139: 197–205.
6. Azarmina M, Soheilian M, Azarmina H, Hosseini B [2011]. Electroretinogram changes following silicone oil removal. *J Ophthalmic Vis Res.* 6(2): 109–113.
7. Karpe G [1948]. Early diagnosis of siderosis retina by the use of electroretinography. *Doc Ophthalmol.* 2(1): 277–296.

4 Anaesthesia: Approaches and Limitations

The primary objective of delivering anaesthesia for surgical procedures elsewhere in the body is to allow the surgeon(s) to carry out the desired procedure in a safe and stable hemodynamic environment without causing pain or discomfort to the patient. The usual forms of anaesthesia used in general surgery include general anaesthesia, regional anaesthesia, and local anaesthesia. While local infiltrative anaesthesia can be administered by the surgeon, for general anaesthesia and regional anaesthesia, the expertise of specially trained physicians is mandatory. Administering anaesthesia during major vitreoretinal surgery, in addition to achieving analgesia, must also ensure akinesia of the extraocular muscles and relaxation of the eyelid muscles. The majority of vitreoretinal procedures can be undertaken using regional anaesthesia, so it is important for the vitreoretinal surgeon to be able to deliver it. Even in situations wherein the patient has other morbidities that increase the risk of a serious systemic intraoperative adverse reaction, such as coronary artery disease or bronchial asthma, ocular anaesthesia of choice remains regional anaesthesia, with continuous monitoring of the systemic parameters by the anaesthetic team. Indications for **general anaesthesia** during vitreoretinal surgery include the paediatric age group, hearing impaired, mentally challenged, and during repair of severe open globe injury.

Preanesthetic evaluation and going through a checklist are as important as administering the anaesthesia itself. Having a relative with the patient is highly recommended on the day of surgery. It reduces patient apprehension and improves their cooperation. Ensure that the patient and close relative comprehend the reason for which surgery is being undertaken and the expected benefits, risks, and limitations. In vitreoretinal surgery, there is commonly a need for repeat interventions such as removal of cataract, removal of silicone oil, or removal of postoperative epimacular membrane, as well as compliance to positioning during the early postoperative period. It is important that these aspects have been thoroughly discussed before the planned surgery and adequate counselling provided. It is the responsibility of the surgeon, and absolutely mandatory, to check that the patient has provided written **informed consent**. [If there is any unanticipated change in the surgical plan intraoperatively, e.g., the need for converting to vitreoretinal surgery from planned scleral buckling surgery, this must be explained to the patient's attendant, and written reconsent for this should also be obtained.] Adequate time must be given to address any additional concerns or queries that the patients may have. Providing a brief on the overall process within the operation theatre, the need for cooperation while anaesthetic agents are being injected, the anticipated discomfort or its absence, the expected duration of surgery and immediate postsurgical aspects [e.g., when the patient can take fluids or solids; how soon the patient can move about; how soon the patient will be able to see; the perception of a floating bubble when air, gas, or silicone oil has been used] would help in improving patient comfort and build confidence in the surgical team.

A note must be made of the blood pressure, blood sugar level, result of any sensitivity tests conducted [e.g., xylocaine sensitivity test], other drug allergies, compliance with preoperative instructions [e.g., nil orally for at least 6 hours prior to surgery], and if the regular medications [e.g., antihypertensive drugs, asthma medication] have been taken or stopped as per recommendation [e.g., of antiplatelet drugs]. Check the recommendations of any consults that have been sent [e.g., to endocrinologist, cardiologist] and adhere to their guidance on appropriate blood pressure and blood sugar values to go forward with the surgery. Also check if a peripheral intravenous access is in place, whether the correct eye has been marked, and if pupillary dilatation has been achieved. In addition, one must be aware if the eye planned for the vitreoretinal procedure has undergone

DOI: 10.1201/9781003179320-5

recent cataract surgery or glaucoma surgery. In this situation, the anaesthesia must be administered with greater caution, and one must avoid any form of pressure on the eyeball.

If surgery is planned under general anaesthesia, it is mandatory to have a prior preanesthetic consultation. All instructions provided by the specialists must be adhered to in order to ensure patient safety, a stable intraoperative and postoperative course, and faster recovery from the effects of the anaesthesia. It is also necessary to have prior dialogue with the anaesthesia team in case intraocular gas is being planned as long-term tamponade, if hypotensive anaesthesia is required for tumour resection, or if the surgical procedure is likely to take more than the anticipated time [e.g., repair of a severe globe rupture]. It is also recommended that one member of the surgical team be present with the anesthetist until the patient has been extubated and wheeled out into the recovery room. If the patient needs some unanticipated special care and prolonged monitoring following surgery under general anaesthesia, it is also the surgeon's responsibility to facilitate this additional care and ensure daily follow-up until the patient can be discharged after complete recovery.

The **anaesthetic agents** generally used include proparacaine for topical anaesthesia and a combination of lidocaine and bupivacaine for regional anaesthesia. By facilitating diffusion of the agent, addition of Hyalase [hyaluronidase] ensures earlier onset of the anaesthetic action. The downside to using Hyalase is that the effect wears off earlier. The normal duration of action is about 60–90 minutes and about 15 minutes shorter without and with Hyalase, respectively. Regional anaesthesia for vitreoretinal surgery must numb both sensory nerves supplying the ocular surface, cornea, and ciliary body [branches of the trigeminal nerve] and the motor nerves supplying the extraocular muscles [oculomotor, trochlear, abducens] and orbicularis oculi [facial nerve]. Traditionally, until about three decades ago, this used to be achieved by a combination of retrobulbar anaesthesia and facial nerve block. This approach has now been almost entirely supplanted by the technique of peribulbar and parabulbar anaesthesia. It makes the surgical procedure more comfortable for the patient if drugs for premedication are given about half an hour prior to administering the anesthetic injection.

Retrobulbar block. In this approach, the anaesthetic agent is injected into the retrobulbar space using a 1½-inch, 23G needle or a specific, commercially available retrobulbar needle. The mechanism of action through which analgesia and akinesia are achieved is by the effect on the ciliary ganglion [wherein parasympathetic fibres relay and sympathetic fibres pass by] and on the nerves supplying the extraocular muscles at the orbital apex. The main advantages of this method were that it is a one-point injection, and a relatively low volume of anaesthesia is needed [about 2–3 cc]. There were innumerable disadvantages, though, some of a very serious nature. These disadvantages include globe perforation, retrobulbar haemorrhage, optic nerve injury, and very rarely the risk of intracranial escape [through the orbital apex] and seizures. In addition, the anaesthesia has a shorter duration of action. Hence, this route of ocular anaesthesia is no longer recommended.

Facial block. For obvious reasons, retrobulbar anaesthesia had no effect on the orbicularis oculi. Without paralyzing the muscles of the eyelids, there would be repeated squeezing and narrowing of the palpebral aperture [creating difficulty in accessing the surgical ports, scleral surface for passage of sutures, drainage of subretinal fluid, and so on], increased patient discomfort, and risk of unsteady intraocular pressure. To achieve akinesia of the orbicularis oculi, the standard procedure in the past was to block the facial nerve by injecting an anaesthetic agent over the mandible, at the site wherein the nerve ramifies into its five divisions. While the method was very effective in consistently inducing paralysis of the orbicularis oculi, it had several disadvantages such as the need for a second injection [in addition to retrobulbar injection], anaesthesia of a larger area and of muscles in no way connected to the ocular surgery, prolonged post-injection numbness and discomfort, and in some cases prolonged ptosis and lagophthalmos. Currently, the only situation wherein a facial block may have a role is during repair of an open globe injury when a general anaesthetic facility is not immediately available.

Peribulbar anaesthesia. This is a form of regional anaesthesia used to obtain anaesthesia and akinesia of the extraocular muscles as well as paralysis of the orbicularis oculi. The method consists of delivering about 6–10 mL of the anaesthetic agent into the peribulbar space by injecting at two

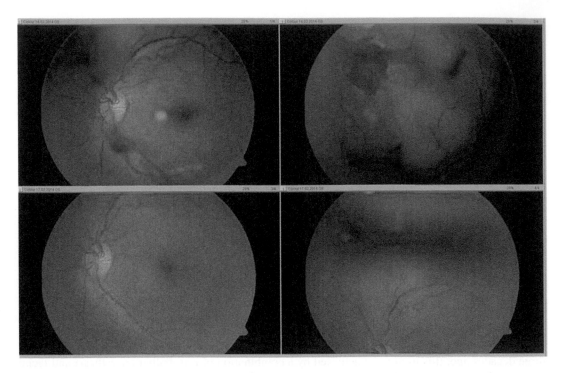

FIGURE 4.1 Large tear in the superior retina on postoperative day 1 of a woman who underwent strabismus surgery under peribulbar anaesthesia. Successful reattachment was achieved with immediate pneumatic reti-nopexy and laser retinopexy.

points using a ½-inch disposable needle. The first point of injection is at the junction of the medial third and the lateral two thirds along the upper orbital margin [close to the supraorbital notch]. The second point of injection is at the junction of the medial two thirds and lateral third along the lower orbital margin. About 2–3 mL of the anaesthetic agent is injected at the upper point and the remainder at the lower point. It is useful to inject some volume of the anaesthetic agent into the orbicularis oculi fibres. Peribulbar anaesthesia achieves its effect peripherally by acting at the neuromuscular junction. This form of anaesthesia has reduced side effects compared with retrobulbar anesthesia, but the threat of globe perforation remains [Figure 4.1].

Parabulbar anaesthesia. To make infiltrative anaesthesia safer, some surgeons prefer parabul-bar anaesthesia. In this approach, the cul de sac is first anaesthetized by instilling topical drops such as proparacaine. Then, a small snip is made using conjunctival scissors into the bulbar conjunctiva and episcleral tissue. Through the access so achieved, the anaesthetic agent is injected into the parabulbar space using a blunt cannula. Although cannulas specially designed for this purpose are available, other substitutes can be safely used [e.g., cannula that comes for injection of viscoelastics]. Parabulbar anaesthesia can also be used to supplement the anaesthetic effect when that from the primary block is found to be wearing off. It can also be given at the end of surgery to reduce pain in the early postoperative period.

Topical anaesthesia is successfully used routinely during phacoemulsification, but it is not rec-ommended for vitreoretinal surgery, except for pneumatic retinopexy, intravitreal injections, and delivery of sustained-drug release implants, such as Posurdex and Iluvien. There are some pub-lished reports on vitreoretinal surgery being performed under topical anaesthesia. Having been an observer to some pars plana vitrectomy surgeries [unreported] under topical anaesthesia, it is opined that one must desist from using this approach. This is because even though the procedure can be completed successfully, the patient would be in visible discomfort and pain compared with being under peribulbar anaesthesia. In addition, there is only marginal benefit to be gained in terms of safety, by adopting topical anaesthesia alone. With the advent of increasingly smaller gauge surgery, recent reports on 27G surgery performed using topical anaesthesia have been described. In comparison with topical anaesthesia, subconjunctival anaesthesia may have a more useful role, particularly in patients at a higher risk of developing haemorrhage following minor interventions [e.g., those on blood thinners].

SUGGESTED READING

1. Malik AI, Foster RE, Correa ZM, Petersen MR, Miller DM, Riemann CD [2012]. Anatomical and visual results of transconjunctival sutureless vitrectomy using subconjunctival anesthesia performed on select patients taking anticoagulant and antiplatelet agents. *Retina*. 32(5): 905–911.
2. Jeroudi AM, Shieh WS, Chen Y, Connors DB, Blinder KJ, Shah GK [2018]. Topical anesthesia in 27-gauge pars plana vitrectomy. *J Vitreoretin Dis*. 2(2): 100–103.
3. Ghosh YK, Goodall KL [2005]. Postoperative pain relief in vitreoretinal surgery with subtenon bupivacaine 0.75%. *Acta Ophthalmol Scand*. 83(1): 119–120.
4. Gombos K [2010]. Techniques and complications of anaesthesia for vitreoretinal surgery and a new technique of local anaesthesia. *Acta Ophthalmol*. 88. doi:10.1111/j.1755-3768.2010.1226.
5. Costen MTJ, Newsom RS, Wainwright AC, Luff AJ, Canning CR [2005]. Expanding role of local anaesthesia in vitreoretinal surgery. *Eye*. 19: 755–761.
6. Rishi K, Venkatesh P, Garg SP [2013]. Management of retinal detachment in block related globe perforation with pneumatic retinopexy. *Ind J Ophthalmol*. 61(3): 131–132.

5 Operation Theatre: Design and Sterilization

There are varying design patterns to an operation theatre, but all of them have four zones to integrate: outer zone, clean zone, aseptic zone, and disposal zone. Another basic necessity in operation theatre designing is to ensure that the path taken by the staff be separate from the path taken by patients. In addition, the path for moving instruments must be different from that meant for the staff and patients. The operating room [OR; theatre] is so planned that the flow of traffic is always maintained from a clean zone to dirty zone, cross contamination is prevented, and there is maximal environmental sanitation. It is most often located in a blind wing or top or bottom floor to facilitate efficient traffic control and allow independent or separate air and water supply from rest of the hospital. In the past, ORs were situated high up in the hospital building to avoid contamination from dust in the air, but with availability of controlled air circulation systems, this is no longer necessary. Circulation of air in the OR should be able to prevent deposition of dust particles and potential aerosols, and this is achieved using a **laminar air flow system**. In this system, outside air is filtered, cooled, and humidified [to recommended standards] and then circulated within the OR. During this process, sufficient air pressure needs to be maintained to prevent a suction effect. The recommended number of air exchanges is 15–25 every hour [optimum being about 16 times]. Within the OR, the area meant for surgery must be clearly demarcated and specified and have restricted access. It should have two regions, restricted and unrestricted. The **restricted area** is subdivided into a sterile area and a sub-sterile area. Restricted area houses the OR, sterile supplies, instrument collection and processing area, autoclaves, anaesthesia supply area, and entrance to the post-anaesthesia recovery room. The **sub-sterile area** is a partially enclosed area, adjacent to an entrance to the OR, where a flash autoclave and utility counter are placed. The sub-sterile area is effectively an extension of the OR because the sterile gowned scrub nurse is often required to retrieve sterile instruments from the autoclave. If there is no adequate barrier, it is hazardous to have scrub sinks located in the sub-sterile area. Offices, posting office, lounges, entrance to dressing rooms, sterile storage areas, and patient transfer areas should be located in the unrestricted area.

Operation theatre sterilization. The routine method consists of washing the theatre with copious amounts of water followed by fumigation. Based on the type of chemical being used, there are several methods of fumigation. Earlier, formalin vapour by aerosol spray was used [30 ml of 40% formalin dissolved in 90 ml of clean water for 1000 cu ft of space]. After sealing the OR for 6 hours, carbolization with 2% carbolic acid is necessary. A major disadvantage of this method is that it takes about 24 hours for the pungent smell of formalin and carbolic acid to dissipate. Aerosol may be obtained using commercially available fumigators [e.g., Oticare]. If this is not available, a basin containing a mixture of 40% formalin [35 ml] and 10 gm. of potassium permanganate [$KMnO_4$] [for 1000 cu ft of space] is placed inside the OR, and the complex is sealed for 24 hours. A new method of fumigation uses Aldekol, a mixture containing 6% formaldehyde, 6% glutaraldehyde, and 5% benzalkonium chloride. To sterilize 4000 cu ft, 325 ml of Aldekol is dissolved in 150 ml of water and sprayed by aerosol for 30 minutes. The room is then closed for 2 hours following which fumes are allowed to clear by putting on the exhaust or air conditioning. With this method, OR sterilization can be completed in about 3 hours.

Housekeeping is an important factor for ensuring proper asepsis in the OR. This involves care of the walls, ceilings, floor, vents, light fixtures, shelves, furniture, and sink areas. Ideally, the floor should be sprayed and a wet vacuum pickup used between surgical procedures and at the

DOI: 10.1201/9781003179320-6

end of the day. An alternative but a less effective method is to mop (with a clean head every time) using a two-bucket system. Spot cleaning of walls and the ceiling should be undertaken as needed every day. Doors and switches should be cleaned with a germicidal detergent. Open shelves need to be cleaned daily with a detergent, whereas closed cabinets may be cleaned once weekly. The sink area should be cleaned several times daily and kept as dry as possible. The spray heads on the faucets should also be cleaned daily. The outside of autoclaves is cleaned daily, and the inside surface is cleaned weekly. Inside cleaning needs use of trisodium phosphate to remove chemical residue. Furniture used during a surgical procedure needs to be wiped with a detergent (germicide) at the end of each case and cleaned thoroughly at the end of the day. The same applies to spotlights and other portable equipment, stretchers, and kick buckets. The laundry bin should be removed immediately after it fills up. Kick buckets should be steam cleaned weekly. Before removing gloves, the scrub nurse should place all soiled linen inside the laundry bin. Soiled linen should never be left on the floor or transported on a trolley used for other purposes, and it must never be handled without wearing protective gloves. Liquid waste materials such as the contents of the suction bottle should never be disposed of in a scrub sink or utility sink but only into a container meant for the purpose.

Strict asepsis is a hallmark of all modern-day surgeries. Asepsis and sterile surgical technique remain the pillars for protecting the patient and for rendering the most satisfactory result from surgical intervention. Aseptic technique is constituted by the series of practices employed to prepare the environment, the personnel, and the patient, since it is near impossible to sterilize these. Practices employed to prepare the instruments, supplies, and other inanimate objects used during surgery are designated as *sterile technique*. The former decreases or abolishes the pathogenic load, while the latter clears all living organisms in both the vegetative and spore state. Previously, sterilization was considered an absolute process by which all micro-organisms were destroyed. This is, however, impossible because micro-organisms die logarithmically. A practical definition implies reduction of micro-organism load to a level below that required to cause infection.

Maintaining stringent asepsis during ocular surgery is of utmost importance because the eye is an extremely delicate organ. Attention has to be paid to the four key sources of contamination: patient, personnel, instruments, and environment. The most important source of organisms producing endophthalmitis after intraocular surgery is the patient's own flora residing in the conjunctival sac. This encourages one to reduce the microbial load within the conjunctival sac by prescribing antibiotics in the preoperative period. However, the role of prophylactic antibiotics in the days preceding surgery and the need for subconjunctival injection at the end of surgery have been constant topics of debate. This practice of prescribing preoperative antibiotics was widely prevalent before cataract surgery began to be performed as a day care procedure by phacoemulsification, despite the lack of high evidence data. Instillation of preoperative antibiotics is not considered mandatory now following the recognition that betadine [povidone-iodine] solution has almost immediate efficacy in eliminating infectious sources within the surgical field. Other preoperative measures that may aid in decreasing the risk of contamination from the periocular skin include facial wash with an antiseptic soap on the night preceding surgery followed by painting of the periocular skin with betadine solution. Betadine paint may be repeated on the morning of surgery hours before shifting into the OR. Povidone-iodine is an iodine releasing polymer [non-stinging, non-staining, water-soluble complex] that has been shown to destroy bacteria in 30 seconds. Its efficacy is considered equivalent to a 3-day course of eye drops containing polymyxin, neomycin, and gentamicin. In addition to strong antibacterial activity, povidone has antifungal and antiviral properties. It has now been shown that placing a solution of half-strength povidone-iodine (5%) in the conjunctival sac for a few minutes before surgery decreases the microbial load comparable with the use of preoperative antibiotic drops. The use of povidone-iodine 5% solution (*not* scrub) is now a strongly recommended practice for all intraocular surgeries. Surprisingly, despite these measures, viable bacteria have been isolated from anterior chamber aspirates obtained at the end of surgery in a large percentage of eyes. Fortunately, the number of these micro-organisms is small enough for the immune system of the anterior chamber to deal with and prevent their colonization. This important finding provides a strong rationale for the use of subconjunctival injections at the end of surgery. Indeed, it has been shown experimentally that subconjunctival antibiotic at the end of surgery reduces the risk of endophthalmitis caused by direct inoculation of organisms into the vitreous cavity. Antibiotic in the infusion fluid is another measure that is used with the aim of decreasing the risk of postoperative endophthalmitis. Commonly used antibiotics for this purpose are gentamicin and vancomycin.

The four sources of contamination during a surgical procedure are environment, personnel, patient, and instruments and supplies. Environment-related factors are concerned with the location of the OR, its water and air supply, traffic patterns, house-keeping practices, laundry processing, and refuse disposal. Factors related to the surgical team and personnel concern personal hygiene, dress code, movement, skin contaminants, surgical scrubbing, and team activity. Patient-related factors include general health, preoperative preparation, transportation to the OR, and preparation of the surgical site. Instrument and supply factors include regular checks on the effectiveness of sterilization equipment; using indicators to ensure adequate sterilization at each cycle; avoiding reuse of items meant for single use; and maintaining a log on the date of manufacture, batch number, date of expiry, and so on of consumables [e.g., suture, viscoelastic, silicone oil, perfluorocarbon liquid, triamcinolone, dyes].

Because they cannot be sterilized, disinfected, or contained, personnel remain the greatest source of contamination. Uncooperative and inappropriate behavior compounds the risk. It is of utmost importance to ensure and implement a strict culture of discipline to be adhered to by all OR personnel. The general health and personal hygiene of individuals working in the OR needs close monitoring. Those with upper respiratory tract infections; draining skin lesions; or infections of the eyes, ear, or mouth should not be a part of the operating team or assisting team. All personnel must change into hospital-laundered scrub attire and don shoe covers [which need to be changed each time the surgeon leaves the restricted area], head covering that adequately covers all scalp hair, and a properly tied high filtration (at least 95%) face mask before entering the OR. Face masks should completely cover the nose and mouth and fit snugly against the face. There should be no venting on the cheeks. Everyone in the OR should wear scrub apparel with long sleeves and tight cuffs at the wrist. Surgical scrubbing is an important aspect of ensuring safety of the operation. The objectives of the surgical scrub are to remove dirt, skin oil, and as many micro-organisms as possible from the hands and forearms and to inhibit the growth and reproduction of bacteria on the skin for as long as possible. Skin of the hands must be free from cuts and abrasions; nails must be short and free of nail polish. There is no consensus on the best method of scrubbing, the most effective antimicrobial solution, adequate duration of scrub time, or the most effective means of applying friction to the skin. Both the timed anatomical scrub (3–10 minutes) and counted brush method are considered satisfactory. Counted brush method has largely been discontinued with the widespread availability of liquid soaps containing polyvinyl pyrrolidine-iodine (PVP–iodine), chlorhexidine, and so on. These scrubs are more effective and accordingly scrub time of 3 minutes for the first scrub of the day and 1 minute for scrubs between cases is considered adequate. Members of the surgical team should be gowned and gloved as soon as they enter the OR. Once gowned and gloved, they should remain in the sterile end of the room until the patient is draped and the sterile set up is moved into place. During any waiting period, gowned and gloved members of the team must keep their hands just above their waist level. They should never sit, place their hands on their lap, or fold their hands. Once the gown is donned, several areas are considered contaminated: the neck and 2 inches below, edges of the cuffs, and below the waist. If a wraparound gown is not worn, the entire back is also considered unsterile.

The furniture on which the sterile packs are to be placed should be placed in the sterile end of the room. These should be clean and dry. Each pack must be examined for holes in the wrapper, watermarks (indicative of area of moisture), expiry date, and integrity of closure. The tops of all furniture should be approximately the same height as the OR table. This level is known as the level of sterility. Unsterile equipment, furniture, and personnel should remain 12 inches from any sterile surface. Unsterile personnel should never walk between two sterile fields. All patients can be a major source of contamination. This can be minimized by providing adequate preoperative instructions to be followed by the patient before the morning of surgery, including evacuation of the bladder and large intestine. The patient must also wear clean attire, a head cap, and shoe covers and must be wheeled into the OR on a stretcher or wheel chair covered with clean linen. It may be useful to premedicate the patient half an hour before the periocular block. Insertion of an intravenous catheter would be of assistance in case of unanticipated systemic adverse events during the surgery. Some surgeons also prefer to have the periocular area cleaned with betadine half an hour before the planned surgical time.

Once the patient is made to lie comfortably on the surgical table [paying attention to the position and inclination of the table and the position of the patient's head], a pulse oximeter is placed on the finger, and then the patient is covered with clean linen from below the neck. Following this, the assistant must paint the periocular region with betadine solution (povidone-iodide 5% solution). The horizontal extent must be from the midline to the beginning of the auricle and the vertical extent from the hair line to a line passing horizontally from the angle of the mouth. Wait for it to dry (about 2 minutes). Scrub the eyelid margin with betadine applicators. Instill betadine drops into the cul de sac. Wash after 1 minute with normal saline. Again, paint the region with betadine solution as indicated earlier and let the region dry. Following this, apply Opsite or other similar adhesive [specifically designed for ocular surgery] over the periorbital area of the eye to be operated. Pay particular attention to ensure its tight adherence at the medial canthus, nasal bridge, and nasolabial fold. Keep the adhesive slightly redundant over the open eyelids while applying. However, prevent corneal touch. Lift the temporal edge of the adhesive at the lateral canthus and make a horizontal slit up to the medial canthus. At the medial canthus, extend the cut in a 'V'- or 'T'-shaped manner. Insert the eyelid speculum through the slit opening in such a manner that the eyelid margin and eyelashes are wrapped beneath margins of the Opsite.

It is useful for the surgeon to be familiar with some important terminology in relation to asepsis and sterilization. The microbial count obtained from the OR environment is known as **bioburden**. Clean air system or **laminar air flow** refers to airflow in which the entire body of air within a confined area moves in one direction. **Surgically clean** implies a state obtained by mechanically removing surface micro-organisms from animate objects. **Terminal sterilization** is sterilization of the instruments and equipment after every surgery, in order to prevent cross contamination. Devices used to achieve sterilization include **autoclave** [uses moist heat in the form of steam under pressure to destroy micro-organisms], **hot air sterilization** [e.g., hot air oven, uses circulating dry air at high temperature], ethylene oxide [ETO] and **cold sterilization** using radiation [cobalt 60 radiation or electron bombardment using linear accelerator, usually for packing disposable items made for single use], or **chemicals** [e.g., Cidex-activated glutaraldehyde, Hibitane-chlorhexidine, Savlon-chlorhexidine and cetrimide]. Manufacturer instructions with regard to uptime, holding time, and down time must be adhered to while using an autoclave. **ETO** is extremely effective and widely used but also carries serious risks if it is not handled with appropriate precautions. It is very inflammable and at concentrations above 3%, highly explosive [hence unsuitable for fumigating OR rooms]. The explosiveness of ethylene oxide is reduced by mixing with an inert gas such as carbon dioxide [85%–90%] or by creating vacuum in the chamber before introducing ethylene oxide. If a leak occurs and it mixes with air, it forms a highly combustible mixture. ETO is effective against all micro-organisms, including viruses and spores, and acts by alkylation and interference with RNA and DNA; thus, risk of biological toxicity also exists. This form of sterilization can be used for a wide range of articles but in particular heat-labile ones. Exposure is maintained for about an hour. Because ETO residues are toxic, desorption of these must be ensured by either storing the goods on an open shelf for at least 24 hours or by using adequate post-vacuum, powerful filtered air rinse under vacuum and at desired temperature. Any apparatus sterilized by the ethylene oxide process should ideally not be used with saline or blood products before it has been flushed with sterile water. This precaution is essential because ethylene oxide residue can react with the chloride radical to form chlorohydrates.

SUGGESTED READING

1. Heather M (Ed) [2016]. *Ophthalmic operating theatre practice: A manual for lower resource settings.* 2nd Edition. International Centre for Eye Health, London.
2. Stallard's Eye surgery [1989]. *Introduction to eye surgery.* Ed. Rooper Hall MJ. 7th Edition. Butterworth, London, 1–42.

6 Surgical Anatomy and Other Considerations

Studies have established that it is possible to project the location of important inner organs [e.g., liver, spleen] and structures [e.g., jugular vein, facial nerve] on to the surface of the body. Knowledge about these landmarks is of significant importance in the diagnosis of varied disorders [e.g., appendicitis] and in the making of surgical incisions in a manner that is safe, least traumatic, and least vascular. Similarly, it is necessary for vitreoretinal surgeons to be aware of certain recognized surface landmarks, anatomical dimensions, distances, strength of adhesion between layers, and locations of blood vessels and anastomosis, irrespective of whether they make a minor or major contribution to the ease and safety of the surgery. Knowledge about surgical anatomy helps the surgeon plan the method of tissue handling, peritomy, traction on the bridle suture, point of trocar-cannula entry, and site of drainage of subretinal fluid etc.

Conjunctival–episcleral attachment. The bulbar conjunctiva is tightly adherent to the limbal conjunctiva and to the episcleral tissue for about 2–3 mm behind the limbus. Thus, incisions for peritomy should preferably be made 3 mm beyond the limbus. This would have several advantages such as minimizing ooze from the episcleral blood vessels [which can hamper visualization under contact lens], preservation of perilimbal neurovascular plexus and stem cells, better closure, and healing. Conjunctiva becomes thinner and fragile with age and so must be handled with greater gentleness in older adults [e.g., by using non-toothed forceps for grasping and round bodied suture, if available, for suturing]. Contrarily, the episcleral tissue is quite exuberant in young patients, and this may increase the risk of side effects such as conjunctival retraction and granuloma formation. To avoid this, one may have to close the episcleral and conjunctival tissue as two separate layers, anchor them to a frill of perilimbal tissue, and in some situations [e.g., very young children] even excise some of the excessive episcleral tissue.

The intermuscular septum [Guerin's ligament] is a loose fascial tissue that sheaths all the extraocular muscles and layers over the scleral surface. It is necessary to retract or move this tissue aside in all four quadrants to gain clear access to the scleral surface. Failure to do so may cause difficulties in placing the scleral mark [for localization of the retinal breaks], passing the scleral sutures, and passing and placing the buckle or band. Separation of the intermuscular septa is achieved using tenotomy scissors. Care must be taken to avoid hinging the blades of the scissors on the sclera; without this precaution, one could inadvertently rupture the sclera. Following this, the septum is further separated by blunt dissection using tissue forceps. In young patients, it may sometimes be necessary to make a cut into the septa with scissors to facilitate its separation. To prevent damage to its fibres, the septa should never be forcefully teased along the margins of the extraocular muscles. Forceful efforts at teasing the septum along the belly of the inferior rectus could damage the Whitnall ligament and sometimes to rupture of the muscle itself. There are seven **muscular arteries**, all recti muscles, except the lateral rectus is supplied by a pair of these arteries. It is important not to injure these vessels, lest one increase the possibility of postoperative anterior segment ischemia. These vessels lie within the facial sheath along the undersurface of each muscle, so the potential for their damage occurs only in the rarest of traumatic tissue dissections.

It is useful to know the distance from the limbus at which the **extraocular muscles** are inserted and the width of these insertions. This enables a more precise approach to passing the muscle hook prior to passage of the bridle sutures. Knowing the usual width of the muscle insertion [generally 10–11.5 mm] helps one to quickly recognize the possibility that only a part of the muscle fibres have been 'hooked'; repeat pass of a second muscle hook would be necessary to prevent further damage

DOI: 10.1201/9781003179320-7

to the muscle and possible difficulties during subsequent steps. The muscles are usually bridled in the order medial, inferior, lateral, and superior rectus [corresponding distance from the limbus is 5.5, 6.5, 7.0, and 7.7 mm]. One must avoid getting fibres of the superior oblique tendon while attempting to hook the superior rectus muscle. There is an increased potential for this to happen because the superior oblique muscle has wide insertion margin on the scleral surface, just beneath the belly of the superior rectus. The risk can be minimized by passing the squint hook from the temporal to the nasal side and staying within the defined distance of the superior rectus insertion (about 7.7 mm) from the limbus and not sweeping the hook too posteriorly [Figure 6.1]. It is important to also remember that the force of action of the rectus muscles is along a plane tangential to the sclera at its site of insertion. So, the surgeon or assistant must apply traction on the bridle sutures along the same tangential plane to achieve the best possible 'control' over movements of the globe. Tangential pull on the bridle also prevents inadvertent corneal abrasion that could result from rubbing of these sutures over the corneal surface during passage of the scleral sutures or placement of the scleral buckle or rotation of the globe. The macula is located about 2.2 mm superior and nasal to the medial insertion of the inferior oblique muscle. This landmark may be useful while planning macular buckle in patients with complicated pathological myopia.

The **sclera** is a relatively avascular protective cover of the eyeball. It has variable thickness and variable orientation of its fibres, awareness of which may help in reducing complications such as scleral perforation and cut-through and also help create appropriate scleral ports during vitreo-retinal surgery. Scleral thickness is maximal at the limbus [0.83 mm] and around the peripapillary zone [1.00 mm]. At the equator, the thickness is 0.5 mm. It is thinnest just beneath and beside the muscle insertion [0.3 mm]. It is also thin just behind the 'spiral' of Tillaux but thicker anterior to this. Scleral fibres are oriented in a circular fashion around the limbus, so the trocar cannula must be oriented so that these fibres are not cut through. Cutting across the scleral fibres while placing the trocar and cannula may contribute to wound leak at the end of a small-gauge surgery. Relationship

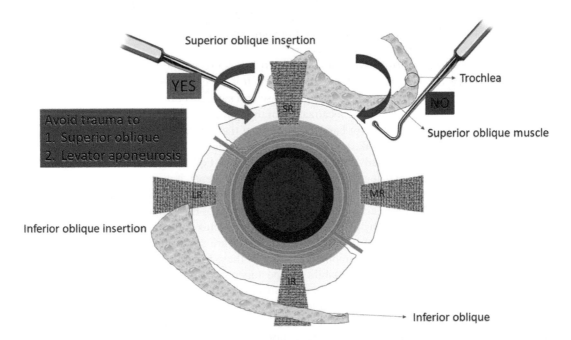

FIGURE 6.1   Relationship between superior rectus and superior oblique muscle and the method to bridle the superior rectus without causing damage to the superior oblique muscle fibres.

Note: SR, superior rectus; LR, lateral rectus; MR, medial rectus; IR, inferior rectus.

of the direction of suture pass and orientation of the scleral fibres explains the increased risk of scleral cut through when buckle sutures are passed circumferentially compared with a radial pass. The reduced risk of cut-through with a radial pass is exploited when the Halstead suture technique is used for buckle placement. Another rarely appreciated property of the sclera [a tissue with a relatively low water content of 68%] is for it to undergo fairly rapid desiccation under the thermal effect of the strong microscope light. This appears as a bluish-black discoloration of the sclera at its most exposed part. Failure to recognize this early is said to have the potential to even rupture the sclera. This complication can be prevented by hydrating the sclera at regular intervals using squirts of saline.

The **spiral of Tillaux** is representative internally of the ora serrata, which in turn is the anterior-most extent of the retina. The distance from the limbus to the ora serrata is different on the temporal and nasal side by about 1 mm [8 mm temporal and 7 mm nasal]. It is marginally less in hypermetropia but may be 1–2 mm more in very high myopia. So, the part of the sclera between the line of muscle insertion and the limbus represents the location of the ciliary body with its components, the pars plicaris anteriorly, and the pars plana posteriorly. The pars plicaris has vascular plexuses and has a width of about 3 mm. The pars plana measures about 4 mm in width and is relatively avascular. It is in continuity with the choroidal layers at the ora serrata. At this junction between the pars plana and choroid [i.e., at the ora serrata] is the vitreous base, the importance of which for vitreoretinal surgeons needs no emphasis. It measures about 3–6 mm in width and straddles anteriorly over the pars plana for 1.5–3 mm and over the peripheral retina for 3–4 mm posteriorly. Being composed of densely condensed vitreous fibrils, it anchors both these tissues, so it is impossible to separate it from the retina without the retina itself tearing first. The dense attachment of the vitreous base posteriorly to the neurosensory retina is the reason why posterior vitreous detachment does not extend beyond this point, why retinal tears often occur here, why only shaving [and not removal] of the vitreous base is attempted during surgery and why it is difficult to remove fixed folds at this region. Attempts at blunt dissection using forceps have a high risk of creating iatrogenic breaks. The relative difficultly of safely removing or shaving the vitreous base [particularly in phakic patients] during surgery can be countered to some extent by providing an external support in the form of a scleral buckle or encirclage. Awareness of the anterior extent of the vitreous base is also important while making a safe entry into the vitreous cavity during standard or small-gauge pars plana vitrectomy. The distance must be such that it reduces the risk of damage to the crystalline lens anteriorly and to the vitreous base [and hence retinal insertion and periphery] posteriorly. Safe distances have been determined to be 3.0, 3.5, and 4.0 mm in aphakic, pseudophakic, and phakic patients, respectively. This distance, however, is different in newborns, infants, toddlers, and young children [Table 6.1] and must be kept in mind while administering anti–vascular endothelial growth factor

TABLE 6.1

Age-adjusted sclerotomy distance from limbus in phakic eyes [derived from morphometric studies]

Age	Sclerotomy distance
0–4 weeks [newborn]	0.5 mm
1–6 months	1.5 mm
6–12 months	2.0 mm
12–24 months	2.5 mm
2–6 years	3.0 mm
6–18 years	3.5 mm
Adults	4.0 mm

injections [for management of retinopathy of prematurity], undertaking pars plana lensectomy or membranectomy, or performing major vitreoretinal procedures in this age group.

Retinal pathologies such as retinal tears are located at or anterior to the equator of the retina, so it is important to be able to identify the equator through some surface landmarks. Since the sclera bulges more on the temporal side, the eyeball is not an ideal sphere. As a result, two equators are considered, anatomical and geographical. The **anatomical equator** represents a circular line, every point of which is equidistant from the anterior pole and posterior pole and lies 13–14 mm from the limbus. Internally, the equator is marked by an imaginary line connecting the posterior margins [ampulla] of the vortex veins. Externally [on the scleral surface], however, there is no visible landmark, so the equator is said to be approximately 7 mm [6–8 mm] posterior to the spiral of Tillaux. Some surgeons prefer to measure the distance from the limbus whence it would be about 14 mm posterior. These external measurements are generally made using an adjustable caliper, one arm of which is placed at the spiral [or limbus] and the other arm is placed with a separation of 7 mm [from the spiral] or 14 mm [from the limbus] posteriorly on the scleral surface. This kind of measurement does not take into consideration the spherical curvature of the globe and in reality is a linear measure. So, there is a mismatch in the distance measured as a curve [length of arc] and as a linear distance [chord length]. But for practical purposes, this discrepancy is not very large and so does not impact the placement of the buckle and encirclage sutures. The vortex veins, usually numbering 4–7, are visible exiting the sclera around the equator, and care must be taken to avoid direct or compressive injury to these veins while placing the buckle and encirclage. The superotemporal, inferotemporal, superonasal, and inferonasal vortex veins leave the sclera 8 mm, 5.5 mm, 6 mm, and 6 mm from the equator, respectively. Before exiting, vortex veins run posteriorly within the sclera [intrascleral part] for about 1–1.5 mm, and scleral sutures should not be passed through these tracks [usually visible as a linear violaceous structure]. If this cannot be completely avoided, one could cut out a notch in the buckle at a site overlying the course of the vortex vein. If vortex veins need to be severed, diathermy must be applied 2–3 mm away from its exit, ligatured, and then resected. Massive intraocular haemorrhage could occur if a vortex vein is cut flush with the sclera [because it tends to retract]. For the same reason, a vortex vein that is accidentally avulsed at its exit must not be coagulated and instead allowed to bleed on the scleral surface. As a landmark, the equator is also important because surgical steps like passing encirclage sutures, drainage of subretinal fluid, drainage of suprachoroidal haemorrhage, and scleral windows for management of nanophthalmos are made in the region between the ora and equator.

With increasing use of scleral fixation of intraocular lens as a method of optical rehabilitation in patients with aphakia and poor capsular support, it is useful to know the surface projection of the **ciliary sulcus**. The ciliary sulcus is a small anatomical space or groove at the junction of the termination of the iris posteriorly and beginning of the ciliary body. Unlike the pars plicata posteriorly and the iris anteriorly, this space is relatively avascular. Hence, instruments, needles, and sutures are manipulated across the ciliary sulcus to achieve a safe outcome during scleral fixation. Ciliary sulcus is said to lie about 1.5 mm behind the limbus. The **limbus** itself has a complex surgical anatomy because it represents the zone of transition from the opaque sclera to the clear cornea. There is a thin line of demarcation, the grey line, about the middle of the transition zone. The region anterior to the line is optically more transparent and that posterior is bluish-greyish. The anterior region is the anatomical limbus and the posterior, the surgical limbus. Incisions to enter the anterior chamber [e.g., during intraocular lens explantation] must be made through the surgical limbus to prevent damage to the Descemet membrane and trabecular meshwork and to reduce the risk of recurrent iris prolapse during surgery.

What has been described is the surgical anatomy of a normal eye. It is important to bear in mind that these guidelines would be inadequate and may even be erroneous while performing vitreoretinal surgery in eyes with buphthalmos, microphthalmos, coloboma, severe ocular trauma, or high myopia. So, it would be important to approach these cases with greater caution and planning.

SUGGESTED READING

1. Silva EEV, Amaya JMH, Cruz JJB, Fernandes DM, Omana REE, Lopez SG [2013]. A morphometric study of the extraocular muscles. *J of Morphometry.* 31: 312–320.
2. Vurgese S, Panda-Jonas S, Jonas JB [2012]. Scleral thickness in human eyes. *PLoS One.* 7(1): e29692.
3. Boote C, Sigal IA, Grytz R et al [2020]. Scleral structure and biomechanics. *Prog Retin Eye Res.* 74: 100773.
4. White MH, Lambert HM, Kincaid MC, Dieckert JP, Lowd DK [1989]. The ora serrata and the spiral of Tillaux. Anatomic relationship and clinical correlation. *Ophthalmol.* 96(4): 508–511.
5. Park DJJ, Karesh J [1998]. Topographic anatomy of the eye: an overview. *Duane's foundations of clinical ophthalmology.* Ed. Jaeger EA, Tasman W. Lippincott Williams, and Wilkins, New York.
6. Verma L, Venkatesh P, Chawla R, Tewari HK [2004]. Choroidal detachment following retinal detachment surgery: an analysis and a new hypothesis to minimize its occurrence in high-risk cases. *Eur J Ophthalmol.* 14(4): 325–329.

7 Machines and Instrumentation

7.1 VITRECTOMY MACHINES

The vitreous machine is truly the heart of every vitreoretinal procedure. Rapid advances in electronic and computer technology, as well those in the field of optics and lasers, have been adapted to the manufacturing of current generation vitreous machines. On the outside, these machines look elegant and produce the desired action with the mere press of a touch button [future machines may have voice control, too] or foot pedal, but within, there is a maze of complex circuitry. Almost all these machines have modules controlling their various functions such as fluid flow, aspiration, and cutting, but they have been seamlessly integrated to function as one unit. Currently marketed vitreous machines have added tremendous precision and safety to our surgeries by introducing several electronic chip– [software-] based sensors to detect, in real time, the stability of the fluidics within the vitreous cavity and then respond and compensate by spontaneously changing the flow rate, the aspiration pressure, and so on. This has greatly reduced catastrophic events such as globe collapse, iatrogenic retinal breaks, and intraocular haemorrhage (suprachoroidal, subretinal, vitreous) that were common occurrences while working with basic vitreous machines of the past that relied largely on gravity-dependent flow and other simple concepts of fluidics and pressure gradients. While the contribution of modern vitreous machines in reducing learning curves, improving reproducibility, and improving patient outcomes is undisputed, it has also significantly increased the economic burden for fledgling surgeons in terms of capital investment needed to start a new venture and for patients in terms of the dent on their savings, borrowings, and insurance premiums.

As clinicians and surgeons, we are well aware of the harm that can result if one neglects the background history, clinical features, and results of the laboratory and other investigations. In a similar manner, we could harm the outcome of our surgical procedure if we fail to comprehend the working principles, recommended settings, controls, limitations, and added advantages of the vitreous machine that we are operating with [e.g., not being aware of how to actuate the reflux function would increase the risk of creating iatrogenic breaks]. What follows is a brief overview of 'vitreo-dynamics' and salient features of some of the high-end vitreous machines that I have had the opportunity of using [Constellation, EVA, Oertli]. All vitreous machines have three basic functions: infusion, aspiration, and vitreous cutting. Integrated into these modules are other adjuvant but critical functions such as diathermy, laser and high-pressure infusion, and removal of viscous fluids. Some machines also have the facility for automated use of intravitreal scissors, auto fill, and injection of air and intraocular gases for intraocular tamponade. In standard phacoemulsification, a single handpiece is designed to allow irrigation, ultrasonic fragmentation, and aspiration. The initial prototype designed by Machemer R, VISC (vitreous infusion suction cutter), was of a similar nature but was very soon replaced by divided-function instrumentation, introduced first by O'Malley. Ever since, this three-port approach has remained the gold standard for the majority of vitreoretinal surgical interventions. Some of the commercially available advanced vitreous machines are Constellation, EVA, Stellaris, and Oertli.

Constellation is a premium machine with which both vitrectomy and phacoemulsification can be performed. The machine is designed with microprocessor circuitry and has a digital interface that is modular and user friendly. Voice confirmations and tones are useful feedback additions. It can be configured using basic or advanced settings. In advanced settings, functions such as flow volume rate can be customized and stored according to surgeon preference. Handpieces needed to accomplish these procedures communicate with the machine console through the cassette to enable

DOI: 10.1201/9781003179320-8

stable intraoperative fluid dynamics during surgery. This is achieved by providing pressurized fluid or air [during air-fluid exchange] through the infusion line, aspirating tissue debris from the vitreous cavity, and maintaining a real-time control of the intraocular pressure [senses outflow through the aspiration line, and reflexly alters the pressure at which fluid or air flows through the infusion line]. There are three types of cassettes: phacoemulsification only, vitrectomy only, and combined surgery; the right cassette must be inserted before the procedure. The combined cassette has several ports [colour coded] for inlet or outlet to enable different functions of the machine. These include pressure source port (1), infusion source port (2), irrigation port (1), aspiration port (2) and low-pressure air source [LPAS] port (1). The lower rim of the cassette has knobs to affix the drainage bag [volume must not be allowed to exceed 500 mL]. For vitrectomy, the machine uses a pneumatically driven vitrectomy cutter that is connected to a pulsed air pressure source. Pneumatic drive is functional at a pressure range of 4–8 Bar [either N2 or clean filtered air can be used]. Aspiration of the cut debris is made possible by vacuum generated across the cassette. Vitreous cutter can operate in three modes: proportional vacuum, momentary, and 3-D. [For phacoemulsification, there are two distinct modes, wet anterior vitrectomy (WetAnt), and dry anterior vitrectomy (VitDry); see section on anterior vitrectomy.] By default, vacuum mode is active when using the posterior or vitrectomy mode [flow mode is active in anterior or phaco mode]. However, using advanced settings, vacuum mode and flow mode can be toggled. The range of pressurized infusion or irrigation is 0–120 mm Hg, flow rate is 0–20 cc/minute [20G], aspiration [vacuum] is 0–650 mm Hg and of LPAS is 0–120 mm Hg. Pressure accuracy is ±2% and is affected by the eye level of the patient with respect to the level of the bottom of the cassette. Hence, before the start of the procedure, the patient's eye level must be aligned with the bottom of the cassette. As the machine forces pressure into the infusion container to force fluid out into the cassette, only glass containers must be used. Use of irrigation or infusion bags could lead to their rupture. Range of cutting possible is 100–10,000 cuts/minute, but the maximum can be achieved only with a compatible probe [ultravit or ultravit+]. Ultravit plus vitreous cutters have a bevelled end to facilitate a closer and safer approach to and dissection of tissue. In momentary mode, a cut rate down to 1 cut/minute is achievable. The duration for which the port of the vitrectomy is open [and closed] can be controlled using the **duty cycle**. There are three modes of duty cycle: core mode, 50/50, and shave mode. In core mode, port opening time is maximal, so there is increased flow towards the port. This mode is used during removal of core vitreous or vitreous that is at a safe distance from the retinal surface. Because of the increased flow rate, the time for removal of vitreous is reduced. However, this mode can increase the risk of traction-induced retinal tears. In shave mode, port opening is minimized, with corresponding reduction in flow rate and retinal traction. This mode is preferred for removal of vitreous over detached retina, peripheral retina, and vitreous base. A 50/50 option is used by some surgeons who prefer to have constant flow rate during the entire procedure. Illumination is provided by two independently controlled ports carrying xenon arc lamp technology [output of 23 ± 13 lumens]. They are generally used for standard endoillumination and chandelier illumination. Two additional auxiliary channels of white light are also available. The machine has a fully integrated diode pumped solid state, green [532 nm, class 4] laser unit with an additional class 2 laser for aiming beam [red, 635 nm]. The laser is functional only when the surgeon's protective filters are in place along the viewing path of the microscope optics [but ensure that the assistant also has a protective filter in place]. Functions and parameters on the console are activated through a multifunctional foot pedal that can be customized according to the surgeon's preference. The foot pedal treadle can also be customized to alter the spans, vibrations, and detent firmness. This machine does not have a wireless foot switch and needs a separate foot switch for the laser.

Modes of function. This describes which function(s) is or are activated and what effect depressing the foot pedal has on that particular function(s). This relationship could be of several types such as single, bimanual (dual linear), 3D mode, linear, proportional reflux, and momentary [Figure 7.1]. In **single mode**, the foot pedal treadle controls only the set function [e.g., inject mode] during its entire travel [start to full depression of the foot pedal] in a linear manner. In **bimanual [dual mode]**,

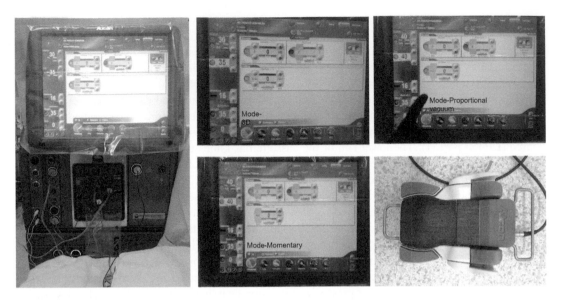

FIGURE 7.1 Modes of vitrectomy possible while using one of the advanced vitrectomy machines [Constellation].

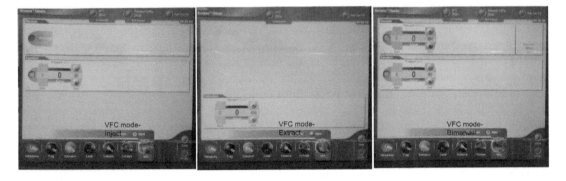

FIGURE 7.2 Modes of viscous fluid controller on the Constellation vitrectomy machine.

the foot pedal controls dual functions, with one function being activated during initial travel and the second function, during later travel. For example, in bimanual mode of viscous fluid controller, initial depression of the foot pedal activates injection and later depression, activates extrusion [Figure 7.2]. This can be extremely useful during manoeuvres such as direct bimanual perfluorocarbon liquid [PFCL] silicone oil exchange, PFCL injection without double-bore cannula, and bimanual dissection wherein initial travel controls pneumatic forceps and later travel pneumatic scissors. It should, however, be remembered that bimanual procedures are generally possible only with a fourth port for chandelier illumination. **Fixed mode** is a kind of dual mode wherein the parameter for one function [e.g., ultrasound power] is fixed from the beginning till the end of the treadle while the other function [e.g., vacuum] is controlled linearly. The term *fixed mode* is applied during fragmatome use. **Proportional vacuum mode** is similar to fixed mode and is applied in relation to the vitreous cutter. In this mode, the cut rate is fixed to the desired preset, while vacuum can be controlled linearly from 0 to a maximum preset value. In **linear mode**, the foot pedal controls two functions linearly—initial travel controlling one function [e.g., vacuum] and later travel, the other [e.g., ultrasonic energy]. This may seem similar to bimanual mode, but there is an important difference between the two. Bimanual mode refers to dual control of two independent, uni-functional instruments inserted through different ports [hence bimanual], while linear mode refers to dual control of multifunctional instrument [inserted through one port] such as vitreous cutter [cutting function and aspiration function] and fragmatome [emulsification and aspiration function]. In **3D mode**, two functions are simultaneously controlled in a linear manner on pressing the foot pedal. For using this mode, two values have to be preset (for both functions separately), one indicating the value when the food pedal is initiated and the other indicating the value when it is fully pressed down. For example, while using the vitreous cutter in 3D mode, the surgeon can achieve ideal vitreodynamic functionality for both core vitrectomy and shave function without having to do so separately on the console. However, this requires fine calibration and constant attention to the treadle of the foot pedal. [In the same manner, the terms *proportional vacuum mode* and *fixed mode* are also applicable only during the use of bifunctional instruments.] **Momentary mode** helps in dissociating the control of the two functions in a bifunctional instrument [e.g., vitreous cutter, fragmatome]. One function [usually vacuum] can be controlled linearly by pressing on the foot pedal while the other can be activated for a momentary period [at a chosen time during surgery] by pressing a vertical plate lying adjacent to the foot pedal. This mode allows the best control and precision over functions such as cutting of membranes with the vitreous cutter [cut rate can be reduced to 1 cpm and hence can be used like scissors] and lens fragmentation [ultrasound can be precisely activated only when full occlusion is obtained]. The author uses this mode regularly during resection of taut membranes [e.g., tractional retinal detachment] and phacofragmentation [Figure 7.3]. **Reflux mode** allows fluid to egress from

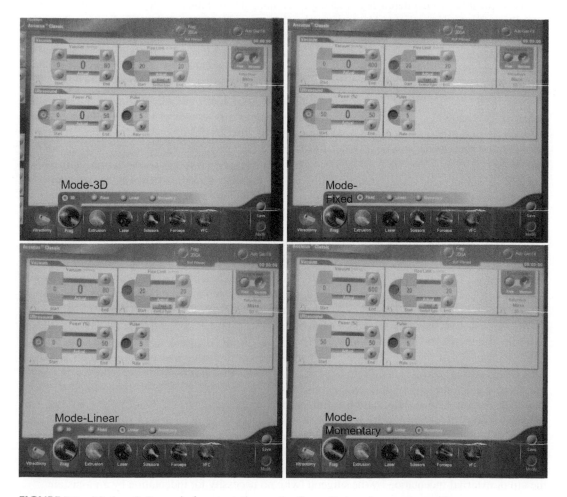

FIGURE 7.3 Modes of ultrasonic fragmentation on the Constellation vitrectomy machine.

the vitrectomy port, thereby pushing away and releasing inadvertent grasp on sensitive tissue [retina]. Two reflux modes are available, proportional [range, 0–120 mmHg] and micro-reflux [range, 10%, 25%, 50%, 75%, or 100%].

Enhancing Visual Acuity [EVA] is an advanced machine that has functions for carrying out both anterior segment and posterior segment surgery. The basic functions integrated into this setup are infusion, vacuum, cutting, illumination, and laser. Unique features include the two-dimensional cutting [TDC] cutter; flow-based aspiration control; a patented trocar cannula system [Aveta]; and a single, wireless foot switch for actuation of instrument parameters, as well as laser delivery. The **TDC cutter** achieves 16,000 [8000 × 2] with the use of compatible probes—those having two openings within the inner tubing of the guillotine cutter. This allows the probe to cut while moving both forward and backward, hence doubling the cut rate. Unlike other vitreous machines, the preferred mode for vacuum to control aspiration in EVA is flow based. **Flow-based aspiration** is said to make the system safer by reducing traction on the retina. However, a disadvantage experienced by the author and generally emphasized is that the probe must be taken closer to the retina to achieve cutting. Hence, flow mode, while reducing the risk of traction induced retinal tear, also has the potential to increase the risk of retinal tear formation from direct contact. **Aveta** is a recently approved, patent-pending trocar-cannula system that uses a push fit infusion connection plus a laser-etched retention feature and a smaller cannula head size [20% smaller]. This is said to allow high flow, reduce the incidence of cannula dislodgement from the port site, and provide more working space. Insertion is also easier, even across a valved cannula, and can be switched to another location without the risk of leak and hypotony. The new trocar has a chamfered edge [having an additional transitional angle] and is claimed to allow smoother, effortless insertion and better wound architecture. The foot switch is wireless, but the author perceives it to be less responsive and needing greater force [despite adjusting the treadle] to depress. The ability to use the same foot switch for the laser is certainly an added advantage.

Both phacoemulsification and vitreous surgery can be performed using Stellaris, a high-end machine that comes in two models, Stellaris PC and Stellaris Elite. Highlights of this machine include a high cut rate 7500 [PC] to 15,000 [Elite- bi-blade technology], hypersonic vitreous liquefaction [Vitesse or HyperV technology], a dual light source [xenon and mercury vapour], and digital filters. **Bi-blade technology** is similar to TDC and allows cutting of the vitreous during movement in both directions [forward and backward]. Similar to TDC, this is said to increase port open time and so improve flow efficiency and at the same time reduce transmission of tractional forces to the retina. **Vitesse** is a patented technology for vitreous 'cutting'. It works by creating a localized vitreous liquefaction zone at the edge of the port. Liquefaction efficiency is said to be equivalent to 1.7 million virtual cuts per minute. The probe has a single-lumen design through which both vitreous liquefaction and aspiration are achieved. The port is fully and constantly open. The light source supports add-ons for even 29G design. Three **digital filters** [yellow, amber, and green] are provided to augment or act as substitute for vital dye staining. The green filter may be useful during membrane peeling and the amber filter at air-fluid exchange. The functions are controlled by a wireless single foot pedal [for vitrectomy and laser].

Oertli's latest model, **OS4**, has certain unique features such as the Caliburn cannula system, tri-pump system, light-emitting diode (LED) illumination source, digital filters, dual infusion–gravity driven or active [gas forced], and continuous flow cutting [10,000 cuts/minute]. The **Caliburn cannula** system has an integrated valve that is located towards the inner opening of the cannula hub rather than the outer opening. This is said to create a tight fit during instrument insertion and withdrawal and hence provide stable vitreodynamics. The **tri-pump** allows the surgeon direct control over both, vacuum, and flow rate. In combination with a new mode, SPEEP [speed and precision], it provides a new feature, HDC (high-definition dynamic direct control). **Goodlight LED** does not dim in brightness with age, has lesser proportion of blue wavelength, and has low irradiance [58 mW/sq cm compared with 140 with xenon at 5-mm distance]. The LED light sources can be customized according to the surgical step [e.g., membrane peeling, spotting a bleeding point]. The endo-illuminator probes can be used with the **ViPer scleral indenter** for peripheral vitreous removal with the aid of external indentation by the surgeon [with no necessity for indentation by an assistant].

VitMan is a portable composite vitrectomy system that is efficient and relatively more afford-able. Basic functions of the surgery such as vitreous cutting, aspiration, endoillumination, and air-fluid exchange can be performed. It is a software-controlled electronic and mechanical system and can be connected to an electric or pneumatic line. Vacuum is generated by a pump with rocking style piston. Illumination is powered by a Tungsten lamp, and three fibre optic cables [each with 35-mV intensity] can be used simultaneously.

Frequency of cutting Max was 1000/minute. As can be seen by the description, this machine was acceptable during the availability of earlier generation of vitrectomy machines such as Accurus and Harmony, which had similar capabilities. With the advent of premium vitrectomy machines [constellation, EVA, Stellaris, Oertli] that provide superior performance using small-gauge instruments, VitMan has lost its advantages and is hence no longer used. A newer portable machine is now available called **Versavit 2.0**. This machine can run on a battery and uses a pneumatic source [compressed air or carbon dioxide] for driving the vitrectomy probe [6000 cuts/minute]. Illumination is provided through dual LED light sources. Endolaser, silicone oil injection, and extrusion are also possible. The cost of the device as well as disposable packs is about 50% to 80% as economical as non-portable vitreous machines.

7.2 SURGICAL MICROSCOPE

The surgical microscope, as the name suggests, is a compound microscope that helps in clear binocular visualization of the surgical field. Like all microscopes, it has optical, illumination, and mechanical components. In addition, unlike simple microscopes, surgical microscopes need a high-input electrical supply to run the lamps incorporated for illuminating the optical path as well as the surgical field. The optical component consists of an objective lens and eyepieces [two, being binocular]. For posterior segment surgery an added optical component is the stereo-diagonal inverter [SDI]. Most operating microscopes currently available also have an assistant's microscope with components similar to the surgeon's microscope. It may be an independent electric or manual zoom [about 5×] or may zoom in parallel with the main microscope. The objective lens is apochromatic [allows better correction of spherical and chromatic aberrations] and helps focus at different operating distances. The eyepiece allows wide field viewing [10× or 12.5×] and has an adjustable dioptric scale [-8D to +5D] and adjustable interpupillary distance. An important performance indicator of a surgical microscope is the depth of field, defined as range of depth that appears sharply defined while an object seen through the microscope is being moved towards and away from the objective. The objective lens could have a focal length of either 200 mm or 175 mm. The focal lengths of the 10× and 12.5× eyepiece are 25 mm and 20mm respectively. The corresponding fields of view are 21 mm and 18 mm, respectively. Magnification obtained [with a 200-mm objective lens and 10× eyepiece] is 3.5× to 21×. The total range of focus is 70 mm [+40 mm upwards and -30 mm downwards]. Some microscopes have a DeepView setting that automatically optimizes the depth of filed and light transmission of the microscope image.

Illumination is delivered as stereo-coaxial illumination [SCI]. SCI illumination has three pre-configured illumination patterns [but the mix ratio of red reflex illumination and surrounding field illumination can be adjusted]—red reflex illumination [100% red reflex, 0% surrounding illumination], mixed light [100% red reflex and 50% surrounding illumination], and surrounding field illumination [0% red reflex, 100% surrounding illumination]. In the past, lamps used for illumination were mercury vapour or metal halide lamps. This has largely been replaced now with xenon lamps and LED lamps because they are considered to be more optically efficient. The xenon light source can be set between 5% to 100% and LED source from 2% to 100% [at 1% increments]. Some microscopes may also carry a back-up lamp. Photic retinal injury from the microscope could occur if the exposure time is beyond 100 minutes. Stereo coaxial illumination provides bright red reflex using very small amounts of light in the central surgical field and higher amounts in the peripheral field, thereby reducing the risk of phototoxicity. Protection from blue portions of the light by using the retina protection filter [blue barrier filter] also helps to reduce phototoxicity. Turning off the micro-scope or covering the eye during pauses in surgery is also a simple way of reducing the risk. Other than retina protection filter, some microscopes have other filters such as a fluorescence filter [485 nm] that makes fluorescent areas visible and a HaMode filter that allows generation of light spectrum similar to halogen light source and grey filter. The last of these reduces the set light intensity to 25% and hence increase the radiation exposure time by a factor of 4.

Mechanical components of a surgical microscope include the massive frame [with a base carrying study wheels that can be locked into position], vertical support, and an oblique mechanical arm that can be used to swivel the optical head into position over the operating field. This arm also carries the main electrical cables within an inbuilt tray and has a magnetic lock to prevent it from inadvertently swivelling away. The main frame may also have provisions for carrying a PC monitor, an intraoperative optical coherence tomography (OCT) monitor, and other controls to remotely control and change the microscope settings. It also houses the illumination lamps through a modular, detachable component. The foot switch, another important mechanical component, has a joystick for XY coupling, rocker switches to adjust the zoom and focus, and multiple other buttons [these are freely configurable] to control some other functions of the device [e.g., pausing the illumination]. XY coupling can be positioned in a 61-mm × 61-mm area. The speed and direction of movement [normal or inverted] can be configured. With the currently available microscopes, it is possible to create and archive surgery profiles for each user.

7.3 VIEWING SYSTEMS

One of the necessities for undertaking good indirect ophthalmoscopy is to have proper illumination. Similarly, there has to be synchrony between illumination and visualization during every step of vitreoretinal surgery. According to Maxwellian principle, 'area illuminated equals area seen'. This principle can be extended into the realm of vitreoretinal surgery as 'area illuminated equals area seen equals area safely operated'. Visualization for posterior segment surgery is obtained using specially devised optical lenses. These are of two kinds, contact lenses and non-contact lenses. Based on the field of view, they could be narrow field lenses or limited view systems and wide-field lenses or panoramic view systems. Contact lenses may be further subdivided into three kinds: lenses held by a handle, lenses retained by a sewn-on ring, and self-stabilizing lenses [with broad extensions or struts at the base; Figure 7.4]. Contact visualization lenses provide sharper and clearer image because they are able to neutralize aberrations at the corneal surface. They also provide a slightly larger field of view with fewer distortions of the periphery compared with non-contact lenses. Disadvantages of these lenses include the need for an assistant to hold or realign the lenses [in self-retaining lenses], the need for coupling fluid or viscoelastic to prevent corneal drying and abrasion, and a reduction in the working space for maneuvers such as scleral indentation. In addition, even a slight pressure on the cornea or tilting of the lens by the assistant can significantly impede visualization. Also, corneal clouding, epithelial defects, and obscuration by blood trapped beneath the lens are potential problems. For corneal wetting, diluted hydroxypropylmethylcellulose should be preferred because the regular viscoelastics may produce disturbing pseudo-refractive surfaces. A standard example of contact, narrow-field lens is the Landers lens. This is of two kinds, on axis and off axis. On-axis lenses provide visualization of the central 20 to 35 degrees of the posterior retina [based on the curvature, planoconcave or biconcave]. Off-axis lenses have one edge that is higher and sloping [short and long] and enable visualization of the equator and beyond. Wide-field lenses have a field of view ranging from 110 to 130 degrees. Earlier, the panfundoscopic lens of Rodenstock [FOV 150 degrees], a contact viewing lens, was reduced in dimensions and used for vitreous surgery as a vitreous panfundoscope. Narrow-field lenses such as the Landers one are usually made of PMMA [polymethyl methacrylate], whereas wide-field lenses are made of glass. One prominent difference while using narrow- and wide-field lenses is that the retinal image gets inverted in the latter. Because very few surgeons are able to operate with an inverted image, corrective optics such as SDI needs

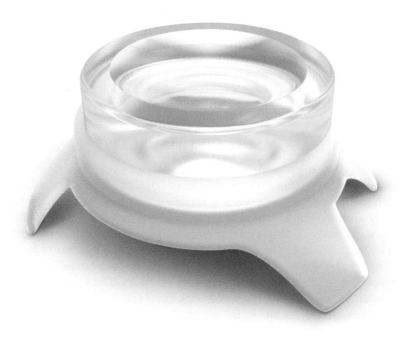

FIGURE 7.4   Self stabilizing contact lens for visualization during vitreoretinal surgery. [Courtesy of Vitreq.]

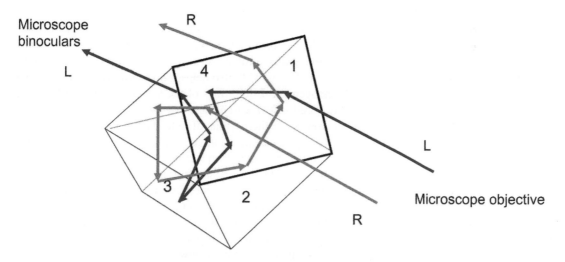

FIGURE 7.5   Optics of the Reinverting Operating Lens System for vitreous surgery under wide-field visualization.

to be placed into the optical path of the microscope visualization axis to reinvert the image. The Reinverting Operating Lens System is a unique type of re-inverter in which inversion of the image is obtained using two prisms [Figure 7.5].

Non-contact lenses are a little more complex and need to be integrated into the operating microscope or surgical field using separate supporting elements. The field of view is slightly narrower, and resolution is lesser [for fine macular surgery such as internal limiting membrane peeling]. Also, corneal dryness needs to be prevented by intermittent fluid jets. The major advantages with these lenses are the lack of dependency on an assistant and the ability to indent the retinal periphery more freely. Non-contact lenses can be manually or automatically swiveled into the viewing axis or moved away. Usually, two types of lenses are available, one for macular or posterior retinal surgery and one for the periphery. Some of the widely used non-contact inverter systems include Resight, AVI, Merlin, EBIOS, and BIOM. Resight has two versions based on the method used for operating these lenses, manual [RESIGHT 500] and electric [RESIGHT 700].

7.4   HEADS-UP VISUALIZATION SURGERY [3D SURGERY]

Traditionally, surgery under a microscope is performed with the neck titled downwards and the eyes [head down] peering into the binocular eyepieces. In 2016, an alternate visualization system for performing both anterior and posterior segment surgery was introduced in which the procedure could be undertaken while looking at a large monitor, placed some distance away. This approach has come to be known as heads-up surgery. Performing surgery while looking into the monitor is not unique to ocular surgery and has in fact already been in practice in other subspecialities for several decades. The concept was well thought out in yesteryears, but available technology at that period was not supportive for carrying out surgery with precision. The limitations were because of poor camera resolution, poor monitor resolution, lack of an optically efficient light source, and glitches and speed of image transmission. Rapid advances in digital, photic, and computer technology over the past decade have overcome these limitations, paving the way for heads-up surgery to quickly gain ground. The chief advantages of heads-up surgery include extremely high magnification, high depth of resolution, 3D visualization using polaroid glasses, and reduced need for tissue illumination. Owing to digital manipulation of the monitor pixels, surgery can be undertaken with almost 10% to 20% levels of illumination compared with standard surgery. In addition, it also allows the possibility of using digital filters [yellow, green, and blue, the exact utility of which is still poorly defined]. For the surgeon, it is considered to be more ergonomic because it reduces strain on the spinal and neck muscles. In addition, it also seems to reduce the ocular strain [author's observation] that could occur while performing surgery for long hours under a standard microscope. Concurrent benefits include the ability of other surgical team members to be able to see the surgical steps in real time and assist efficiently. It also helps fellows and residents to grasp the concepts and nuances of surgical management. Limitations of the system include added cost, delicate maintenance, need for special licensed software to be able to view the surgical recordings, unnatural color values, inexplicable shadowing of the peripheral field during vitreous surgery at times, and most important, in case of difficulty in visualization, having to replace the entire digital camera-mounted microscope with a standard microscope. Initial attempts at amalgamating digital imaging technology into the optical pathway [by placing a beam splitter] for dual viewing through eyepieces, as well as on the monitor, failed because the amount of illumination was found to be grossly reduced. To resolve this, the microscope eyepieces were done away with, and images from the surgical field were directly captured by high—resolution digital cameras and relayed to a large monitor. Initial monitors were 2K, so image resolution was only just adequate to undertake the procedure. By replacing 2K monitors with the 4K monitors that are now routinely available, resolution improves significantly [however, it still remains lower than the resolution achieved under a standard surgical microscope]. Loss of some resolution is compensated to a certain extent by increased digital magnification.

The first commercially available visualization system for heads-up surgery was **Ngenuity** [Alcon, 2016]. This system incorporates a patented 3D technology by TrueView for stereoscopic 3D visualization on a 4K 55-inch monitor. Ngenuity consists of three components: a digital camera [image capture module (ICM), which replaces the standard visualization head on the microscope], an embedded processing unit [EPU], and a visualization monitor [3D flat-panel display]. EPU and the monitor are located on a movable workstation [mobile cart]. The digital camera allows capture of images in high definition and 3D using the inbuilt light of the microscope itself.

It has two 3MP sensors, which convert the analog signals into digital signals for video stream-ing to the EPU [at a rate of 3GB/s]. Camera resolution is placed at 1920 × 1080 for each eye. The latency between image capture and display on the monitor is less than 100 ms. The ICM also has an iris slider to control the amount of light entering the camera [recommended being 20%–60%]. The higher the opening on the iris slider, the lower the depth of field. The EPU uses a digital video interface to deliver high-resolution, high–refresh rate [60 fps simultaneously for each eye] stereoscopic images to the display monitor. The monitor has a resolution of 3840 × 2160 pixels [1920 × 1080 for each image of the stereopair]. It also has a circularly polarized, micro-polarizing filter that displays the right and left images alternately. Corresponding circularly polarized glasses that have to be worn by the surgeon allow the right eye to visualize only the right image and left eye only the left image. The recommended distance of the monitor to achieve the best 3D visualization is 4–6 feet away from the surgeon, just beside the surgical bed. The distance can, however, be adjusted as per the surgeon's comfort and perception. Adjusting the white balance of the ICM image sensor to the microscope light before the start of the surgery each day is neces-sary to obtain a colour-balanced, good-quality image. Image properties such as colour, bright-ness, contrast, gamma, hue, and saturation can be digitally adjusted. Camera orientation can be toggled between standard [upright] and inverted [while using an inverting lens during posterior segment surgery] using a button on the foot switch or remotely on the wireless keyboard. Focus of the surgical field is achieved in a manner similar [but looking at the image on the monitor] to that of a standard surgical microscope. A 2-TB storage drive within the EPU allows 100 hours of recording in 3D. In the automatic recording mode, the maximum length of continuous recording possible is 20 minutes. After this, the software automatically starts recording another clip lasting 20 minutes, then another 20 minutes, and so on.

ARTEVO 800 is a surgical microscope [Zeiss] designed for 3D visualization of the ophthalmic field during both anterior and posterior segment surgery. It provides wide magnification, illumina-tion, and visualization possibilities. The digital microscope has integrated 4K cameras, inverter-tube E, eyepieces for the surgeon and assistant [optional], and an objective lens. It enlarges and illuminates the surgical field and displays it on the 3D monitor. The digital camera consists of two integrated 4K cameras [three sensor chips] and provides the same resolution as Ngenuity [3840 × 2160]. Video resolution is also similar to that of Ngenuity. The camera head carries an infrared filter and laser filter [532 nm]. Invertertube E rotates inverted images into an upright position. Artevo is usually integrated with RESCAN 700, an intraoperative high-resolution spectral domain [SD]-OCT [840-nm superluminescent diode source] that allows applicability of OCT functionality to surgical procedures. Both can be controlled via the foot pedal or remotely by an assistant through a touch interface. The device has been contraindicated for diagnostic use. It is composed of a range of illumination sources, stereo-coaxial illumination (SCI) system, fibre slit illuminator (Visolux), and attachable fundus viewing systems (RESIGHT 500 and 700). For viewing and training, the surgeon can alternate between two modes, hybrid [viewing is possible through the eyepiece as well as 3D monitor] or digital [viewing is possible only on 3D monitor]. Polaroid 3D glasses are necessary for heads-up surgery or viewing on the monitor. For posterior segment surgery, specific contact lenses for RESIGHT must be used. When OCT scanning is in use, images are displayed as picture in picture on the monitor. Hardware and interfaces on the CALLISTO [PC monitor attached through a separate arm support] allows visualization, modification of the image, positioning of the OCT scan, taking a snapshot, recording, and review and transfer of images or surgical videos [for archiving]. Callisto software settings are optimized for the RESIGHT 700 fundus viewing system with 60D and 128D ophthalmoscopy lenses. Images may not be of satisfactory quality with use of other lenses. For flat contact lenses, the system has been tested only with a DORC 1284 flat lens. Similar to Ngenuity, white balance [as per manufacture recommendations] is needed at the begin-ning of surgery each day. When white balance is initiated, the device adjusts the 4K cameras so that white areas in the surgical field also appear white on the monitor. This helps to provide a natural colour to the images.

7.5   INTRAOPERATIVE OPTICAL COHERENCE TOMOGRAPHY

Over the past two decades, optical coherence tomography has revolutionized the diagnosis, decision making, treatment, and follow-up of patients with innumerable macular and retinal disorders. Speed and comfort of image capture, tissue resolution, and depth of penetration as well as eye-tracking ability have steadily improved from the days of time domain OCT to the current era of SD and swept source OCT. It is hence no wonder that efforts have been made to exploit and apply the ability of OCT to provide vivid details of vitreoretinal relationships, in real time, during vitreoretinal surgery. Initial models of intraoperative optical coherence tomography (iOCT) were stand-alone units and hence the surgical step had to be paused before intraoperative imaging could be undertaken. Models in current use are integrated into the operating microscope and can be used in real time, while performing a surgical step, such as ILM peeling. There are several iOCT options available commercially, each adapted to a particular model and type of operating microscope. The objective lens of the OCT is co-axially aligned with the microscope and can be introduced or removed from the visualization axis at the surgeon's discretion. Alignment of the image on the capture window, degree of focus, and clarity have to be frequently monitored and adjusted on the monitor by an assistant using the available touch buttons.

The role of iOCT has been explored during surgical intervention for macular hole, epimacular membrane, vitreomacular traction, optic disc pit maculopathy, myopic foveoschisis, and a few others. Most observations seem to suggest that iOCT does improve the detection, documentation, and manipulation of surface membranes to achieve a more definitive anatomical configuration. However, its ability to correspondingly improve surgical and visual outcomes has not been irrefutably established. One of the limitations of realizing the full potential of real-time iOCT imaging is the bothersome shadowing from the shaft or tip of the intravitreal instrument. Currently, instruments made of material that can offset this limitation are under evaluation. Some of the applications of iOCT would include the ability to discern the presence of a safe cleavage plane between the retinal surface and aberrant membrane [e.g., in diabetic surgery, surgery for removal of epimacular membrane], identification and safer removal of the Weiss ring during posterior vitreous detachment induction, detect residual membrane after epimacular membrane surgery, and refine the placement of inverted ILM flap, free flap, or submacular amniotic membrane graft during macular hole surgery. Future applications after integration of iOCT with heads-up vitrectomy could include subretinal injection of therapeutic agents with precision, placement of retinal prostheses, and in being able to perform retinal endovascular interventions.

7.6   ILLUMINATION IN VITREOUS SURGERY

Quality illumination of the operative field is an important prerequisite to successful surgery. Unlike anterior segment surgery, illumination for posterior segment surgery has to be entirely delivered through the endoillumination probe and/or chandelier light source. Several factors of the illumination have a bearing on the quality of visualization, including colour, spectral wavelength, amount of blue light, beam width, closeness to the retinal surface, and presence of extraneous light sources. Several light sources for illumination have been used and include metal halide, mercury vapour, halogen, xenon arc, and LED. Currently available high-end vitreous machine use either xenon arc or LED and most have a dual light source that are completely independent. Xenon arc light is the most widely used source to power illumination for small-gauge vitreous surgery. Studies seem to, however, indicate that, in terms of safety, LED sources may be better because they have lower irradiance. In addition, LED sources do not dim in intensity even after significant usage. A complication that is uniquely linked to illumination during vitreoretinal surgery is macular phototoxicity [see section on complications]. The ease of visibility during surgery is also determined by the cone angle of the endoilluminator probes [varies from 50–100 degrees]. Some probes are bevelled and have a sheath to reduce glare and improve visualization [Figure 7.6]. Chandelier light probes are self-retaining and inserted directly into the sclera [after making a trocar entry]. Although they are designed to provide wide-angle diffuse illumination, the tip of chandelier light may need to be directed manually [by the assistant] towards an area of dissection. To overcome this limitation, a new directional chandelier illumination has been introduced [Figure 7.7]. Other forms of illumination available are

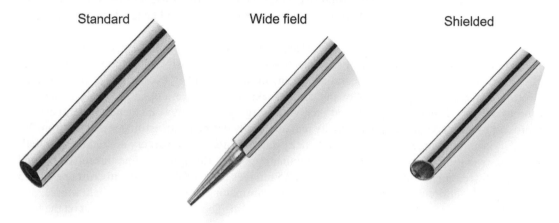

Standard   Wide field   Shielded

FIGURE 7.6 Types of endoilluminators based on the cone of visualization. [Courtesy of Vitreq.]

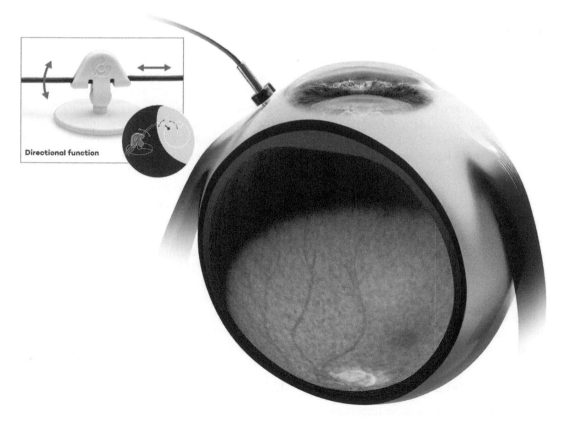

Directional function

FIGURE 7.7 Chandelier illumination with directional function. [Courtesy of Vitreq.]

lighted intravitreal instruments [including infusion] and twin-light chandelier [minimizes shadows seen with single fibres]. Chandelier light is best suited to perform endoillumination-assisted scleral buckling surgery [EASB; see section on EASB] and biopsy of intraocular mass. While chandelier light is routinely used to carry out bimanual procedures, the distant location and diffuse nature of the light makes membrane dissection more difficult than under focal illumination of a light pipe. Reflexes also get exaggerated after air-fluid exchange. Some machines use a filter in the path of the illumination to reduce delivery of harmful wavelengths to the retina and hence decrease the risk of phototoxicity.

Photic retinopathy results from the toxic effects of photochemical, photothermal, and mechanical interaction between light and retinal tissue. Tso first reported the possibility of retinal phototoxicity from artificial light under experimental conditions in rhesus monkey eyes in 1973. Subsequently, several other reports appeared following cataract extraction, epikeratophakia, triple procedure, vitreous surgery, Molteno implant, and pterygium surgery. The actual incidence from operating microscope–induced macular phototoxicity remains poorly defined with estimates ranging from 3% to 28%. The main sources of retinal phototoxicity during vitreoretinal surgery are indirect ophthalmoscope, operating microscope, and endoilluminator probes. Recognized time thresholds beyond which photic retinopathy could occur are 4.0 to 7.5 minutes for a 30W operating microscope and 15 minutes for the indirect ophthalmoscope. For endoilluminators, it depends on the light source, distance from the retina, diameter, and divergence of the beam. The shape and size depend on the light source. Operating light–induced lesions are sharply defined and are rarely more than 1–2 disc areas, while endoilluminator lesions are larger and have less distinct margins. The location of the lesion in operation microscope–induced photic maculopathy is typically superior or inferior to the fovea. This is determined by the effect of the bridle suture and because the coaxial light is normally 1.5–6 degrees off normal. Because phototoxicity has a cumulative effect, reducing surgical time under the microscope and endoilluminator would reduce the risk of this 'invisible' and delayed complication.

Clinically, photic maculopathy is usually not visible for 1–2 days, and features depend on the severity and stage of phototoxicity (early or late). In the early stages, there is well-circumscribed outer retinal whitening. Within a few days, mild pigmentary disturbances become evident, and in the subsequent 1–2 weeks, the pigmentation becomes coarse and may also take on a targetoid appearance. After a period of about 4 weeks, the lesion appears smaller, and epiretinal membrane formation may occur. At 3–6 months, the only remnant may be a yellow-white plaque. Choroidal neovascular membrane and cystoid macular edema are rare sequelae. Visual outcome is usually favourable. It has been recommended that patients taking photosensitizing drugs such as hydroxychloroquine, allopurinol, retinoic acid, phenothiazines, and psoralen compounds be asked to discontinue them several days before any surgical procedure under the operating microscope. Measures that have been described to decrease foveal irradiance are use of an eclipse filter, injecting an air bubble temporarily into the anterior chamber, and avoiding direct foveal exposure by tilting the microscope about 10 degrees and infraduction of the globe. The eclipse filter described by McIntyre consists of an opaque disk placed at an appropriate plane along the illumination path of the operating microscope so as to project a sharply focused opaque spot of 11 mm on the cornea to decrease retinal irradiance. Use of corneal covers such as Gelfoam, and opaque soft contact lenses, have also been reported to protect against photic maculopathy. Prophylactic use of dexamethasone and mildly cool infusion fluid have also been suggested as protective measures. Studies on the role of ultraviolet-absorbing intraocular implants in protecting against the occurrence of cystoid macular edema [and hence photic maculopathy] have shown conflicting results.

7.7 HANDHELD TOOLS, SUTURES, AND NEEDLES

Vitreous cutters are the most important component of a vitrectomy kit and enable cutting of vitreous fibrils and aspiration of the debris simultaneously. Vitreous cutters could be powered through pneumatic drives, dual pneumatic drives, or electrical drives. The **lighting cutter** was a very efficient cutter driven by electricity. However, it is no longer available because the handpiece was heavily built and hence considered ergonomically inefficient. Cut rates have steadily increased from 750, 1000, 2500, 4000, 5000, 7500, 10,000, 15,000, and 16,000 cuts/minute over the past several decades, more so after the advent of small-gauge vitrectomy systems. The mechanism of vitreous fragmentation could be rotatory [initial vitreous cutter introduced by Machemer], guillotine [most widely used], bi-blade, two-dimensional cutting, dual pneumatic cutting, or hypersonic vitreous removal [Vitesse]. The **TDC cutter** achieves 16,000 [8000 × 2] with the use of compatible probes (i.e., those having two openings within the inner tubing of the guillotine cutter). This allows the probe to cut while moving both forward and backward, hence doubling the cut rate. **Bi-blade technology** is similar to TDC and allows cutting of the vitreous during movement in both directions [forward and backward]. Similar to TDC, this is said to increase port open time and so improve flow efficiency and at the same time reduce transmission of tractional forces to the retina. **Vitesse** is a patented technology for vitreous 'cutting'. It works by creating a localized vitreous liquefaction zone at the edge of the port. Liquefaction efficiency is said to be equivalent to 1.7 million virtual cuts/minute. The probe has a single lumen design through which both vitreous liquefaction and aspiration is achieved. The port is fully and constantly open.

Fragmatome has a stainless steel shell housing the ultrasonic crystal [piezoelectric]. An ultrasound needle [20G or 23G] is attached to its distal end before the procedure, while the proximal end is connected to the aspiration line. Depending on the control setup and type of machine, ultrasound energy is delivered as continuous mode or pulse mode. Fragmatome can be used in four modes, 3D, fixed, linear, and momentary mode [see section on vitreous machines]. Micro-reflux or proportional reflux is available during fragmatome use and can be activated when necessary by pressing the control button on the foot pedal. An important precaution that needs to be taken during phacofragmentation is to increase the flow volume rate by 15% to 90%. This is because aspiration volume across the ultrasound handpiece is significantly higher [owing to the port being open before occlusion and because of caliber mismatch if a 25G system is being used]. The range of pulse discharge is between 0 and 100 pps. Tip stroke at 100% power is between 2.5 and 3.5 mils. After autoclaving, the handle must be allowed to air cool for at least 15 minutes. The needle tip must be fully secured into the handpiece; without this, adequate power is not delivered. The ultrasonic handpiece must never be cleaned ultrasonically because it can be irreparably damaged.

A unique complication associated with the ultrasound handpiece is the risk of thermal damage to the incision site as well as intraocular structures. This results from excessive heating of the handpiece secondary to one or more of the following factors: high ultrasound energy, low flow rate, low vacuum, excessive duration [continuous], tight incision, clogged aspiration line, presence of significant viscoelastic, or poor tuning [before surgery]. Tuning of the handpiece must also be carried out with the tip immersed in fluid. Dry tuning leads to irreversible and severe damage to the device. Tissue damage [e.g., to the retina or iris] could occur because of direct contact [mechanical injury] or by exposure to high ultrasound energy [thermal injury]. A rare occurrence is dispersion of metal fragments into the surgical field caused by micro-abrasion of the tip from the ultrasonic energy.

A **pneumatic handle** is used for tissue manipulation with automated forceps or scissors [these tips can be connected to the handle as needed]. Two handles can be used for bimanual surgery [with console setting on corresponding bimanual mode]. In this mode, initial travel of the foot pedal enables forceps activation and later travel, scissors activation. Two types of control are possible, multiple cut and proportional.

Diathermy tips are made of high conductive, non-stick alloy such as titanium and provide unimanual, bipolar coagulation. Several designs are available, including straight, curved, tapered, and wide stroke. [Diathermy is defined as introducing an electric field, at a low radiofrequency (1.5 MHz), to a body part to produce heat.]

Small-gauge instrumentation has added safety to vitreoretinal surgery in multiple ways. One of these, which is often poorly emphasized, is the declining need for using multiple intravitreal instruments such as forceps, scissors of different curvatures [based on the pathoanatomy], membrane

scrappers, or bent picks. One of the key reasons for this is the design change in small-gauge vitreous cutters. In the newer designs, not only has the diameter reduced, but the port opening is also
much closer to the end of the shaft than with 20G cutter. This allows the small-gauge cutter to be
used as a multipurpose tool; other than cutting and aspiration, they can also be efficiently used to
lift fine membranes [like forceps], detect and create tissue cleavage planes, and cut abnormal tissue
in a controlled manner [like scissors]. In addition, the use of preoperative intravitreal injection of
bevacizumab in complex proliferative vitreoretinopathies allows maintenance of a clear surgical
field and allows precise tissue dissection without the need for multiple or repeated instrumentation. Hence, intravitreal instruments that were vital to surgical success some years ago are only
rarely needed nowadays. Nevertheless, awareness about the design features and utility of some of
these instruments would be beneficial. While 20G instruments were largely designed to be reusable,
small-gauge intravitreal instruments are predominantly manufactured as disposable units meant for
single use.

Small-gauge instruments include curved scissors, vertical scissors, serrated forceps, micro
pick [for lifting ILM edge], and fine-gripping forceps. Different materials are used to manufacture
intravitreal instruments, and these include stainless steel, titanium, and kryptonite. Kryptonite is
a non-ferrous alloy that is incapable of rusting. It is seven times more resistant to damage than
stainless steel, when dropped. It is not a coating alone, so there is no risk of flaking. Kryptonite is
also glare free. The handles to operate these instruments could be anyone of the following types:
squeeze handle, small squeeze handle, enterprise handle, lever action handle, or universal handle
[Figure 7.8]. Most of these instruments are available in different sizes such as 20G, 23G, 25G,
and 27G. Some instruments are customized for surgery in young children, highly myopic patients
[long-handled tools], and submacular surgery. **Forceps** [Figure 7.9] are used for holding, grasping,
peeling, and removing tissue by means of blunt dissection [exclusive shear], and scissors are used
for incising, cutting, separating, and resecting tissue by means of fine dissection [inclusive shear].

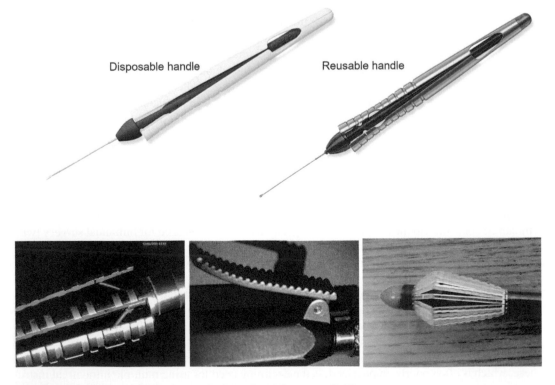

Disposable handle   Reusable handle

FIGURE 7.8 Types of handle designs for intravitreal forceps and scissors.

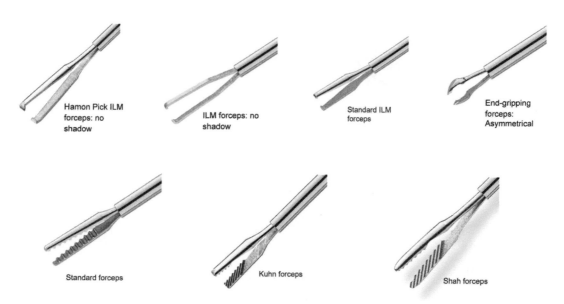

FIGURE 7.9 Types of intravitreal forceps designs. ILM, internal limiting membrane. [Courtesy of Vitreq.]

During bimanual surgery, both of these instruments [forceps and scissors] are used hand in hand, while illumination is provided by chandelier light source. Forceps could be symmetric or asymmetric [based on design of the jaws] and may also be recognized by eponymous names [based on the name of the designer] such as Thomas, Lambert, or Tano. Forceps are generally characterized by the nature of their jaw and tip design—straight, slightly tapering with broad platform [e.g., ILM forceps]; straight, appreciable tapering with fine platform [delicate grasping forceps]; pick forceps with an angulated tip [e.g., Naito ILM forceps]; and straight forceps with serrated jaws. Subretinal forceps have an angulation of 120–135 degrees, 3.5–4.5 mm proximal to the tip. [e.g., Thomas forceps have horizontal, diamondized jaws. Tips of the forceps close first, followed progressively by the length of the long narrow jaws; Lambert forceps has one fixed jaw and one moving jaw pivoted at the angulation. This is said to improve safety of manoeuvring and also reduce the chance of enlargement of the retinotomy while grasping subretinal membranes; Ducournau forceps has a fine pick at the tip]. Subretinal forceps are available only in 20G and so may be used, when necessary, through a separate standard MVR scleral incision. **Scissors** [Figure 7.10] have the same general features excepting that their inner edges are sharpened to allow cutting of tissues. In small-gauge, curved [jaw length, 1.25 mm], angled-horizontal [30 degree angulation with 3.15-mm blade length], and vertical scissors [45 degree angled with 1.75-mm distal blade] are available. Most small-gauge intravitreal instruments have a shaft length between 32 and 40 mm. In addition to forceps and scissors, small-gauge tissue manipulators [Figure 7.11] may sometimes be of use in finding the edge of pathological membranes etc.

Special-purpose intravitreal tools include **magnets** [intraocular, 19G, 20G; extraocular] and **foreign body forceps** [20G]. The latter has a locking mechanism to allow firm grasp on the foreign body while it is being manipulated out of the eye. Intraocular magnets are made of stainless steel and a small amount of rare earth metal such as neodymium. [These elements are unique because the magnetic fields in their atoms do not cancel each other and so they behave as magnets. Their discovery led to designing of handheld magnets for intraocular foreign body removal by Parel. The availability of handheld magnets enabled ophthalmic surgeons to do away with the huge, cumbersome, and heavy giant electromagnets that were in use in the past.] Still infrequently used tools could include Arumi **retinal diamond blade** [for radial optic neurotomy, arteriovenous sheathotomy, and microvascular dissection such as embolectomy]. In addition to forceps and scissors, there

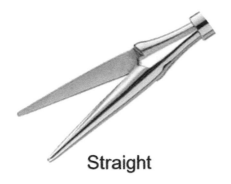

Straight

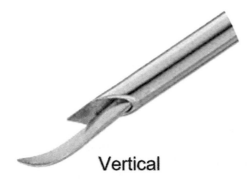

Vertical

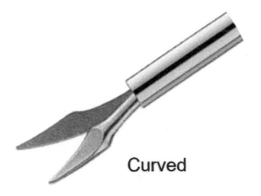

Curved

FIGURE 7.10 Types of intravitreal scissors designs. [Courtesy of Vitreq.]

are additional instruments that are used infrequently but may of be of use such as **retractable MVR blades** [prevents accidental pricks and may be of particular use in patients with HIV/ hepatitis; has a locking mechanism also], membrane scrapers [blunt and serrated, diamond dusted], and membrane spatulas.

The **finesse flex loop** [Figure 7.12] is an innovative, retractable membrane scraper introduced recently as an aid to fracture the ILM before peeling. It has fine micro-serrations along one edge of the loop and gently scraping the retinal surface along this edge induces fracture of the ILM. The

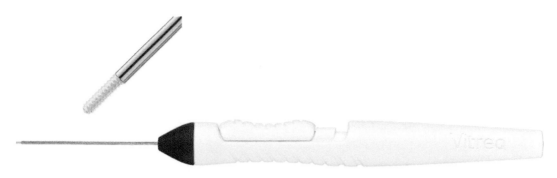

FIGURE 7.11   One type of tissue manipulator [retractable]. [Courtesy of Vitreq.]

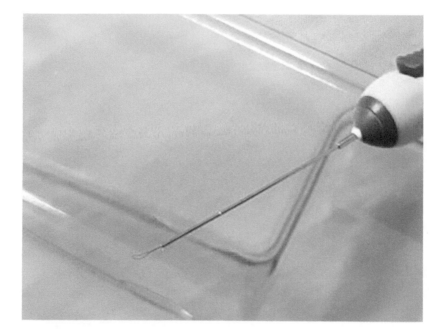

FIGURE 7.12   Finesse loop for internal limiting membrane peeling.

author finds that the opposite edge of the loop is useful in gently massaging a large macular hole from outside in. The loop is made of nitinol [nickel-titanium, naval ordinance laboratory-developed intermetallic compound; flexible material routinely used for removal of ureteric stones]. The force of the scraping can be controlled by the length to which the loop has been opened or retracted. It can freely be inserted though valved cannulas.

Backflush handles are an important part of intravitreal instrumentation. They are of two types, manual use or automated use by connecting to the machine console [Figure 7.13]. The former is of the rigid type with a control hole [Charles] or soft squeeze with control hole [Packo]. These handles are used with plain soft tip [silicone-coloured or translucent], brush soft tip [useful to remove blood layered on the retinal surface and for gentle tissue massage], and a diamond-dusted soft tip [to scrape fine epiretinal membrane]. **Backflush cannulas** can be used to remove layered blood by gently sweeping over the surface or by using the squeeze handle to actively dislodge the layered blood or triamcinolone [by squirting a jet of fluid]. A dual-bore cannula is necessary for simultaneous injection of PFCL and egress of intraocular fluid [this maintains steady intraocular pressure].

Trocar-cannula systems. When 25G microincision vitreous surgery was first introduced, the trocar entry was a two-step system. In the first step, the globe was stabilized with the Eckardt plate and

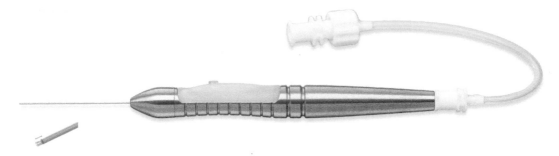

FIGURE 7.13   Cannula with retractable tip for automated extrusion of intraocular fluid. [Courtesy of Vitreq.]

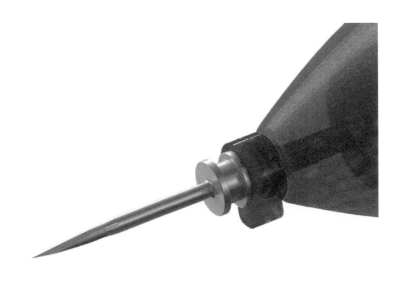

FIGURE 7.14   Trocar with beveled cannula for small-gauge vitreoretinal surgery.

entry made with an angled blade. In the second step, a round-bodied trocar-cannula was inserted through the opening made in the first step. This was soon replaced by one-step insertion systems. Currently available trocar-cannula systems may be valved or non-valved. In addition, there are variations in the trocar design, cannula design, and location of the valve. Trocar designs include back bevel, lancet bevel, spear bevel, and spatula bevel types. Cannulas can be made of metal completely or metal in combination with inert material such as polyimide. Valves can be an integral part of the cannula or placed on the hub, like a cap [the latter design allows them to be easily removed when necessary]. Caliburn is a trocar-cannula design in which the valve is located closer to the inner opening of the hub. Most cannulas have an end-on opening, and this may increase the risk of subretinal or choroidal positioning of the cannula. More recently, bevelled cannulas have become available and may provide greater safety [Figure 7.14]. The opaque shaft of the cannulas may also create a zone of darkness around the region of the port and make removal of the vitreous at this region, unsafe. This could possibly be overcome by designing cannula systems that have a transparent shaft [Figure 7.15a-c].

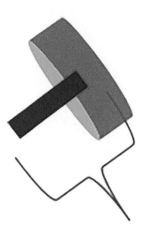

~3-mm shaft

FIGURE 7.15A   Small-gauge cannula with an opaque shaft.

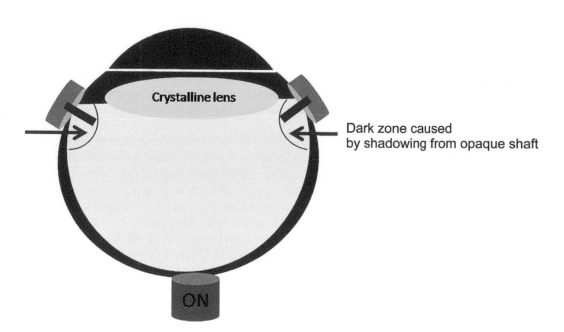

FIGURE 7.15B   Limitation of an opaque shaft: the dark zone around the cannula.

General-purpose instruments that are required during vitreous surgery are a speculum [e.g., Barraquer standard wire, heavy (1 mm) wire or solid blade; Kratz-Barraquer (open blades); Kraff solid blade adjustable; Lieberman open blade adjustable]; Castroviejo calliper [straight or curved, measuring 1–20 mm in 1-mm increments]; scleral depressor [Schepens, Schokett, Packo (has marker)]; muscle hook [Gass, Green]; suture holding and tissue forceps [Lim, Bishop-Harman]; tissue forceps [serrated or non-serrated]; suturing forceps [Castroviejo]; tying forceps that are

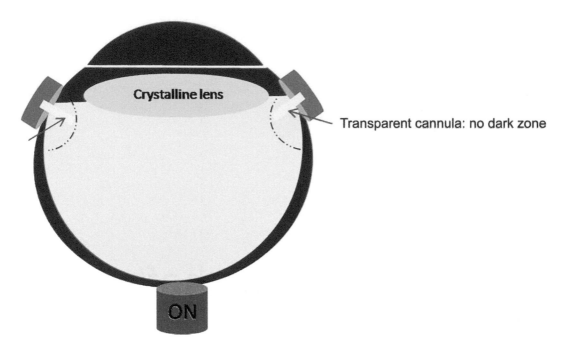

FIGURE 7.15C Transparent shaft design with a reduction in the dark zone.

straight, angled, or curved [McPherson/ Jaffe]; needle holder [Castroviejo with or without a lock; Barraquer, McPherson, Sinskey]; conjunctival scissors; and tenotomy scissors [Westcott-spring handle, Stevens-ring handle]. Scleral plugs or cannula plugs and plug-holding forceps are rarely necessary with valved instrumentation. A 10-mm polyimide tip is necessary to inject viscous fluid [silicone oil] under high pressure.

Sutures may need to be passed through three tissues—conjunctiva, sclera, and cornea [rarely]—during retinal detachment or vitreoretinal surgery. Very rarely, one may use non-absorbable sutures to anchor an intraocular lens [scleral fixation] or intraocular implant [e.g., Retisert]. There are four categories of **needles** available: round bodied, straight cutting, reverse cutting, and spatulated. For all ophthalmic tissues, the recommended needle type for suturing is a spatulated needle because it allows smooth, stable, and predictable tissue penetration at a desired depth. If available, a diaspatulated needle should be preferred over a spatulated needle. The normally used suture for closure of conjunctival peritomy is absorbable 7-0/8-0 polyglycolic acid [PGA–synthetic, braided on 3/8 curve needle], scleral port is absorbable 6-0/7-0 PGA [on a 3/8 inch curve needle], and the corneal incision is 10-0 nylon [3/8 inch curve needle]. Preferred suture for placement of scleral buckle or encirclage is polyester [5-0, braided] on ¼ curve diaspatulated or spatulated needle.

7.8 CRYOTHERAPY AND ENDOLASER

The tissue-damaging effects of extreme temperature are easy to comprehend. Both high and low temperatures induce instantaneous cellular damage, which is then followed by subclinical or clinical features of inflammation and finally tissue atrophy and the evolution of abnormal adhesions between the surviving cellular and acellular elements. When mature, these abnormal adhesions have been experimentally found to be extraordinarily strong. This property of thermal–tissue interaction has been routinely used to seal retinal tears or barricade areas of retinal weakness, such as lattice degeneration, in high-risk patients.

After years of pioneering work, it was Harvey Lincoff who introduced tissue freezing [cryotherapy] as a method for inducing sterile chorioretinal adhesions during retinal surgery. Cryotherapy works on the principle of Joule-Thompson effect, which states that 'rapid cooling results when there is high flow and sudden expansion of a gas'. The cooling is a result of instantaneous absorption of the higher temperature within the surrounding tissue and air. The nature of freezing that results during cryotherapy is influenced by multiple factors such as the gas being used [nitrogen, nitrous oxide, carbon dioxide, Freon]; pressure, velocity, and duration of gas flow; design of the probe tip; temperature differential; and tissue and material resistance. The source of gas generally used for cryotherapy is nitrous oxide or carbon dioxide. For retinal surgery, nitrous oxide is preferred. Traditional equipment for retinal cryotherapy includes a gas source from a cylinder, input tubing with a pressure gauge, a gas console, output tubing, a cryo probe, and a foot pedal. More recently compact, handheld cryo probes have been introduced for retinal surgery [Figure 7.16]. These probes allow about 20–25 freeze and thaw cycles. The probe used for retinal cryopexy is curved and has a bulbous tip 2.5 mm in diameter [the intraocular cryoprobe tip is 1 mm, that for cataract extraction is 1.5 mm, and the cyclocryopexy probe is 4 mm]. The temperature at the probe tip during a freeze is between -50 degrees and -60 degrees. Based on the intensity of reaction, four grades of cryotherapy have been categorized. Grade 1 is mild and appears as an intense orange or red colour, grade 2 is moderate and appears as a greyish reaction, while grade 3 is an intense white reaction [Video 7.1]. In grade 4 reaction [heavy cryopexy], ice crystals form within the tissue [and enlarge into the vitreous]. While grade 1–2 reaction is adequate for treating retinal lesions as prophylaxis, grade 2–3 reaction is necessary for treating retinal tears during retinal detachment surgery. The cryoreaction usually appears within 10 sections, and failure to do so must raise the following possibilities: the probe is overlying the eyelids, silicone sleeve is covering the probe tip, input cylinder pressure is inadequate, or the indentation is being caused by the shaft and the probe tip is in the posterior orbit. The latter is a serious complication because it could damage the macula or optic nerve, and it must be avoided. It is important to remember that during the initial 5–7 days after cryotherapy, tissue adhesions may become weaker because of inflammation and edema. It is only during and after the healing phase that the adhesion becomes strong. This is unlike retinopexy with laser, when the adhesion becomes strong within 24–48 hours.

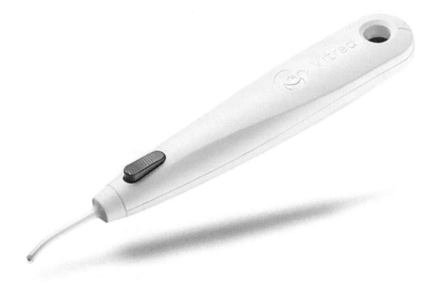

FIGURE 7.16 Hand-held disposable cryoprobe for retinal surgery. [Courtesy of Vitreq.]

FIGURE 7.17   Directional, retractable endolaser probe.

Endolaser probes are used to deliver laser energy to the retina. The usual laser source in use currently is a frequency-doubled neodymium-doped yttrium aluminum garnet (Nd: YAG) laser. Laser probes have a red [helium-neon] beam to identify the site at which the laser would be delivered. Laser probe designs include straight or curved and rigid or retractable [Figure 7.17].

7.9   PRINCIPLES OF PHYSICS

Vitreous surgery is one of the most complex surgeries because the surgeon must separate the vitreous meshwork that is tightly adherent to the delicate neurosensory retina without injuring the latter. Oftentimes the procedure has to be performed with a detached, mobile, and fluttering retina. Hence, the machinery used for the surgery must provide the highest quality of technological stability in terms of infusion flow, aspiration control, and cutting of the vitreous fibrils. In addition, retinopexy [laser, cryopexy], thermal coagulation [diathermy, cautery] to stop bleeding or create retinotomy, fragmentation of the crystalline lens, removal of a magnetic foreign body, gas dynamics, and injection or removal of highly viscous fluids are also based on fundamental laws of physics, and some of these are briefly described here.

Poiseuille's law. A practical observation is that volume flow rate decreases as the tubing gets narrower. Poiseuille's law helps to determine the volume flow rate of a fluid through a circular tube of constant cross section and factors that influence the flow rate. It is important in relation to the amount of irrigating fluid that flows into the vitreous cavity through the tubing of 20G surgery vis a vis small-gauge surgery. According to Poiseuille's equation, flow rate is inversely proportional to the fourth power of the inner radius of the tube [other variables remaining constant]. Hence, if the diameter of the tubing is reduced by half, then fluid flow reduces by a factor of 16. In addition, this law also states that fluid flow is also inversely proportional to the length of the tubing and viscosity of fluid flowing through the tubing. Fluid flow is, however, directly proportional to the pressure gradient across the two ends of the tubing. In small-gauge surgery, the tubing size is reduced, leading to significant drop in volume flow rate. However, this is compensated by increasing the pressure gradient across the two ends, using vented forced infusion, or increasing the height of the bottle [in gravity-dependent systems]. In addition, lower volume flow rate across the reduced tube diameter of the aspiration or extrusion line and reduced leak of fluid [due to valved cannulas] also balances the volume flow rate of irrigating fluid flowing into the vitreous cavity. This fine balance can be disturbed when using the fragmatome, making a larger incision [e.g., removal of retained intraocular foreign body, dropped intraocular lens], or during hybrid instrumentation. These situations lead to increased outflow of fluid in the vitreous cavity across the aspiration line or increased wound leak, and hence care must be taken to correspondingly ensure increase in the volume flow rate through the infusion line [with advanced machines, software automatically compensates to a certain extent]. A sudden or continued mismatch in the amount of fluid flowing into and out of the eye would otherwise lead to collapse of the globe and its associated serious sequelae.

Bernoulli's principle. This is based on the law of conservation of mass and is important in understanding the pressure and velocity relationship when fluid flows from a tubing with larger diameter into a tubing of smaller diameter [as seen with small-gauge devices], all other factors such as static fluid pressure, and fluid height remaining constant. According to this principle, when fluid flows from a tubing of larger diameter into a narrower one, the velocity of flow automatically increases, but there is also a corresponding decrease in the pressure gradient across the two tubes.

Ohm's law [fluidics]. While Ohm's law in electricity is well known, the corresponding law for fluidics is rarely discussed. It states that the pressure gradient across two points is equal to the resistance to flow multiplied by the fluid velocity. As mentioned earlier, narrower tubing used in small-gauge surgery significantly impedes fluid flow, so the pressure gradient also becomes low. This is not conducive to fluidic stability during surgery. To overcome loss of pressure head due to use of narrower tubing, infusion of fluid into the tubing at a much higher pressure is necessary. This is achieved by increasing the infusion pressure setting on the vitreous machine to a much higher level [40–60 mmHg] compared with settings in 20G surgery.

Joule-Thompson principle. According to this law, when a gas flowing under pressure suddenly and rapidly expands, it absorbs heat from the surrounding. This principle is used in the design of cryoprobes and cryopexy. The approximate drop in temperature for each 100 psi of pressure change is about 6–8 degrees.

Hooke's law. This law is applied to explain the effect of a scleral buckle on vitreous elastic forces [which is perceived to act like an elastic slinky] and successful retinal reattachment. Hooke's law states that the amount of force necessary to expand or compress a spring by a certain distance is directly proportional to the distance. Scleral buckle by shortening the circumference of the globe at the region of the break compresses the vitreous fibrils and thus reduces the effective forces acting on the tear [keeping it open]. By doing so, it reduces the flow of liquefied vitreous into the subretinal space and so promotes retinal reattachment.

Ohm's law [electric conduction]. This law is applicable during the use of wet-field cautery [*cautery* is a misnomer because no passive heat is being used] and diathermy. It states that the current flow across two points of a conductor is directly proportional to the voltage difference across the points. Current flowing through the tissue causes a raise in temperature resulting in coagulation [e.g., stop intraocular bleed] or focal tissue necrosis [e.g., create retinotomy].

SUGGESTED READING

1. Williams GA [2008]. 25-, 23-, or 20-gauge instrumentation for vitreous surgery? *Eye*. 22(10): 1263–1266.
2. Ohji M, Tano Y. [2007]. New instruments in vitrectomy. In: Kirchhoff B, Wong D (Eds) *Vitreo-retinal surgery: Essentials in ophthalmology*. Springer, Berlin, Heidelberg.
3. Diniz B, Ribeiro RM, Fernandes RB, Lue JC, Teixeira AG, Maia M, Humayun MS [2013]. Fluidics in a dual pneumatic ultra-high-speed vitreous cutter system. *Ophthalmologica*. 229(1): 15–20.
4. Fang SY, DeBoer CMT, Humayun MS [2007]. Performance analysis of new-generation vitreous cutters. *Graef Arch Clin Exp Ophthalmol*. 246(1): 61–67.
5. Ehlers JP, Uchida A, Srivastava SK [2017]. Intraoperative optical coherence tomography-compatible surgical instruments for real-time image-guided ophthalmic surgery. *Br J Ophthalmol*. 101(10): 1306–1308.
6. Hadi TM, Knight DK, Aggarwal S, Mehta MC [2020]. Improving the view in vitreoretinal surgery. *Int Ophthalmol Clin*. 60(3): 91–101.
7. Tso MO, Woodford BJ [1983 Aug]. Effect of photic injury on the retinal tissues. *Ophthalmology*. 90(8): 952–963.

8 Adjuncts in Vitreoretinal Surgery

8.1 VITREOUS SUBSTITUTES

The vitreous, either normal or abnormal, has to be removed in a safe manner during vitreoretinal surgery. Hence, it is imperative that the loss of vitreous is replaced at the conclusion of surgery using substances that would immediately restore ocular volume and in the majority of situations also be able perform a few other functions. These substances, known as vitreous substitutes, must possess the following qualities: they must be biologically inert, optically clear, non-toxic, sterile, and easy to inject [and if necessary, remove] and must have minimal risk of inducing complications. Once the vitreous substitute spontaneously gets absorbed or is surgically removed, the vitreous cavity gets finally filled with aqueous humor secreted by the ciliary body. If the ciliary body is dysfunctional, either due to chronic inflammation or due to long-standing anterior proliferative vitreoretinopathy [PVR], aqueous production alone is incapable of replacing the lost vitreous. Hence, the eye becomes hypotonus. Small volumes of gas, categorized as vitreous substitutes, are also used in the management of fresh retinal detachment through a procedure called pneumatic retinopexy.

Vitreous substitutes may be classified based on the physical nature of the substance as well as the duration of stay within the eyeball. Based on the physical nature, they could be gases [e.g., air, sulphur hexafluoride, perfluoropropane] or liquids [e.g., silicone oil, perfluorocarbon liquids such as perfluorodecalin, perfluoro-n-octane-perfluoron, perfluorophenentherene, vitreon, and synthetic gels (still in experimental stages)]. Gaseous vitreous substitutes are self-absorbing over variable amounts of time. In contrast, liquid substitutes have to be surgically removed. Short-acting vitreous substitutes stay for a few days to about 10 days, while long-acting substitutes stay for several weeks. It is interesting to note that many of the vitreous substitutes were actually being used earlier, either in industry or for non-ocular medical purposes.

Each vitreous substitute has a particular indication and risk profile and must be chosen accordingly. In general, air is chosen when uncomplicated surgery has been performed for non-resolving vitreous haemorrhage, removal of dropped intraocular lens [IOL] or lens, or removal of epiretinal membrane [ERM] without retinal detachment. More recently some surgeons claim good results in macular hole surgery with air tamponade alone. Short-acting gases such as SF6 are chosen when there is iatrogenic break formation during these procedures, macular hole surgery, or surgery for optic disc pit maculopathy or at the completion of vitreoretinal surgery for retinal detachment and mild to moderate PVR. Long-acting gases are chosen when managing complex retinal detachment with severe to advanced PVR or advanced proliferative diabetic retinopathy. In the latter conditions, it may be preferable to use silicone oil because it helps earlier rehabilitation due to its optical clarity, allows earlier documentation of abnormalities, and allows the ability to carry out secondary procedures such as laser photocoagulation with greater ease. These advantages sometimes outweigh the disadvantage of having to perform another surgery to remove the silicone oil. Perfluorocarbon liquids are frequently used in large quantity for managing retinal detachment secondary to giant retinal tear, during retinectomies, and while undertaking endoresection of intraocular tumours. A small quantity of perfluorocarbon liquid [PFCL] is used during internal limiting membrane (ILM) peel in macular holes associated with retinal detachment and to act as a buffer for protecting the posterior pole while removing a dropped IOL or lens. As a rule, PFCL needs to be removed at the conclusion of surgery and replaced with the other vitreous substitutes

DOI: 10.1201/9781003179320-9

mentioned earlier. However, it may be advantageous to retain the PFCL [and maintain the patient in supine position postoperatively] for 7–10 days in patients with giant retinal tear and severe PVR, in endoresection of intraocular tumours [wherein it could reduce the risk of early choroidal and intraocular haemorrhage], and in the management of large and chronic macular hole managed with a free flap or graft. After this interval, it can be safely removed and replaced with long-acting gas or silicone oil.

It is useful to be aware of some physical properties of vitreous substitutes such as specific gravity, surface tension, interfacial tension, buoyancy, miscibility, viscosity, and vapourization pressure. It is also important to know the stages in the dynamics of a gaseous vitreous substitute and the dynamics of silicone oil degradation and emulsification.

Specific gravity is the density of a substance relative to the density of a reference substance [usually water for liquids and solids and air for gases]. The lower the specific gravity, the higher the tendency of a substance to float above water, and vice versa. This is the reason that silicone oil with a specific gravity of 0.97 tends to float above water while PFCL with a specific gravity of 1.7–1.9 sinks under the irrigating fluid, within the vitreous cavity. [Note that specific gravity has no units of measurement because it is the relative density of one substance against the relative density of another substance.]

The integrity of a substance is maintained by molecular and atomic forces of interaction, both within the body and on the surface of the substance. It has been observed that for gases and liquids, these forces are stronger at the surface than within the body of the substance. This implies that the molecules at the surface of a liquid or gas tend to attract and bind to one another with a certain force [usually through van der Waals forces]. This force of interaction between molecules at the surface is known as **surface tension**. The higher the surface tension, the greater the force of attraction. A substance is able to maintain its structure and shape [e.g., gas bubbles assume a spherical shape or shape of a flat-bottomed cap within the vitreous; water droplets assume a tear drop shape] as long as the surface tension is not disturbed. Surface tension can be reduced by surfactants, chemical impurities, products of biological interactions, and inflammatory reactions, an evident effect of breakdown of surface tension is emulsification of silicone oil [both non-fluorinated and fluorinated]. Surface tension is also dependent on the radius of the gas bubble. Hence, small bubbles have a lower surface tension and risk travelling into the subretinal space across an open break.

When two immiscible compounds interact, there is a force of interaction between the two at the area of contact. This force, generated by the surface of one substance against the surface of another substance at the area of contact, is known as **interfacial tension**. Interfacial tension is the reason why a gas bubble is able to tamponade a retinal break and PFCL is able to unfold and maintain the retina in a stretched position. Interfacial tension is dependent on the buoyancy as well as specific gravity of a substance.

When two immiscible substances with differing specific gravity are mixed, the substance with the lower specific gravity occupies the space above the one with a higher specific gravity. In addition, there is force exerted by one on the other, and this force is known as **buoyant force**. Buoyant force is the reason that a gas bubble apposes itself to the retinal surface, including the retinal break. This apposing force prevents currents of liquefied vitreous from flowing into the subretinal space across the tear and enables the retinal pigment epithelial pump to remove the already accumulated subretinal fluid, resulting in retinal reattachment.

The **viscosity** of a substance is the resistive force that is encountered when a liquid is forced through a narrow tube. It is dependent on the molecular weight and degree of polymerization of the substance. It is measured as centistoke (cs). Generally, the higher the molecular weight, the greater the viscosity. During vitreoretinal surgery, the role of viscosity is most evident during injection and removal of silicone oil. The higher the viscosity of silicone oil, the greater the force necessary to inject and remove the oil from the vitreous cavity. This is the reason that 5000 cs of silicone oil is more difficult to inject and remove than 1000 cs of oil. Hence, 1000 cs of oil is preferred during uncomplicated surgery. However, higher viscosity oil has a lower risk of emulsification. Hence, in situations wherein it is deemed necessary to retain oil for longer periods [e.g., resurgery in one-eyed patients, choroidal coloboma–associated retinal detachment, retinal detachment in patients with oculocutaneous albinism], 5000 cs of oil is preferred.

Vapourization pressure is the pressure at which a liquid changes into a vapour phase. It is dependent on the mass of the substance and ambient conditions of the surrounding, such as temperature. The lower the vapourization pressure, the greater the ease with which a residual bubble of an element vaporizes. Vapourization pressure is important while discussing management of residual PFCL following vitreoretinal surgery. PFCL has a relatively low vapourization pressure, so if the residual bubbles are small, they may not have to be removed [as they could spontaneously vapourize into the surrounding milieu]. Vaporization does not occur if the bubble is trapped under the neurosensory retina.

Unlike liquid vitreous substitutes, which maintain their volume, gaseous substitutes [except air and inert gases] undergo dynamic changes over a variable period of time. These changes occur imperceptibly but are categorized into three phases, the phase of expansion, phase of equilibration, and phase of dissolution. The predominant element involved in this, in relation to gaseous vitreous substitutes, is the concentration of ambient nitrogen. In the phase of expansion, nitrogen moves into the injected gas bubble and continues to do so until an equilibrium is reached between its volume inside and outside the bubble. After this phase is reached, the rate at which other elements of the gas were exiting the bubble outweigh the amount of nitrogen moving into the bubble. This is the phase of dissolution, whence the volume of the gas bubble gradually begins to decline. Most of the expansion occurs in the initial 4–6 hours followed by a more gradual increase until equilibrium is reached. At this time, the bubble size is maximal. The amount of expansion is dependent on the nature of the gas injected, and generally, the lower the molecular weight, the lower the expansion [e.g., maximal expansile volume of SF_6 is twice the injected volume and of C_3F_8, four times]. Monitoring intraocular pressure during this phase of expansion is very critical to prevent acute elevation of intraocular pressure and central retinal artery occlusion.

The dynamics of the gas bubble expansion are also important in two other situations. The first is when use of a gaseous substitute is planned at the end of a vitreoretinal surgery being performed under general anaesthesia. The second is when a patient with intraocular gaseous vitreous substitute inadvertently travels by air or ascends rapidly to a mountain top. In the first situation, nitrous oxide and nitric oxide [due to higher solubility] used for anaesthesia rapidly enters the gas bubble and equally rapidly exits the bubble when anaesthesia is stopped. Owing to the later, the volume of the gas bubble rapidly decreases, leading to hypotony and inadequate tamponade. In the second situation, owing to different partial pressure of air mixture within a pressurized cabin of an airplane and air at higher altitudes, the gas bubble rapidly expands, leading to dangerous elevation of intraocular pressure and risk of retinal artery occlusion.

Two gaseous concentrations are used during vitreoretinal surgery, expansile and non-expansile, depending on the objective. Pure (100%) gas is injected when its expansile properties are used to achieve retinal attachment during pneumatic retinopexy [in nonvitrectomized eyes or in post-vitrectomy early retinal detachment], displacement of subretinal haemorrhage [e.g., secondary to trauma, PCV], and induction of posterior vitreous detachment [PVD; contentious]. Nonexpansile mixture [gas mixed with a certain percentage of air] is used as a vitreous substitute at the end of vitreous surgery for retinal detachment and complications of diabetic retinopathy. Nonexpansile concentrations are 20% [20%-40%] and 14% [12%–18%] for SF_6 and C_3F_8, respectively.

8.2 VITAL DYES IN VITREOUS SURGERY

To ensure unhindered transmission of light rays to the retinal photoreceptors, the optical path is anatomically designed to maintain a high degree of transparency. This includes the vitreous body, posterior vitreous cortex [posterior hyaloid], and ILM. These are also the structures that need to be removed surgically during all basic and some advanced vitreoretinal procedures. Although the transparent vitreous body and detached hyaloid can be visualized by eliciting the Tyndall effect during surgery, this is tedious and not always reliable. So, methods have been described to improve visualization of these structures at surgery, either using intravitreal injection of triamcinolone suspension or specialized dyes such as trypan blue, brilliant blue, or indocyanine green (ICG). Use of digital filters for the same purpose is a relatively new concept, but there is as yet no consensus on the utility of this approach.

The primary function of the visual apparatus is to enable clear vision, and this is possible only when all the structures in the optical path are transparent; this includes the vitreous body, posterior hyaloid, ILM, and neurosensory retina. One of the basic and most important components of every vitreous surgery is removal of the vitreous from the port site, posteriorly [core] and periphery. In advanced vitreous surgery, as for macular hole, there is need to remove the ILM. Visualization of the vitreous as well as the ILM is difficult owing to their transparent nature. Although dyes for staining of epimacular membrane are also available, their utility is less critical because these membranes are better recognized, being more well-formed and relatively opaque. Performing surgery assisted by vital dyes is also attested to as **chromovitrectomy**. It is a practical observation that **visualization of the vitreous** is easier in patients with vitreous haemorrhage due to the presence of dehemoglobinized or fresh blood. Vitreous can also be visualized without aid of any dye by eliciting the Tyndall effect using the beam of the endoilluminator light. However, this is tedious and increases the surgical time. In recent years, difficulty in visualization of the transparent vitreous and ILM has been significantly overcome by intraoperative injection of triamcinolone [a synthetic non-soluble steroid- $C_{24}H_{31}FO_6$] suspension and synthetic dyes, respectively. Although the use of preservative-free triamcinolone is recommended, we have found no adverse effect using commercially available systemic preparation. Injection of triamcinolone is generally carried out after removing some amount of the core vitreous. The most common practice is to inject triamcinolone over the posterior pole in order to identify the posterior hyaloid [see section on PVD induction] and decipher the absence or presence of PVD; however, it is also useful when directly injected close to the equator or peripheral retina. This is the region where residual vitreous can produce serious complications in the postoperative period and hence needs to be removed. It is important to remember that triamcinolone improves the visibility of the vitreous and posterior hyaloid not by staining but indirectly by getting enmeshed within the vitreous fibrils, as the drug is in the form of a suspension, and its particles are relatively insoluble and large. Visualization of the vitreous base, however, remains poor because the collagen fibrils are tightly packed here and do not trap any triamcinolone crystals. Injection of diluted triamcinolone in amounts barely necessary is recommended. Injection of a large amount of triamcinolone [particularly undiluted] must be avoided because it tends to layer over the posterior hyaloid and may completely mask the anatomical details beneath. Sometimes it may be useful to inject triamcinolone more than once, as in patients with suspected vitreoschisis and during vitreoretinal surgery in paediatric patients. Some surgeons report triamcinolone-assisted peeling of ILM, but this is less efficacious.

The ILM may be considered as a supporting membrane for the basal processes of Mueller cells, as well as a delimiting layer [separating posterior hyaloid from the neurosensory retina]. Like other basement membranes, it is acellular and composed predominantly of type 4 collagen. Its thickness varies across the retina and ranges between 2 and 4 µm [being thickest at the parafovea]. It also seems to have an inherent elasticity, so it tends to scroll spontaneously when incised. ILM thickness increases with age, while its elasticity decreases. The idea that ILM peeling may not have any deleterious effect was first observed following surgery for premacular haemorrhage in which the blood was behind the ILM and so had to be removed. There is an increasing trend towards peeling of the ILM as it has been shown to improve the success of macular hole closure, reduce the risk of EMM recurrence, and prevent formation of macular pucker after vitreoretinal surgery for retinal detachment. Although widely discussed, the safety of ILM peeling in patients with diabetic macular edema, vitreomacular traction, myopic foveoschisis, and optic disc pit maculopathy needs further confirmation in prospective trials.

Peeling of the ILM is one of the most challenging steps in vitreoretinal surgery for multiple reasons: it is stretched out as an invisible layer, measures only a few microns in thickness, and overlies the delicate neurosensory retina. Staining of the ILM with dyes significantly improves safety of the procedure by transforming it into a visible layer. It is less taxing to incise, fracture, or pinch and peel a visible membrane than an invisible one. Some of the dyes that have been used for ILM or ERM staining include ICG (0.05%), infracyanine (0.05%), trypan blue [0.05%–1.12%], brilliant blue G [0.025%; G because the blue has a slightly greenish tint], and membrane blue [0.15% trypan blue]. Brilliant blue G is a molecular modification of a dye, Coomassie blue, used widely in protein electrophoresis. Factors that determine the intensity of staining include tissue affinity, dye concentration, contact time of the dye with the tissue, contrast of the native tissue, presence of early cataract, and method of staining [dry or wet]. Dyes that stain tissue blue or green are chosen because these colors are said to provide the best contrast against the normal fundus reflex. Even with the same dye concentration, the intensity of staining shows significant interindividual variability. In the presence of nuclear sclerosis, the staining appears much lighter than a pseudophakic eye as the lens acts like a 'blue minus' filter. Sometimes, staining is also noted to be patchy within the same person [even in the absence of EMM]. In general, ICG provides the most consistent, intense, rapid [within 30 seconds], and uniform staining but is generally not preferred as first choice because of theoretically higher risk of retinal toxicity. In patients with senile choroidal atrophy and high myopia wherein the contrast is poor, ICG may be preferable to other dyes. Trypan blue does not stain acellular tissues. Hence, it is not suited for staining of ILM but better suited for staining ERM.

As most dyes are water soluble, they instantaneously disperse into the vitreous cavity when injected into a fluid-filled eye. Hence, in the past, it was standard procedure to inject the dye over the posterior pole in an air-filled eye [after fluid-air exchange] and leave it for a few minutes for tissue absorption to occur. Following this wait period, air was again replaced with fluid, and further steps were then carried on. More recently, 'heavy' dyes have become commercially available, and these are able to stain the ILM even on injection into a fluid-filled eye. These dyes are made 'heavy' by adding compounds such as polyethylene glycol [PEG] [e.g., ILM blue, combination of 0.025% brilliant blue G with 4% PEG]. Membrane blue-dual is a commercially available dye [trypan blue 0.15%, brilliant blue G 0.025%, and PEG] that allows simultaneously staining of ILM and ERM. Staining of tissue with dyes in an air-filled eye is called 'dry' staining, and that in a fluid-filled eye as 'wet' staining. Some precautions to be used while injecting dyes is to use the basic minimum amount, avoid direct injection over the macular hole, and minimize exposure to endoillumination light [as the risk of macular phototoxicity is augmented during dye-assisted surgical maneuvers]. It is also useful to use a Luer-Lock syringe or hold the hub of the soft tip [and have the assistant press the plunger] prior to injection [to prevent the risk of harpooning and injury to intraocular tissues]. Newer dyes that are under evaluation as potential dyes for facilitating vitreous surgery include lutein and zeaxanthin.

SUGGESTED READING

1. Romano MR, Xu X, Li KKW. [2014]. Vitreous substitutes: From tamponade effect to intraocular inflammation. *Biomed Res Int.* 1–2.
2. Schramm C, Spitzer MS, Henke-Fahle S, Steinmetz G, Januschowski K, Heiduschka P et al [2012]. The Cross-linked biopolymer hyaluronic acid as an artificial vitreous substitute. *Invest Ophthalmol Vis Sci.* 53(2): 613. Doi:10.1167/iovs.11-7322.
3. Stolba U, Binder S, Velikay M, Datlinger P, Wedrich A [1995]. Use of perfluorocarbon liquids in proliferative vitreoretinopathy: Results and complications. *Br J Ophthalmol.* 79(12): 1106–1110.
4. Barca F, Caporossi T, Rizzo S [2014]. Silicone oil: Different physical proprieties and clinical applications. *Biomed Res Int.* 1–7. Doi:10.1155/2014/502143.
5. Wong IY, Cheung N, Wong D [2014]. Physiology of vitreous substitutes. In: Sebag J (Ed) *Vitreous: In health and disease.* Springer, New York, 537–549.

6. Cekic O, Ohji M [2000]. Intraocular gas tamponades. *Semin Ophthalmol.* 15(1): 3–14.
7. Alovisi C, Panico C, Sanctis U de, Eandi CM [2017]. Vitreous substitutes: Old and new materials in vitreoretinal surgery. *J Ophthalmol.* 1–6. Doi:10.1155/2017/3172138.
8. Wu Y, Zhu W, Xu D, Li YH, Ba J, Zhang XL et al [2012]. Indocyanine green-assisted internal limiting membrane peeling in macular hole surgery: A meta-analysis. *PloS One.* 7(11): e48405.
9. Schumann RG, Haritoglou C [2013]. Chromovitrectomy and the vitreoretinal interface. *Ophthalmologica.* 230(s2): 3–10.
10. Enaida H, Hisatomi T, Nakao S, Ikeda Y, Yoshida S, Ishibashi T [2014]. Chromovitrectomy and vital dyes. *Dev Ophthalmol.* 120–125.
11. Rodrigues EB, Maia M, Meyer CH, Penha FM, Dib E, Farah ME [2007]. Vital dyes for chromovitrectomy. *Curr Opin Ophthalmol.* 18(3): 179–187.

9 Surgical Approaches and Steps

9.1 RETINAL DETACHMENT SURGERY

9.1.1 Conjunctival Peritomy and Tenotomy

Peritomy is the surgical step of incising the conjunctiva and gaining access to the tenons fascia and subtenon space. Handling of the conjunctiva is the first and last step during scleral buckling surgery, combined scleral buckle– band and vitrectomy, and standard 20G pars plana vitrectomy. It is also important while performing rare procedures like drainage of suprachoroidal haemorrhage, scleral fixation of intraocular lens (IOL), macular buckle in myopia, and scleral resection in nanophthalmos. Peritomy helps to gain access into the subtenon space, and there onwards, to the intermuscular septum. Several approaches to peritomy can be considered [Figure 9.1], and each has its own advantages and disadvantages. These approaches include limbal peritomy, para-limbal peritomy, and bulbar peritomy. In general, it is recommended that the conjunctiva be held with non-toothed forceps and that relaxing cuts be made before starting the circumferential cuts. The smallest opening through which the procedure can be completed is made, and a 2–3 mm frill of conjunctiva is left at the limbus. Relaxing cuts must be avoided over the horizontal meridian as they could extend into the medial or lateral canthus. While closing the peritomy, conjunctiva-to-conjunctiva closure must be achieved without exposing the episcleral tissue. The proximal ends of the conjunctiva must be approximated through an anchoring bite at the limbal frill. Poor closure of the peritomy could result in complications like retraction of the conjunctiva, granuloma and abscess formation, buckle exposure and infection, shortening of the fornix, and poor ocular surface.

Tenotomy is the surgical step of incising the tenons capsule [and intermuscular septa] to gain access to the muscle insertion and scleral surface [Figure 9.2]. This is followed by bridling the recti muscles [see section on surgical anatomy], taking precautions to not split the muscle, the muscular arteries, and fibres of the superior and inferior oblique [Figure 9.3]. Thick cotton thread or silk suture could be used to for this purpose. Bridle suture must be about 10 cm in length [after doubling] and is knotted proximally at about 10 mm from the muscle insertion and distally close to the ends of the suture. Knots at about 10 mm from the muscle insertion allow the surgeon to have better control on the muscles, thereby allowing precise globe rotation and preventing sudden slippage [while passing scleral sutures].

9.1.2 Scleral Inspection, Marking of Tears, and Cryotherapy

Once the scleral surface is exposed, it must be meticulously inspected in all four quadrants to identify areas of thinning and ectasia. This is achieved by retracting the tenons fascia with the aid of Desmarres retractor, one quadrant at a time [Figure 9.4]. Neglecting this step may result in inadvertent perforation of the globe during scleral indentation to locate and mark the retinal tears. [If sclera is evidently ectatic, it would be preferable to convert to primary vitrectomy.] Following this, one or more tears in the retina are located by indentation under indirect ophthalmoscopic visualization or chandelier-assisted endoillumination [see section on endoillumination-assisted scleral buckling [EASB]. All the breaks are precisely marked on the scleral surface using a surgical pen or gentian violet paint. If there is a cluster of breaks very close by, then the most posterior break should be marked [Figure 9.5a], if the break is in the form of a horseshoe tear, the posterior extent and both anterior horns need to be marked [Figure 9.5b], and if a large circumferential tear or dialysis is present, then the lateral extremities, as well as the posterior extent should be marked [Figure 9.5c].

DOI: 10.1201/9781003179320-10

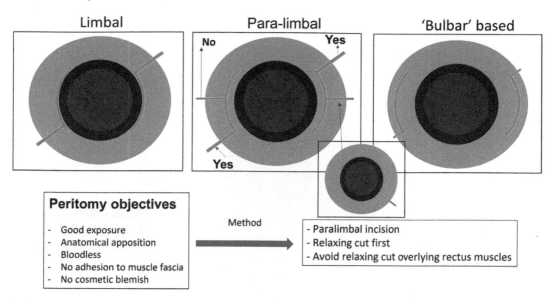

Peritomy objectives

- Good exposure
- Anatomical apposition
- Bloodless
- No adhesion to muscle fascia
- No cosmetic blemish

Method →

- Paralimbal incision
- Relaxing cut first
- Avoid relaxing cut overlying rectus muscles

FIGURE 9.1   Various patterns of conjunctival peritomy.

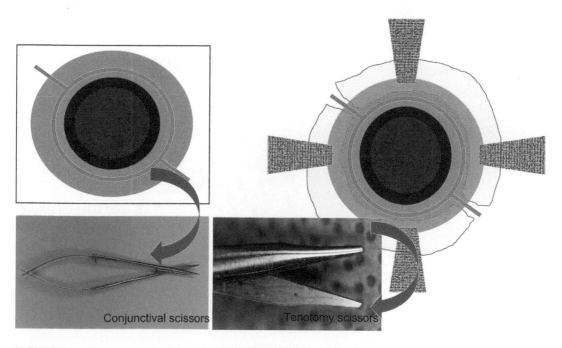

FIGURE 9.2   Tenotomy using blunt-tip [rounded] scissors.

Once all the breaks have been marked, cryotherapy is undertaken to induce retinopexy. Functioning of the cryomachine or probe must be checked just before the procedure. For tears in detached retina, grade 3 reaction must be achieved and for tears in attached retina, grade 1 or grade 2. Grade 4 reaction must be avoided [see section on instrumentation and cryotherapy]. For a break that is small, a solitary freeze centred on the break is adequate. But for larger breaks, confluent cryoburns are placed to cover the entire margin of the tear [Figure 9.6]. Care must be taken to avoid

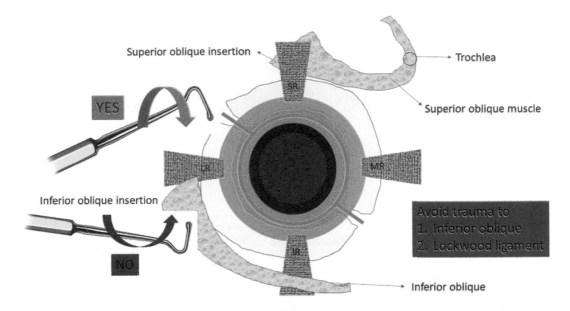

FIGURE 9.3   Avoiding trauma to the inferior oblique muscle during muscle bridle.

Note: SR, superior rectus; LR, lateral rectus; MR, medial rectus; IR, inferior rectus.

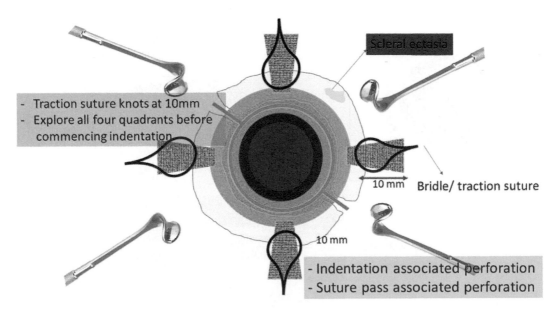

FIGURE 9.4   Importance of scleral inspection before indentation.

wrongly indenting the globe or tear with the shaft of the probe. If this is not promptly recognized, it could result in inadvertent application of freeze to the macular or peripapillary region. Indentation of the globe by unrecognized placement of the cryoprobe on the eyelid would result in lid burn [that could sometimes lead to permanent depigmentation], and this, too, must be avoided. Other risks involved during this step are inducing subretinal or choroidal bleed by sudden withdrawal of the probe [before thawing] and excessive pigment release [hence postoperative PVR].

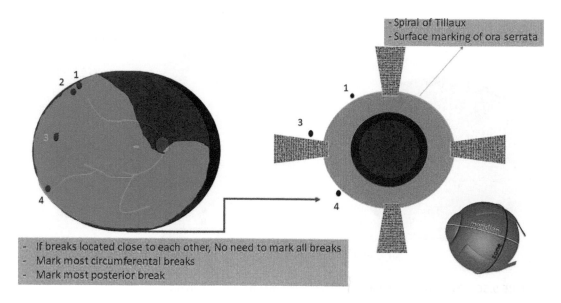

FIGURE 9.5A Method of scleral marking in the presence of multiple breaks.

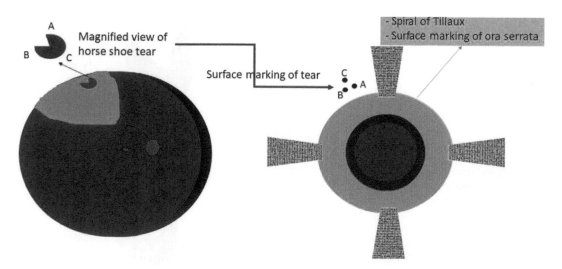

FIGURE 9.5B Method of scleral marking in the presence of a horseshoe tear.

9.1.3 Scleral Sutures and Buckle Placement

The sclera is a tough, collagenous outer protective coat of the eyeball with a thickness varying from 0.3 mm beneath the muscle insertion to 0.8 mm adjacent to the site of exit of the optic nerve. For the purpose of passing scleral sutures before placement of a scleral buckle or encirclage, scleral thickness at two regions—the circle of Tillaux and the equator—is important. The thickness along the spiral is 0.6 mm and along the equator is 0.5 mm. The objectives of a scleral suture are its safe passage without causing a perforation or scleral cut-through, wide and deep enough to hold and generate desired indentation of the sclera, and avoiding compression of the vortex veins. In addition to the thickness of the sclera, other factors that contribute to safe passage of scleral sutures are type of suture [spatulated, cutting, reverse cutting, round bodied; Figure 9.7], thickness of the needle,

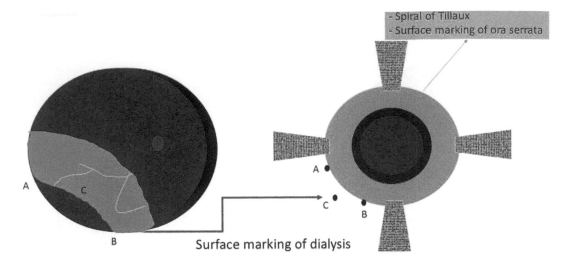

FIGURE 9.5C Method of scleral marking in the presence of retinal dialysis.

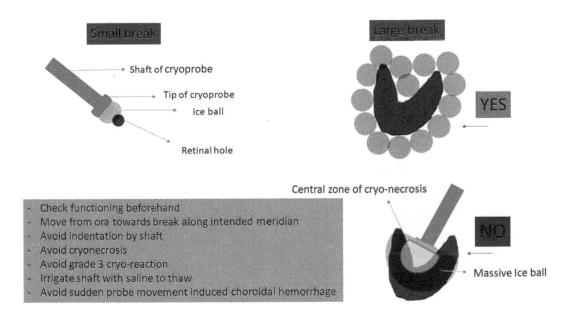

FIGURE 9.6 Technique of applying cryopexy and precautions to be taken.

orientation of the needle, grasp on the needle, positioning of the surgeon, positioning of the eyeball, stability of the eyeball, initial depth of entry, firmness of the globe [intraocular pressure (IOP)], and needle orientation while exiting.

Several components of the suture need planning before passing the suture. These include ease of exposure to the suture site, IOP, thickness of the sclera, width of the scleral bite, depth of needle passage, and type of explant [encirclage, broad buckle, standard buckle, radial explant; Figure 9.8a–c] to be used. Standard scleral suture is essentially a mattress suture with four points of entry and exit, two each for anterior and posterior intrascleral pass [Figure 9.9a]. The intrascleral pass must be at least 5 mm in length and have a uniform depth of penetration between 60% and 75%. The width of the suture pass must be 3 mm more than the width of the planned buckle [e.g., 10 mm wide for a

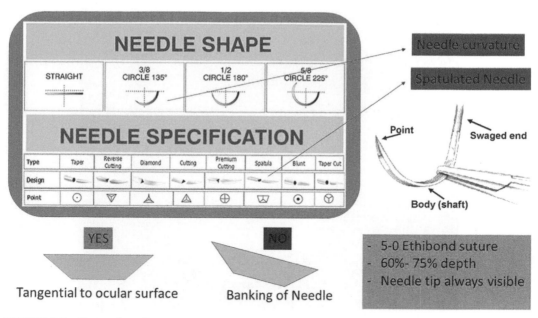

FIGURE 9.7   Types of needles and passage of scleral sutures.

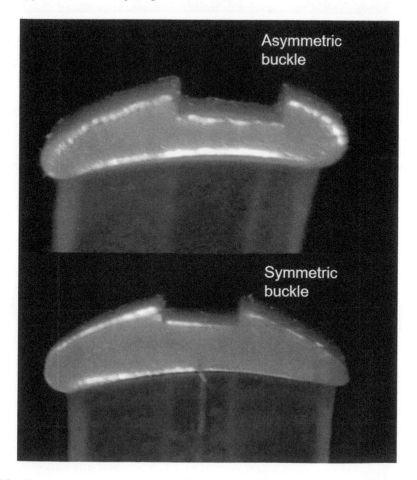

FIGURE 9.8A   Symmetric versus asymmetric solid silicone scleral buckle [cross section].

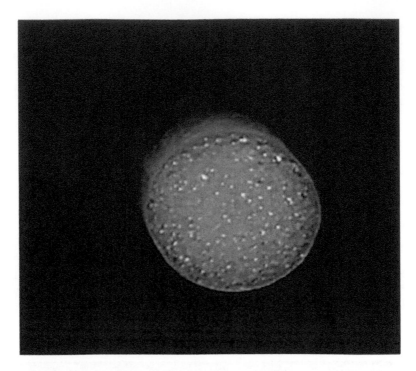

FIGURE 9.8B   Cross section of silicone sponge showing air pockets.

Tires	Sponges
Solid, not compressible	Solid, compressible
Circumferential, segmental (with or without encirclage)	Radial (stand alone or no encirclage)
Area of support is large	Area of support is narrow
Indent is broad and shallow	Indent is focal and high
Needs 90% precision in break localization	Needs 100% precision in break localization

FIGURE 9.8C   Differences between solid silicone buckle [tire] and silicone sponge.

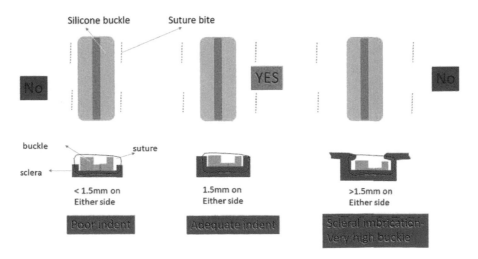

FIGURE 9.9A   Method of passing scleral sutures to obtain proper buckle indent.

Orientation of Scleral Suture Pass

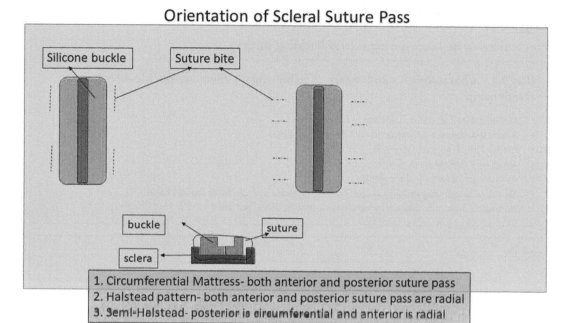

FIGURE 9.9B   Types of scleral buckle sutures in relation to orientation of scleral fibres.

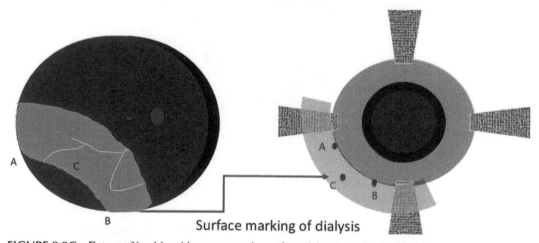

FIGURE 9.9C   Extent of buckle with respect to circumferential extent of retinal break.

7-mm buckle] or encirclage [e.g., 5 mm for a 2.5-mm silicone band]. It is useful to also be aware of a few variants of scleral suture pass such as the Halstead suture and semi-Halstead suture. In standard scleral suture placement, the anterior and posterior pass is circumferential to the limbus, while in Halstead suture, the pass is radial, both anteriorly and posteriorly. In semi-Halstead suture, the posterior bite is circumferential, while the anterior bite is radial [Figure 9.9b]. Radial scleral bites for both Halstead and semi-Halstead sutures are short and deep. In circumferential pass, a significant part of the suture is within the sclera [intrascleral], and this is unlike that with Halstead suture. Because Halstead suture bites run perpendicular to the direction of scleral fibres, there is lesser risk of cheese wiring. Short, radial bites may also be useful in the presence of significant scleral thinning. The buckle must extend at least 1 clock hour on either side of the break [Figure 9.9c]. Currently, the suture that is most often used for retinal detachment surgery to hold the explants is 5-0 Ethibond (polyester) on a spatulated needle (8 mm, ¼c) or diaspatulated needle. [Ethibond is a synthetic, braided, non-absorbable suture. Ethibond suture in green colour is more freely available,

TABLE 9.1

Precautions to be taken during scleral buckling surgery

Box 9.1   Characteristics and means of achieving an adequate buckle–break relationship

- Meridional (radial) and circumferential relationship
- Scleral indentation relationship (up to 3 mm of separation)
- Extend 1 clock hour on either side
- Avoid very shallow and very high indent
- Always consider non-drainage surgery
- Tie scleral sutures sequentially (assistant depresses buckle and also holds the first knot)
- Normalize intraocular pressure by paracentesis (usually more than once)

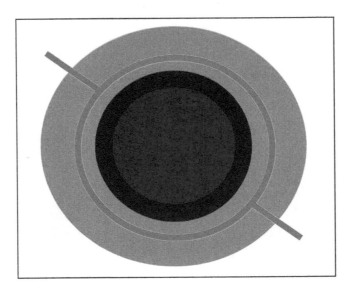

FIGURE 9.10   Ideal appearance of the eye after closure of the peritomy and need to check for induced pulsation [in non-drainage surgery].

but this could be cosmetically unacceptable to the patient. To prevent this, one could use Ethibond (w) that is white in colour, but it may be difficult to obtain commercially.] Silicone buckle or band is then passed beneath the recti muscles and scleral sutures and tied in place so as to achieve the desired height. [Some surgeons prefer to first place the buckle or band and then pass the scleral sutures.] Characteristics and means of achieving an adequate buckle–break relationship are depicted in Table 9.1, Box 9.1. The final step before closure of the peritomy is to repeat indirect ophthalmoscopy and observe the colour of the optic nerve head and elicit induced pulsation. Absence of induced pulsation indicates dangerously high IOP, which must be immediately lowered by paracentesis and indirect ophthalmoscopic evaluation repeated. Peritomy closure is best achieved by realigning the relaxing cuts made in the conjunctiva during the earliest step of surgery [Figure 9.10].

9.1.4 Drainage of Subretinal Fluid

In selected cases, the outcome of retinal detachment surgery without drainage of subretinal fluid could be excellent. In non-drainage surgery, however, it is important to prevent high IOP during

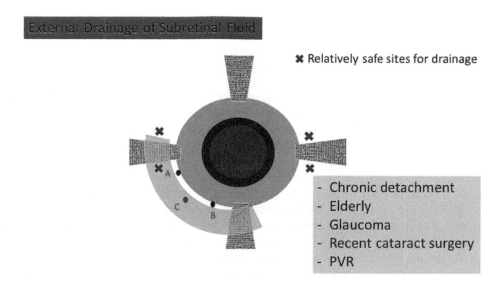

FIGURE 9.11   Indications for drainage of subretinal fluid and site of drainage.

surgery [using intravenous mannitol and one or more paracenteses] as well as immediate postoperative period [using Acetazolamide]. The decision to drain subretinal fluid must be taken judiciously as it can lead to severe vision-threatening complications like haemorrhagic choroidal detachment, subretinal haemorrhage, retinal perforation, vitreous incarceration, and retinal incarceration. Traditional indications to drain subretinal fluid included chronic detachment, bullous retinal detachment [when it is difficult to obtain adequate buckle break relationship], inferior retinal detachment, glaucoma, recent cataract surgery, and high myopia. [Currently, however, with advances in vitrectomy machines and equipment, it is prudent to undertake primary vitrectomy in these conditions rather than risk the consequences of subretinal fluid drainage.] There are several methods described for subretinal fluid drainage, including scleral cut-down, the Prang method [using 10-0 needle point], and needle drainage [Charles, modifications]. More recently, a retractable and calibrated cannula for subretinal fluid has been introduced. The most appropriate sites for drainage are just above and below the horizontal rectii muscles [with adequate amount of subretinal fluid located in this region] [Figure 9.11]. One must avoid draining around the following: shallow detachment, long ciliary and choroidal vessels, areas of cryotherapy, and over a large tear [increases risk of vitreous drainage].

9.2   ENDOILLUMINATION- [CHANDELIER-] ASSISTED SCLERAL BUCKLING SURGERY

Until about a decade ago, rhegmatogenous retinal detachment was being managed by conventional scleral buckling, pneumatic retinopexy, or vitreoretinal surgery. Vitreoretinal surgery was initially advocated for patients with complex retinal detachments such as giant retinal tear (GRT) or higher grades of proliferative vitreoretinopathy [PVR]. With increasing experience with vitreous surgery and advances in surgical instrumentation, vitreoretinal surgery began to be more frequently used in the primary management of even simple retinal detachments. However, vitreoretinal surgery also has the risk of attracting unanticipated and serious intraoperative complications. To overcome the disadvantages of a full-fledged vitreoretinal surgery in patients with simple retinal detachments, endoillumination-assisted scleral buckling surgery using chandelier illumination was first described by the author at an ophthalmological meeting at Udupi [Karnataka, India] in 2010. Initial attempts at publication in a few peer-reviewed journals was unsuccessful with reviewers surprisingly stating that there was nothing new in the approach. As a result, this approach was published the next year in *Retinal Physician*, and the surgical video was released on YouTube [in public domain; <u>Video 9.1</u>]. Subsequently, we published our 2-year follow-up outcomes using this procedure. Since the initial description, this procedure has been recognized as a useful alternative in the management of retinal detachment using scleral buckling, as is evidenced by a surfeit of subsequent publications in peer reviewed literature.

Success of conventional scleral buckling surgery is dependent on accurate localization of retinal break(s) and its subsequent closure using silicone buckle sutured to the scleral surface. Accurate localization of retinal breaks during this surgery is dependent on skill of the surgeon with indirect ophthalmoscopy. Indirect ophthalmoscopic localization of the retinal break(s) during buckling surgery is, however, considered tedious. This is because surgeons have to move around the operation table with the indirect ophthalmoscope mounted on the head. Moving from the operating microscope time and again tends to make the surgery more cumbersome. To do away with the need for indirect ophthalmoscopy, surgeons are now more inclined towards primary vitreoretinal surgery even in simple retinal detachment. Accurate localization of the break may also be impeded by other factors such as non-dilating pupil, posterior capsular opacification, mild vitreous haemorrhage and opacities in the crystalline lens, and presence of a bullous retinal detachment. Lesser emphasis on teaching the 'art of buckling', medical insurance issues, and market forces have also driven the movement of surgeons from preferring primary vitreous surgery over scleral buckling. While it is true that vitreoretinal surgery decreases the risk of missing any retinal breaks, it also carries with it disadvantages like progression of cataract, creation of iatrogenic tears, placement of long-acting vitreous substitutes like intraocular gas or silicone oil, silicone oil glaucoma, and silicone oil keratopathy. In addition, visual rehabilitation time following vitreoretinal surgery is more prolonged than that following scleral buckling surgery.

In EASB, instead of using an indirect ophthalmoscope, visualization of the internal operative field is achieved using self-retaining endoilluminator [chandelier] or cannula-supported endoillumination and wide-angle viewing lens [contact or non-contact]. Technological advances have enabled commercial availability of small-gauge (23G, 25G, 27G) powerful light sources for endoillumination, and these can be placed at a desired location through the pars plana. Our initial surgeries were performed using the Awh 25G self-retaining endoilluminator connected to a Photon (Synergetic) light source. Reinverting Operating Lens System [Volk] lenses were used for wide-angle viewing. Once there is endoillumination, wide-angle-viewing lenses enable visualization of the retina up to the ora serrata. Scleral indentation can be performed by the surgeon sitting at the microscope without having to wear an indirect ophthalmoscope and move around the operating table. Visualization is excellent even in the presence of non-dilating pupil, posterior capsular opacification, or early cataract. With this approach, it is not only possible to locate the number and location of breaks more accurately while seated at the microscope but also to undertake cryopexy of the breaks, drainage of subretinal fluid at a site where the height of detachment is maximum, and titrate the buckle height to achieve an ideal buckle–break relationship. The self-retaining endoilluminator can be removed at the end of the procedure after looking for induced retinal arterial pulsation. The site where the endoilluminator was placed may need to be closed with a single stitch in some patients. The surgical steps are highlighted in Figure 9.12a-d. Figure 9.13 shows preoperative and postoperative fundus photos of an early patient with retinal detachment repaired successfully with this technique.

EASB combines the advantages of visualization provided by vitreoretinal instruments (endoillumination and wide-angle viewing) and safety and simplicity of conventional scleral buckling surgery. This is likely to improve surgical results even in eyes with rigid pupils or capsular opacification. The new technique allows every step of conventional buckling surgery to be performed entirely under the microscope. It removes the disadvantages of the current approach—that of using an indirect ophthalmoscope to view the retina, to localize and cryo the break, and for drainage of subretinal fluid. This technique, being a truly microscopic retinal detachment surgery, is more likely to gain wider acceptance amongst younger retina specialists as they are more attuned to modern vitreoretinal approaches to retinal repair than conventional scleral buckling surgery.

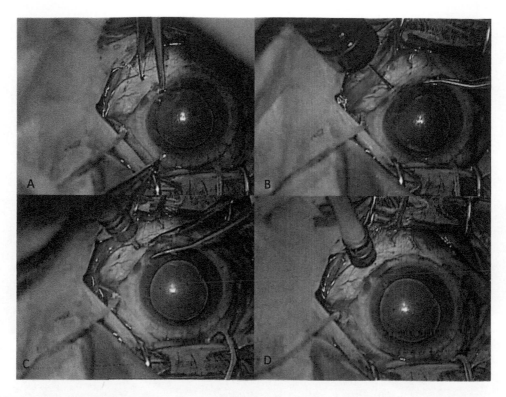

FIGURE 9.12A Endoillumination-assisted scleral buckling. Initial steps: placing the chandelier light source.

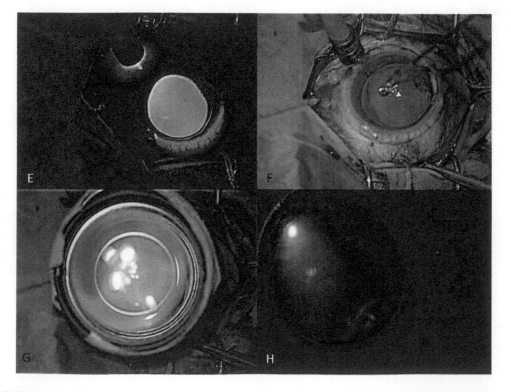

FIGURE 9.12B Endoillumination assisted scleral buckling: scleral indentation under wide-angle visualization lens.

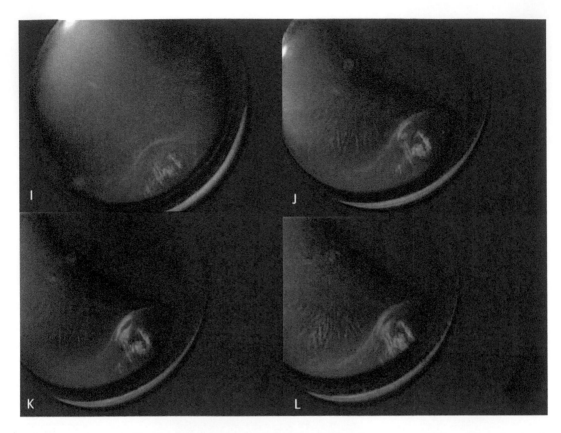

FIGURE 9.12C   Endoillumination-assisted scleral buckling. Performing cryopexy under wide-angle visualization lens.

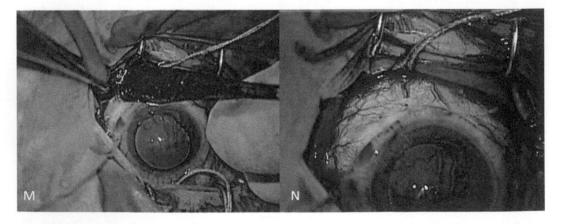

FIGURE 9.12D   Endoillumination assisted scleral buckling: removal of chandelier light after localization of retinal break(s) and cryopexy.

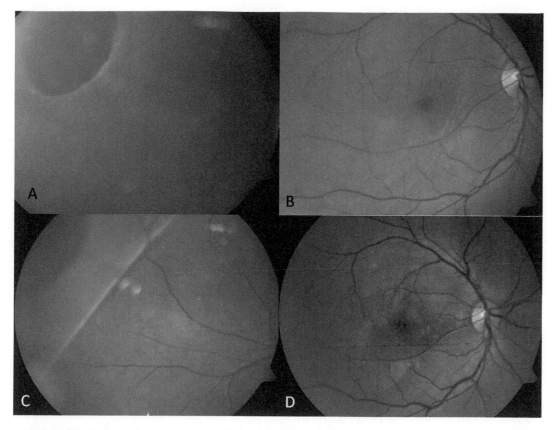

FIGURE 9.13 Preoperative and postoperative images of retinal detachment treated by endoillumination assisted scleral buckling.

9.3 VITREORETINAL SURGERY

9.3.1 CONSTRUCTION OF THE SCLERAL PORT AND EARLY STEPS

Wound construction is an important component of all surgical interventions, and this is true for vitreoretinal surgery as well. The objectives while making the scleral ports are to ensure that the gauge chosen would help to achieve the desired surgical objective. Circumferential location of the port allows adequate manoeuvrability and access to sites of tissue dissection, while radial location and direction of entry into the vitreous cavity averts any damage to the crystalline lens, vascular pars plicata, vitreous base, and ora serrata. A well-constructed port allows sutureless and safe closure at the end of surgery and prevents a direct tract to the surface of the globe across the overlying conjunctiva [reducing the risk of posterior vitreous wick syndrome]. The most frequently recommended circumferential location to make the scleral ports is just below the lower margin of the lateral rectus for the infusion port and about 160 degrees apart for the active port and endoillumination port, above the upper margins of the medial and lateral rectus. Wide spacing between the upper ports is important to reach the peripheral vitreous and abnormalities [like PVR membranes], located between 11.00 and 1.00 o'clock. Modifications to this guideline may, however, be useful in resurgeries, removal of dropped IOL, phacofragmentation, endoillumination-assisted biopsy of intraocular mass, removal of retained intraocular foreign body [RIOFB], and a few others. A temporal approach may also be considered in some cases. Radial location of a port that is too anterior increases the risk of trauma to the crystalline lens, as well as inducing haemorrhage from the relatively more vascular part of the ciliary body, pars plicata. Port entry that is posterior increases the risk of drag on the vitreous base and induction of iatrogenic trauma to the ora serrata and peripheral retina. For these reasons, the recommended radial distances of the scleral ports from the limbus are 3.0 mm, 3.5 mm, and 4.00 mm in aphakic, pseudophakic, and phakic eyes, respectively. In phakic eyes, 4.00 mm instead of 3.5 mm reduces the risk of iatrogenic trauma to the crystalline lens. These measurements do not hold true while operating on infants and toddlers [see section on surgical anatomy]. Even if the distance from the limbus is well measured, such iatrogenic injuries may still occur if the entry of the trocar into the vitreous cavity is not directed towards the optic nerve [with the eyeball in primary position]. Anteriorly directed entry results in injury to the lens, while a very tangential entry risks injury to the peripheral retina and choroid. It is often observed that there is a natural tendency to push the eyeball deeper into the orbit while making the port entries. This must be avoided as it tends to result in ballooning of the conjunctiva and masking of the anatomy at the entry site, loss of precision on wound construction, and inadvertent globe rotation and injury to the lens or other tissues. This can be avoided by gripping the globe at the limbus, relatively in a meridian adjacent to the site of entry, and consciously applying a counterforce directed upwards. Some surgeons prefer to hold the globe in the opposite meridian. Unlike the bevelled and two-step trocar cannula systems of the past, current generation lancet-shaped trocars slice through the sclera with minimal force and so reduce this occurrence. However, one may still encounter this situation while operating on children [in whom the sclera is more tough], in deep-set eyes, and when there is prior hypotony.

The collagen fibres within the sclera run in a circumferential manner in the anterior sclera. Hence, the blade of the trocar must also be circumferential to the limbus to achieve entry to the vitreous cavity by displacement of these fibres. Failure to follow this would result instead in the trocar cutting across these fibres. The latter could increase the risk of port leakage at the end of surgery and force the surgeon to use a suture to close the leak. If this is not recognized intraoperatively and the port is left sutureless, persistent hypotony from delayed spontaneous closure of the scleral opening may be noted in the early postoperative period. Poor scleral port construction could also tend to increase the risk of loss of gas that has been injected for long-term tamponade, with resultant failure of retinal surgery. When silicone oil is used for long-term tamponade, poor scleral port could result in entrapment of silicone oil in the subconjunctival space, either as solitary or as multiple globules. Poor wound construction may also expose the patient to postsurgical endophthalmitis. This occurs if a direct tract is present between the outer surface of the globe and the vitreous cavity, across a scleral port that is poorly covered by the conjunctiva [posterior vitreous wick syndrome]. This complication can be mimimized by displacing the conjunctiva by a few millimeters before making the port entry. Conjunctival displacement could be lateral or anteroposterior. Sliding the conjunctiva from posterior to anterior using the reverse end of another, capped trocar allows simultaneous displacement of the conjunctiva as well as measured entry of the trocar at 3.5—4.0 mm.

Several types of insertion techniques have been described for 25G trocar-cannula entry, including Eckardt incision [straight], Hagemann's incision [oblique-perpendicular], Rizzo incision [parallel], and modified Rizzo [oblique-parallel]. Similarly, several methods have been described for 23G trocar-cannula entry, including Eckardt incision [two-step], Zorro direct incision [30-degree obliquity], Zorro oblique incision [10- to 15-degree obliquity], Pollack incision [5-degree entry up to 50% depth and then 30-degree obliquity at entry], and Rizzo incision.

While placing the infusion cannula, it is important to ensure that the hub is in tight contact with the scleral surface with no part of the steel shaft showing through. This would indicate that the entire 4 mm shaft of the cannula is in the sclera and vitreous cavity. Incomplete penetration of the cannula induces the risk of choroidal and subretinal placement of its inner opening and its associated complications, not only at the beginning of surgery but more so in the midst of other steps such as indentation vitrectomy. It is also important to ensure that the tip of the infusion line is snuggly 'locked' within the infusion port cannula. Failure to do so may increase the chances of the infusion line coming away from the cannula even with a minor, inadvertent tug. Before switching on the infusion line, ensure that the machine has been primed beforehand, the lowest part of the suction cassette is in line with the eye level, there is no air bubble within the tubing, and the tip of the cannula is clearly identified as being within the vitreous cavity. The latter can be achieved by momentarily indenting the infusion port into the vitreous cavity and simultaneously visualizing [either under the microscope or from outside, with the naked eye] the tip of the cannula while shining a bright beam of light from an endoilluminator from the opposite meridian. While indenting the infusion port at this step, directing it anteriorly increases the risk of lens injury in phakic eyes. In pseudophakic eyes, however, the direction of indentation should be more anterior as this makes it easier to observe the location of the internal opening of the cannula. Even when no air is seen to be trapped within the infusion line, it is often seen that a small bubble shows up in the vitreous cavity on switching on the infusion. This may be innocuous and could be easily removed in pseudophakic and aphakic eyes. In phakic eyes, however, attempts at its removal may put the clear lens in jeopardy of a lens touch or increase risk of peripheral vitreous traction. Hence, it is best to prevent such bubbles from showing up at all. One normally checks the free flow of fluid from the infusion line, outside the surgical field, before it is placed into the infusion port cannula. Having checked this, the flow is stopped. On stopping the flow, a minimal negative pressure gets created within the tubing, so some air gets sucked into the hub of the infusion line. Being only a small amount of air, it stays within the opaque steel part of the infusion line and remains unnoticed. It is this trapped air that dislodges into the vitreous cavity when the infusion fluid is switched on. So, to the avoid this from happening, it is useful to pinch the infusion line at its tip [and hence prevent negative pressure from developing] before switching off the fluid flow during the test run. The infusion line can then be placed into the cannula, with the firm pinch still in place. Some surgeons place the infusion line into the cannula while the fluid is still flowing. While this avoids the occurrence of air bubbles within the vitreous cavity, it increases the risk of subretinal or choroidal infusion [as the location of the cannula tip internally has not been ascertained at this stage].

Despite taking all these precautions, there are a few situations wherein the risk of incomplete penetration of the infusion cannula into the vitreous cavity is high. These include hypotony, anterior PVR, non-dilating pupil, peripheral capsular opacification, dense vitreous haemorrhage, significant vitreous membranes [e.g., in endophthalmitis], cilioretinochoroidal detachment, and bullous retinal detachment. In these situations, it may be prudent to place a 20G, 6-mm cannula beforehand. When the infusion cannula is noted to be subretinal, in some patients, particularly those who are pseudophakic, it may be managed by carefully incising or teasing the tissue [not retina] over the cannula, using 23G or 25G microvitreoretinal (MVR) blade, tapered tip of the diathermy probe, or trocar. During this step, there is risk of inducing intraocular bleeding from the choroidal blood vessels, but this occurs relatively infrequently and is usually mild. In phakic eyes, there is a risk of lens injury during this manoever, and so it may be prudent to move the infusion cannula adjacent to either of the superior ports. Location of the internal opening of the infusion can be ascertained with certainty by internal visualization [under wide angle lens and endoillumination] before switching on fluid flow.

9.3.2 Induction of Posterior Vitreous Detachment

Posterior hyaloid face [PHF] is part of the vitreous that assumes the features of a membrane owing to condensation and characteristic orientation of the posterior cortical fibrils. Hyalocytes are also located within the fibrils of the posterior hyaloid. In thickness, the posterior hyaloid measures about 5 μ and has a firm attachment to the internal limiting membrane (ILM). Attachments around the optic nerve head, vitreous base, retinal vasculature, and along abnormal retinal pathologies such as lattice degeneration are particularly very firm. ILM and PHF interactions become weaker with age, and this, with the increasing vitreous liquefaction [synchesis] occurring alongside, results in natural and spontaneous PVD. In relation to surgical interventions on the retina, the posterior hyaloid holds significant importance owing to multiple reasons. PHF could behave like a contractile membrane exerting traction on the retina or act as a scaffold for the ingrowth of proliferative vessels [in proliferative vascular retinopathies] as well as proliferative membranes [in proliferative vitreoretinopathy]. These properties have a bearing not only on the pathogenesis of primary retinal pathologies like epiretinal membrane, macular hole, vitreomacular traction, tractional retinal detachment, retinal tear, and retinal detachment but also on the success and outcomes of surgical interventions to treat these pathologies. Failure to remove the posterior hyaloid at surgery increases the risk of redetachment and the development of postsurgical epiretinal membranes. So, removal of the posterior hyaloid is an important and critical step of most vitreoretinal interventions. There are several classifications of PVD based on slit lamp evaluation, ultrasonography, and optical coherence tomography. However, for the purpose of surgical planning, relationship of the PHF and retina could be categorized into the following situations [Box 9.2].

Understanding the varied relationships would help in better informed planning of the preoperative, as well as intraoperative approach, to handle the pathology in a safer and more effective manner. The selection of instruments, direction of membrane peel, use of perfluorocarbon liquid (PFCL), choice of tamponade, and need for 360 peripheral laser are likely to be impacted by the status of the PHF–retina relationship. The surgical step of PVD induction can be broken down into several mini steps, including stage of visualization of the hyaloid, stage of engagement of the hyaloid, stage of occlusion of the probe opening or silicone tip, stage of initiation of separation of Weiss ring, stage of Weiss ring separation from the optic nerve head, and stage of hyaloid separation from the posterior retinal surface followed by stage of completion [Box 9.3]. Usually, these steps proceed imperceptibly during actual surgery but, it may be useful in the learning stages to be attentive to the tissue-instrument interaction throughout the process. This approach would be particularly useful when one is unable to induce PVD in an expected manner or when one encounters a complication [such as formation of a retinal tear]. Reasons for not being able to induce PVD may be related to strong adhesion between the PHF and ILM [e.g., children, familial vitreoretinopathies], inadequate build-up of vacuum [incomplete occlusion of the probe; inadequate preset vacuum on the machine] or to a combination of these. In some situations, it is inherently more difficult so induce PVD safely, as in the presence of a bullous retinal detachment, GRT, choroidal detachment, overlying dropped nucleus or IOL, and impacted RIOFB. Certain times, one may need to be more cautious while inducing PVD with high suction. Some of these conditions include vitreomacular traction, cystoid diabetic macular edema, Kranenberg syndrome, endophthalmitis, and acute retinal necrosis. In some situations, it may be easier to first induce PVD at the macula or at the site of the pathology itself [e.g., impacted foreign body] and then extend it further. The necessity, effectiveness, and safety of manoevers like hydrodissection, viscodissection, and perfluorodissection during PVD induction remain a matter of discussion.

Visualization of the posterior hyaloid that is still attached to the optic disc and retina is as difficult as visualizing the vitreous, owing to its translucent nature as well as its end on alignment. To visualize the posterior hyaloid, it would be useful to use triamcinolone suspension injected into the vitreous

---

Box 9.2   Relationship between posterior hyaloid face [PHF] and retina

1. Retina attached with or without peripheral lesions

   a. No posterior vitreous detachment [nPVD]
   b. Partially attached PHF [incomplete PVD-icPVD]
   c. Complete PVD [cPVD]

2. Retina detached

   a. Partially attached PHF [incomplete PVD-icPVD]
   b. Complete PVD [cPVD]
   c. Abnormal retina–hyaloid interaction [abPVD]: retinal stiffness, focal and diffuse folds, circumferential contraction, retinal shortening
   d. Aberrant proliferation of glial and metaplastic cells [proliferative vitreoretinopathy PVR]

Box 9.3   Stages in PVD induction

- Stage of visualization
- Stage of occlusion
- Stage of initiation
- Stage of extension
- Stage of completion

Box 9.4   Patterns of tricort 'staining'

- Suspended or enmeshed in the vitreous
- Sprinkled on the retinal surface
- Sheet-like deposition on the retinal surface
- Linear deposition on the retinal surface
- String-like attachment to the retina

---

cavity. Some surgeons may prefer to use chromovitrectomy. An indirect evidence to the presence of PHF and posterior vitreous fibrils is the observation of transmitted movement to the underlying structures [e.g., detached retina]. After aspirating out the excess, several patterns of tricort distribution may be observed [Box 9.4].

The next step in the process is engagement of the posterior hyaloid followed by its elevation from the retinal surface. For reasons of safety, the preferred location for engagement of the posterior hyaloid is just adjacent to the nasal margin of the optic nerve head. Three approaches are described for this step based on the instrument used—silicone tip, vitreous cutter, and bent pick. This is the firmest area of attachment and so while using the silicone tip or suction mode of the vitreous cutter, higher vacuum and higher infusion flow are needed to engage and induce PVD around the optic disc. Successful separation of the PHF from the optic disc is heralded by the appearance of the Weiss ring. Before increasing the vacuum to high levels, it is important to ensure that there is complete occlusion of the silicone tip by the hyaloid or dense posterior cortical fibres. The fish strike sign while using a silicone tip is indicative of complete occlusion. For the purpose of inducing PVD, one must refrain from trimming down the soft silicone tip. Sudden loss of occlusion may result in hypotony and rarely to engagement and pull on adjacent structures such as major blood vessels over the optic disc. Before increasing the suction, it is also important to ensure that the neurosensory retina is not a part of the tissue occluding the silicone tip or cutter port. Failure to take this precaution would result in the creation of a posterior retinal tear. Use of a bent pick to engage and lift the posterior hyaloid may be tried when attempts using vacuum fail. PVD induction using a bent pick is only safe when there is at least a minor plane of separation beforehand. Once the Weiss ring forms, it is relatively easier to extend the PVD all around. As the posterior hyaloid lifts up from the retina surface, the foveal-macular hyaloid becomes well delineated as a horizontal oval sheet, attached to the Weiss ring. The most efficient way of extending the PVD farther peripherally is by obtaining complete occlusion with the silicone tip or vitreous cutter and directing the pull along the pupillary axis [but taking care to avoid lens touch]. Direction along this axis would induce a uniform ring of separation spreading outwards from the disc [seen initially as a shadow of the leading edge; Video 9.2]. Application of tangential traction instead of axial traction is likely to result in asymmetric spread of PHF separation and to incomplete PVD induction. Tangential and clock-hour separation may be needed during PVD induction in the presence of retinal detachment.

9.3.4 Internal Limiting Membrane Peeling

The approach to peeling of ILM is probably one of the most 'non-standardized' steps in all of vitreoretinal surgery. There are multiple variables such as choice of staining [no staining, trypan blue, indocyanine green, triamcinolone, brilliant blue, membrane blue, dual stain], instrument to initiate the peel [ILM forceps, MVR blade, diamond dusted membrane scraper, Finesse loop], instrument to complete the peel [ILM forceps, end-grasping forceps], preferred site to initiate the peel [nasal, superior, inferior, temporal; adjacent to a blood vessel, avascular region], area of peel [arcade to arcade, lesser], amount of peel [complete circumferential peel with removal (no flap), complete circumferential peel with multilayer inverted flap, temporal flap], use of mechanical force on the edges of the hole [none, massager, removing adhesions beneath the hole], drainage of residual fluid through the hole, use of adjuvants [none, blood, serum, transforming growth factor-beta], and preference of vitreous tamponade [air, SF6, C3F8, silicone oil]. Postoperative advice about patient positioning is also highly debated [a few hours, a few days, 1 week]. One trend in macular hole surgery that seems to be gaining wider acceptance is combined surgery [with phacoemulsification and IOL implantation]. The most taxing step in ILM peeling is creation of an edge; once this is achieved, further steps are akin to capsulorrhexis [circumambulatory movement around the macular hole with multiple mini-steps of grasp-regrasp; Video 9.3]. It is a matter of curiosity as to why initiation of ILM peel is not done at the already well formed edge of the macular hole itself. The author perceives this to be a safer and simpler approach to initiating ILM peel, and it does away with the likely risks associated with creating an ILM flap over the retinal surface. A gentle approach would prevent perceived risks of hole widening and retinal pigment epithelial loss.

General guidelines to improve the safety of ILM peeling in uncomplicated cases [with high myopia, with retinal detachment, chronic macular hole, large macular hole, failed macular hole] include use a lens that provides good stereoscopic visualization with minimal distortion [irrigating lens, self-retaining lens such as Landers lens], staining of ILM, initiating peel after incising or fracturing ILM surface with finesse loop or appropriate-gauge MVR, avoiding peel initiation close to large blood vessels and thin retina [nasal retina preferred], continuing peel with end grasping forceps [reduces easy fragmentation of ILM], minimizing proximity of endoilluminator to the fovea, using short-acting gas, and at least few hours of postoperative prone positioning. In addition, it may be best to avoid maneuvers that are likely to increase the risk of subfoveal retinal pigment epithelium loss and whose efficacy is not fully established. These maneuvers include drainage of fluid over the macular hole and massage of the hole margins. Management of complicated macular hole also has surgeon preferences like the type of flap [inverted-multilayer, temporal], choice of free flap [ILM, neurosensory retina, lens capsule, amniotic membrane], use of adjuvants, vitreous tamponade, and postoperative positioning.

9.3.5 Fluid–PFCL Exchange and PFCL–Silicone Oil Exchange

Perfluorocarbon liquid [PFCL] serves as a useful intraoperative tool during vitreoretinal surgery, particularly in the management of giant retinal tears, in which they help in unfolding the flap. However, injecting PFCL into the vitreous cavity in a fluid-filled eye requires simultaneous egress of the infusion fluid. When the intraocular fluid does not exit the eye as PFCL is being injected, there occurs a dangerous increase in IOP as well as anterior ballooning of the peripheral retina due to subretinal fluid shifting anteriorly. While the former can lead to compromise of the optic disc perfusion, the latter increases the risk of iatrogenic tear formation and vitreoretinal incarceration. The most widely recommended means to enable safe injection of PFCL in a fluid-filled eye is to use a double-bore cannula, first described by Dr. Stanley Chang. However, this instrument is not widely and freely available to all retina surgeons. So, in the absence of a double-bore cannula, surgeons achieve PFCL injection by intermittently leaving one of the pars plana ports open to allow some fluid to flow out of the vitreous cavity. This approach is, however, fraught with risks as there is significant fluctuation in the IOP. Microincisional vitreous surgery [MIVS] has rapidly become the standard procedure of choice for vitreous surgery over the past decade. One of the key advantages of MIVS is that it allows the IOP to be maintained at all times due to the tight fit between the cannula and the vitreous instruments or from the use of valved cannula. For this reason, during MIVS, the risks of PFCL injection mentioned are significantly enhanced if no double-bore cannula is available. Use of mismatch between a 23G cannula and 25G injection cannula is a useful technique that allows PFCL injection with simultaneous and spontaneous egress of the intraocular fluid without the need for any specialized instrumentation. In cases like giant retinal tears and complex retinal detachments, in which PFCL is often required, the infusion port and endoilluminator port should use a standard 25G trocar and cannula. For the third (active) port, however, the sclerotomy should be made using a 23G trocar and cannula. After completing vitrectomy, PFCL injection is performed using a syringe carrying a 25G cannula. Before the start of PFCL injection, infusion pressure is lowered to about 15 mmHg. Then, as PFCL is injected into the vitreous cavity, IOP rises, and the vitreous fluid spontaneously and passively egresses from the active port due to mismatch in diameters of cannula and soft tip. This enables better control of the IOP and eliminates the need for having to intermittently keep one of the ports open or stopping the infusion. This technique helps in maintaining the IOP gradients constant, thereby adding safety to the surgery by reducing the risk of anterior ballooning of the peripheral retina and by maintaining optic disc perfusion. The rationale behind this added safety is that the 23G cannula has a diameter of 0.69 mm, while the 25G cannula has a diameter of 0.53 mm. The resulting small difference between the port and injection cannula creates adequate space for simultaneous and equivalent egress of the infusion fluid out of the vitreous cavity, with no rise or drop in the intraocular pressure [Figure 9.14].

After the completion of PFCL-assisted retinal attachment and laser, in the management of a large GRT, it is necessary to replace PFCL with a long-acting tamponade, preferably silicone oil. This can be achieved in two ways: first to replace PFCL with air and then inject silicone oil [a two-step

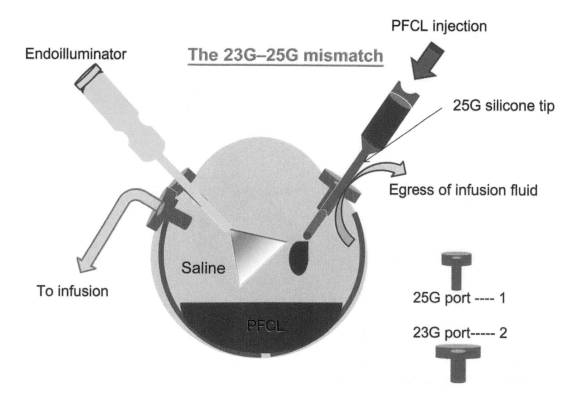

FIGURE 9.14 Injection of perfluorocarbon liquid using 23G–25G cannula mismatch.

approach]; the second is to perform a direct PFCL–silicone oil exchange [a one-step approach]. The latter approach is to be preferred as it reduces the risk of retinal slippage. While undertaking direct exchange, the surgeon can use the viscous fluid controller module and alternate between injection of silicone oil and extrusion of PFCL using automated extrusion cannula [PFCL extrusion may also be undertaken using a flute handle and using the control hole] or use of the bimanual sub-mode [see section on vitreous machines]. During direct exchange, silicone oil in the high-pressure injector can be inserted directly into the infusion line and hence a fourth port for chandelier illumination would not be necessary. An important precaution to take during this step is to ensure that the silicone tip of the extrusion cannula is always within the PFCL bubble [placement even momentarily into the silicone globule could result in the tip getting clogged by silicone oil; Figure 9.15a and 9.15b].

9.4 PNEUMATIC RETINOPEXY

Pneumatic retinopexy is the surgical procedure of injecting an expansile [pure, long-acting] gas into the vitreous cavity to achieve retinal reattachment. Concurrently, retinopexy has to be achieved using either cryotherapy before injection of the gas or by laser photocoagulation as soon as reattachment is noted [laser indirect ophthalmoscope delivery]. Owing to its simplicity, the procedure is considered extremely useful by some surgeons. Many others shun the approach entirely owing to lower one surgery success rate [70%], stringent need for postoperative positioning, and higher incidence of new break formation and proliferative vitreoretinopathy. Patients who respond better to pneumatic retinopexy are those who are phakic and have fresh detachment caused by a solitary tear in the upper and horizontal confines of the retina. It is carried out under strict asepsis and topical

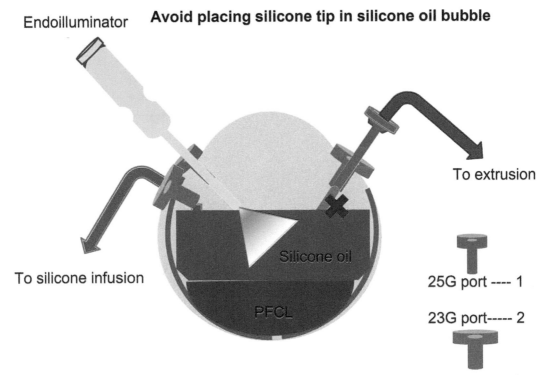

FIGURE 9.15A Technique of direct PFCL–silicone exchange.

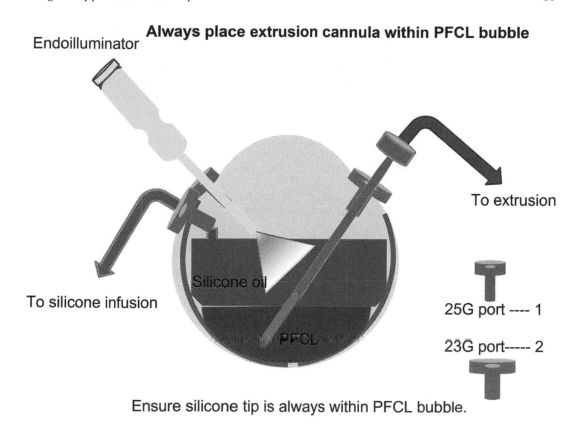

FIGURE 9.15B Technique of Direct PFCL–silicone exchange.

anaesthesia. Either SF6 [0.6 cc] or C3F8 [0.3 cc] gas is injected using a 30G needle [see section on vitreous substitutes] in a quadrant devoid of bullous detachment and away from the tear. Prior to injection, a degree of lowered intraocular pressure is achieved by paracentesis. However, this may create undue hypotony, reduce scleral rigidity, and make gas injection slightly more difficult. Hence, it may be safer to perform paracentesis after gas injection. Post-injection, patient is advised to maintain prone position for 6–8 hours and then asked to adopt a posture that places the tear [and the gas bubble] into the most superior location. If the macula was on before the procedure, the steam-rolling manoeuvre is said to prevent macular detachment by preventing displacement of subretinal fluid into the posterior pole. Reasons for failure other than poor case selection, missed breaks, and new break formation include loss of injected gas volume by escape into the subconjunctival space [across the injection site], intravitreal bubble failure [injected gas bubble fails to expand and maintain adequate volume for at least 3–5 days], positioning failure [poor compliance to positioning], and sometimes late migration of gas bubbles into the subretinal space. Tornambe recommends performing 360-degree barrage laser to improve the overall success of pneumatic retinopexy. Despite the lower single surgery success rate, the final anatomical reattachment rate recovers to more than 95% after the second intervention [scleral buckle or pars plana vitrectomy].

SUGGESTED READING

1. Venkatesh P, Verma L, Tewari H [2002]. Posterior vitreous wick syndrome: A potential cause of endophthalmitis following vitreo-retinal surgery. *Med Hypotheses*. 58(6): 513–515.
2. Venkatesh P, Garg SP [2012]. Endoillumination-assisted scleral buckling: A new approach to retinal detachment repair. *Retinal Physician*. 9: 34–37.

3. Gogia V, Venkatesh P, Gupta S, Kakkar A, Garg SP [2014]. Endoilluminator-assisted scleral buckling: 2 year results. *Ind J Ophthalmol.* 62(8): 893–894.
4. Temkar S, Takkar B, Azad S, Venkatesh P [2016]. Endoillumination (chandelier) assisted scleral buckling for a complex case of retinal detachment. *Ind J Ophthalmol.* 64(11): 845–846.
5. Eckardt C [2005]. Transconjunctival sutureless 23G vitrectomy. *Retina.* 25: 208–211.
6. Rizzo S, Genovesi-Ebert F, Vento A, Miniaci S, Cresti F, Palla M [2007]. Modified incision in 25-gauge vitrectomy in the creation of a tunneled airtight sclerotomy: An ultra-biomicroscopic study. *Graefes Arch Clin Exp Ophthalmol.* 245(9): 1281–1288.
7. Tomita Y, Kurihara T, Uchida A et al [2015]. Wide-angle viewing system versus conventional indirect ophthalmoscopy for scleral buckling. *Sci Rep.* 5: 13256.
8. Anaya JA, Shah CP, Heier JS, Morley MG [2016]. Outcomes after failed pneumatic retinopexy for retinal detachment. *Ophthalmol.* 123: 1137–1142.
9. Tornambe PE [1997]. Pneumatic retinopexy: The evolution of case selection and surgical technique. A twelve-year study of 302 eyes. *Trans Am Ophthalmol Soc.* 95: 551–578.

10 Common Vitreoretinal Procedures

10.1 DIABETIC VITREOUS SURGERY

Diabetic retinopathy is one of the major end-organ complications secondary to chronic hyperglycaemia and tissue hypoxia. It is a progressive microvascular disease that is driven by hypoxia-induced overexpression and secretion of vascular endothelial growth factor (VEGF). It proceeds at a variable pace from mild retinopathy to severe retinopathy and then to advanced diabetic eye disease. It is a major cause of moderate to severe vision loss in patients with type 1 and type 2 diabetes mellitus. Vision loss from diabetic retinopathy can be prevented in the majority of patients by following recommendations for screening set up by various national and international societies. However, screening programs have been far from successful, so it is common, even today, to see patients presenting for the first time to a retina specialist, when the retinopathy has progressed into advanced stages. In its most advanced grades, diabetic retinopathy is characterized by non-resolving vitreous haemorrhage, tractional retinal detachment, and combined traction–rhegmatogenous detachment. In addition to these traditional indications for vitreoretinal surgery in patients with diabetic retinopathy, some newer indications have been recognized. These indications include persisting or advancing fibrovascular proliferation despite adequate retinal photocoagulation, diabetic tractional papillopathy, tractional diabetic macular edema, and non-tractional but resistant diabetic macular edema.

The outcome of vitreoretinal surgery depends not only on meticulous planning and intraoperative tissue dissection but also on careful perioperative assessment and management. Important considerations before subjecting a patient with diabetes to surgery are age and gender; type and duration of diabetes mellitus, quality of diabetes control; presence of other comorbidities [severe hypertension, nephropathy, cardiovascular, cerebrovascular, or peripheral vascular disease]; recent prolonged hospital admission/major surgery; duration of ocular symptoms; visual acuity and grade of retinopathy in the fellow eye; past history of retinal laser; intravitreal injection, or surgery; extent of pupillary dilatation; status of the crystalline lens; presence of neovascularization of the iris or angle; evidence of macular ischemia or global retinal ischemia [as suggested by the extent of sclerosed vessels and confirmed by fluorescein angiography]; presence, absence, or completeness of posterior vitreous detachment (PVD); presence of vitreoschisis, intraocular pressure (IOP); and status of the optic nerve. A more detailed informed consent covering the risk-to-benefit ratio, risk of no light perception, and need for further interventions such as laser, cataract surgery, glaucoma surgery, or anti-VEGF therapy, after the main procedure, must be obtained and checked by the surgical team prior to surgery. In the absence of media opacity or vitreous haemorrhage, slit lamp fundoscopy or detailed inspection of high-quality fundus images and optical coherence tomography (OCT)/ OCT angiography images would be most useful in understanding the pathoanatomy of the given situation. In the presence of vitreous haemorrhage, one has to rely on a well performed ultrasonography [USG] examination to decipher the pathoanatomy. Prior knowledge of the pathoanatomy assists in minutely planning the surgery and locating sites of safe separation of membranes away from the retina [cleavage], as well as sites of microvascular attachments.

Surgery for patients with advanced diabetic retinopathy is amongst one of the most challenging. The surgery is fraught with a higher risk of intraoperative events like variable degrees of haemorrhage and iatrogenic breaks, increased risk of corneal epithelial edema, worsening of lens opacity, and compromised perfusion of the optic nerve. The increased surgical risks are related to several

DOI: 10.1201/9781003179320-11

pathoanatomic features such as absent or partially separated posterior hyaloid; vitreoschisis; multi-layered haemorrhage; ischemic, thin, and atrophic retina; multiple, firmly adherent, opaque epiretinal membranes with focal or diffuse microvascular attachments [Figure 10.1a]; active or regressed neovascular proliferation; atrophic and small retinal breaks; tightly adherent hyaloid to areas of dense laser scars and proliferation; presence of variable degree of macular and extramacular exudation; macular drag; and dense fibrovascular stalk attached to the optic disc with tractional papillopathy.

Removal of the vitreous and posterior hyaloid during surgery for complications of diabetic retinopathy is usually very different from almost all other commonly performed procedures. Vitreous degeneration, liquefaction, and PVD are said to occur at an earlier age in patients with diabetes. However, in patients who develop proliferative retinopathy before the onset of these changes, the situation becomes complex. The vitreous tends to retain its gel configuration more often, vitreoschisis becomes inevitable, and the posterior hyaloid phase becomes firmly anchored to the neovascular ingrowth at multiple points and also diffusely to a large surface of the retina. When this complex of posterior hyaloid and epiretinal membrane contracts, it results in tractional retinal detachment, retinal drag, macular ectopia, tractional papillopathy, and combined traction–rhegmatogenous detachment. Based on the surgical pathoanatomy, three broad situations could be evident—complete absence of PVD [nPVD, least common], incomplete PVD [icPVD, most common], and complete PVD [cPVD]. When PVD is absent, the type of hyaloid–retinal relationship could be of several types—few points of focal attachment, extensive points of focal attachment, combination of focal and limited diffuse attachment, and diffuse broad area of attachment, extending into the vitreous base. The last pattern is very difficult to dissect, but fortunately, it is also the least common situation encountered during surgery. Focal attachments tend to tent the retina, creating retinal folds with crests and troughs. Diffuse attachments tend to drag the retina into a table-top configuration and may also cause macular ectopia. It is important to identify the type of hyaloid–retinal relationship that is present at each point of surgical dissection. Failure to do so may result in application of faulty steps and hence significantly increase the risk of iatrogenic breaks and intraocular bleed.

Many times during diabetic vitreous surgery, multiple membranes are encountered while proceeding with vitreous removal in the mid and posterior vitreous cavity. This is indicative of vitreoschisis. A sign that the posterior hyaloid is still intact is the presence of a layer of trapped (not getting dispersed) blood over the retinal surface. The hyaloid can also be recognized by the presence of a

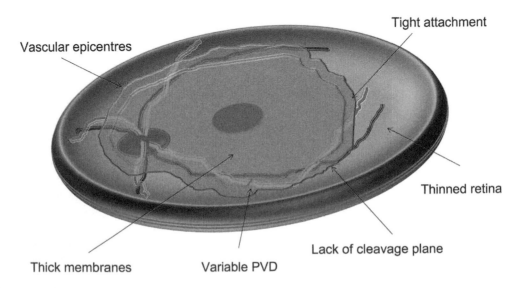

FIGURE 10.1A Characteristics of diabetic tractional retinal detachment.

shimmering (due to reflected light) membrane over the layered blood. Careful creation of an opening in this membrane releases the trapped blood into the vitreous cavity. At this point, the hyaloid becomes more clearly visible along with anatomical details of the underlying retina, and the hyaloid can be removed more safely using the vitreous cutter. In some patients, a similar appearance can be noted due to the presence of a thin layer of subretinal bleed overlying a thin, atrophic, dull-appearing, and avascular retina. This should not be mistaken for the posterior hyaloid, and failure to do so would result in the creation of an iatrogenic break and add to the complexity and chances of surgical failure. To avoid this situation, it is important to closely look for any blood vessels [perfused or sclerosed] and, when present, the nature of the vascular divisions (dichotomous or irregular) before cutting any membrane.

Several approaches have been described for the handling and removal of the hyaloid and tractional membranes in complex diabetic surgery. Traditionally, they have been identified as segmentation, delamination, and en-bloc dissection. In segmentation, the surgeon uses vertical scissors to meticulously cut down wide areas of attachment of the hyaloid and tractional membranes into smaller islands (segments) of tissue. This relieves tangential and overall traction on the retina and may be sufficient to allow the retina to settle. Islands created in this manner could be made further small, either by trimming them with the vitreous cutter or by shrinking them further with diathermy. In delamination, as the name suggests, the tractional membrane is disconnected and removed from the underlying retina in the form as a sheet or lamina by cutting the microvascular pegs connecting the two. As is evident, this maneuver is possible only with a horizontal or curved scissors and reduces anteroposterior traction on the retina. In en-bloc dissection, early entry is gained into the sub-hyaloid space at the equator using the cutter and then scissors are used to cut all the tissue tethering the underlying retina to the hyaloid in a sequential manner, without breaking down the hyaloid into multiple segments. Hence, the entire dissection occurs beneath the hyaloid and progresses from the periphery towards the most central attachment (usually the optic nerve head or peripapillary retina). Although these three methods are described, surgeons normally apply a combination of these approaches to successfully release all the traction on the retina. With the advent and widespread acceptance of small-gauge vitreous surgery, the need for separate instruments such as scissors to segment and delaminate the tissue has reduced. This is because the opening of the port in small-gauge vitreous cutters is much closer to the tip of the probe. In addition, currently available vitreous machines and control systems allow controlled grasping of a tissue followed by precise actuation of the cut function, so much so that the cutter itself can be used as a fine scissors [Figure 10.1b–i]. This approach is best possible by using the vitreous cutter in the momentary mode and setting the cut rate to 100/minute. Another advantage of using the cutter for segmentation and delamination instead of scissors is the ability to be able to simultaneously aspirate any induced intraocular bleed.

Tissue dissection in diabetic vitreoretinal surgery can proceed from inside out (centrifugal) or from outside in (centripetal) and can be performed using standard three-port approach or using a bimanual approach, with a chandelier light source placed into a fourth port. In the inside-out approach, dissection begins from or around the optic nerve head and moves progressively outwards using a combination of segmentation and delamination. Contrarily, in the outside-in approach, dissection moves from outside the retinal vascular arcade towards the optic nerve head. Both approaches have advantages and disadvantages. The advantage of the inside out approach is that a large area of the tractional attachment loosens once the strongest point of attachment at the disc is released. This facilitates creation of cleavage planes to carry forward further dissection in a safer manner. Also, the retina is thicker posteriorly and less likely to contain hidden folds, both of which reduce the risk of creating an iatrogenic tear. In addition, the inside-out approach favors tissue removal by using the plane or path of least resistance (akin to removal of Velcro from the right and the wrong directions). Disadvantages with this approach are that the attachment is the strongest at this location, it is difficult to find a natural edge with which to grasp the tissue or commence dissection, and the neovascularization is likely to be most profuse and bearing

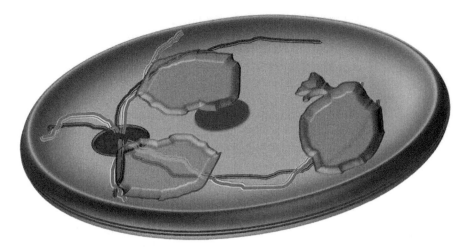

FIGURE 10.1B Surgery for diabetic tractional retinal detachment: segmentation into small islands using a small-gauge vitrectomy probe.

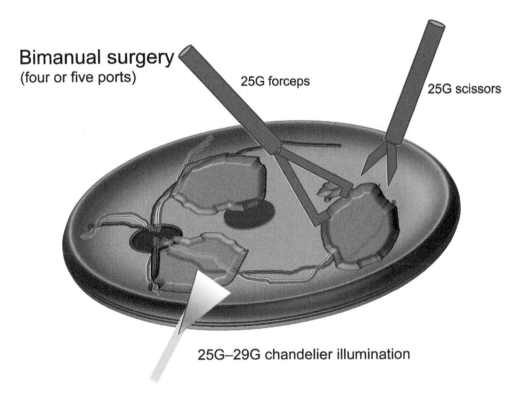

FIGURE 10.1C Surgery for diabetic tractional retinal detachment: removal of traction using bimanual resection [note the need for the fourth port for chandelier illumination].

large-caliber blood vessels [which enhances the risk of significant intraocular haemorrhage]. The main advantage of the outside in approach is the presence of a natural edge, in most cases, from which to commence tissue dissection. But this approach is more likely to result in an iatrogenic tear as the retina in this region is thinner (and sometimes atrophic), and the direction of surgical dissection and pull on the tissue is from anterior to posterior. Also, this location, being usually the

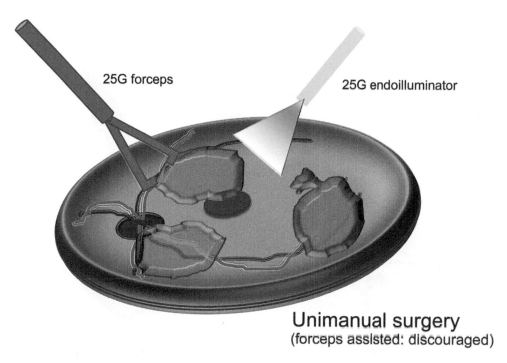

25G forceps

25G endoilluminator

Unimanual surgery
(forceps assisted: discouraged)

FIGURE 10.1D   Surgery for diabetic tractional retinal detachment: removal of tractional tissue using blunt dissection [forceps, exclusive shear] is discouraged.

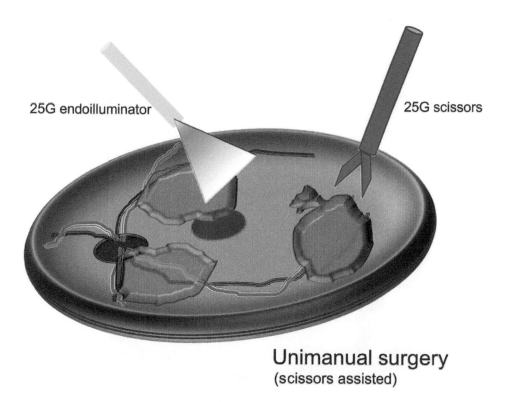

25G endoilluminator

25G scissors

Unimanual surgery
(scissors assisted)

FIGURE 10.1E   Surgery for diabetic tractional retinal detachment: removal of tissue using sharp dissection [scissors, inclusive shear] is preferred.

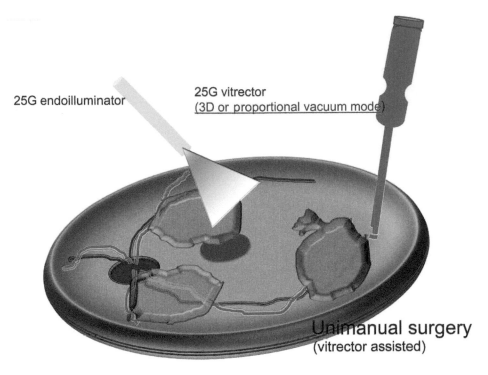

25G endoilluminator

25G vitrector
(3D or proportional vacuum mode)

Unimanual surgery
(vitrector assisted)

FIGURE 10.1F   Surgery for diabetic tractional retinal detachment: removal of traction using a small-gauge probe in proportional vacuum or 3D mode. This is successful but may be associated with increased risk for iatrogenic breaks.

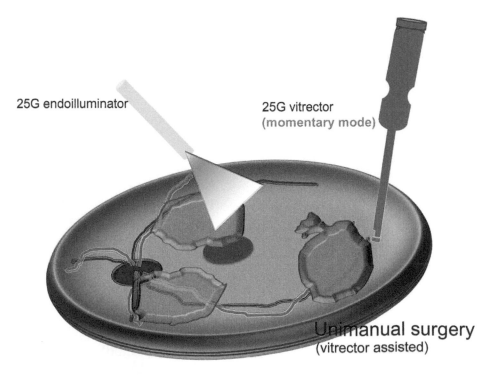

25G endoilluminator

25G vitrector
(momentary mode)

Unimanual surgery
(vitrector assisted)

FIGURE 10.1G   Surgery for diabetic tractional retinal detachment: removal of traction using a small-gauge probe in momentary mode is successful and allows precise control.

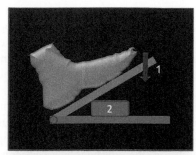

Proportional and linear mode

- Only downward force on footswitch (1) (red arrow)
- Simultaneous actuation of suction and
  cutting (ultrasound) are active
- Decreased safety margin

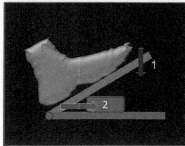

Momentary mode

- Downward force on footswitch (1) (red arrow)
  causes actuation of suction alone
- Lateral movement of vertical footplate (2) actuates
  cutting (ultrasound)
- Improved safety margin
- Controlled cutting of tissue possible (1 cut/ sec)

FIGURE 10.1H Method of actuating momentary mode function on the foot pedal in comparison with proportional vacuum or 3D mode.

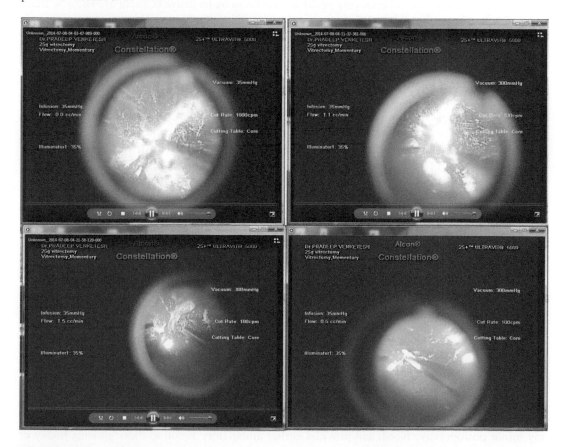

FIGURE 10.1I Intraoperative sequential screen shots during surgery for diabetic tractional retinal detachment using momentary mode. Note the cut rate at 100/minute.

distal attachment site of the proliferative growth, creates a form of ridge, the attachment of which to the underlying retina is very dense and difficult to safely dissect. Hence, the safest approach would be to begin dissection in the peripapillary zone. To obtain a safe edge to begin dissection, one could use an MVR blade [small-gauge blades are available] to make an incision into the hyaloid at this location or achieve the same using the vitreous cutter in a controlled manner (see momentary mode).

Similar to managing tractional membranes, managing intraocular haemorrhage during surgery for complex diabetic retinopathy surgery remains a challenge. These haemorrhages are sometimes so severe that they quickly spread and obscure the anatomical details, hampering further safe dissection and completion of surgery. In addition, the clot becomes very tenacious and strongly adherent to the underlying retina. Removal of such clots not only adds to the surgical time but also increases the risk of further iatrogenic complications such as creation of a retinal tear. Hence, it is best to take all preoperative and intraoperative precautions to minimize the chances of having to face an intraocular haemorrhage. Preoperative control of hypertension, stoppage of anti-platelet therapy [in consultation with cardiologist], and prior history of panretinal photocoagulation [PRP] completion assist in reducing the risk. More recently, the risk of intraoperative bleed has been significantly minimized by the practice of giving an intravitreal injection of bevacizumab a few days prior to surgery. The sclerosing effect of the injection is sometimes noted within 12–24 hours. There are several precautions that need be taken during tissue dissection so as to reduce the risk of intraocular haemorrhage. First, it is necessary to understand that even when a neovascular frond appears regressed, the proximal ends remain patent and perfused. It is hence necessary to avoid removing proliferative tissue by inclusive or exclusive shear without first inducing thermal occlusion of the proximal ends using diathermy. For the same reason, if microvascular pegs under a tractional membrane are being cut using scissors or vitreous cutter, it is important to do so along the apex of the peg [being flush with the under surface of the membrane] and avoid its proximal end. Diathermy of predisposed neovascular fronds and increasing the IOP before carrying out tissue dissection at a site that is prone to or anticipated to bleed is more safe and helpful rather than increasing the IOP and applying diathermy after the bleeding commences. Use of the cutter instead of separate instruments such as intravitreal scissors has also reduced the risk of intraocular haemorrhage during tissue dissection. As mentioned earlier, this approach also allows instantaneous aspiration of any induced bleed, so it helps maintain good visualization of the surgical field. In addition, to stop the arrest of an ooze, the blunt end of the cutter itself can also be sometimes used to apply direct but gentle pressure on the bleeding vessel. Injecting a sufficiently sized perfluorocarbon liquid [PFCL] bubble, is also useful to tamponade minor intraocular bleed/ ooze from the optic disc vessels. In this situation, PFCL also helps to maintain clarity of the surgical field. When elevated IOP [preset of 60 mmHg] is used to control bleeding, it is of utmost importance for the surgeon and her or his team to remember this and bring it down to acceptable levels at the earliest possible [but never beyond 60–90 seconds]. Failure to do so could result in permanent damage to the optic nerve [which in patients with diabetes could already have been compromised].

Once tissue dissection is complete and the retina is attached, it is best to complete PRP intraoperatively using endolaser. If there is a high risk of intraocular haemorrhage during complex tissue dissection, it may also be prudent to first complete endolaser over regions of attached retina and then proceed with the dissection. Before air-fluid exchange, it is again important to check the port site and retinal periphery for any breaks and manage these. For vitreous tamponade, one could use air if the patient had only vitreous haemorrhage and the tissue dissection needed was not very extensive or complicated. In all other patients, it is useful to use a long-acting gas or silicone oil as long-term tamponade [Figure 10.2]. Silicone oil is preferred as it maintains optical clarity, compartmentalizes any minor postoperative bleed, and provides earlier ambulatory vision to these patients [many of whom are absolutely blind before the surgery]. In patients with diabetes, it would be safe to close the ports with a suture even when a small-gauge procedure has been performed.

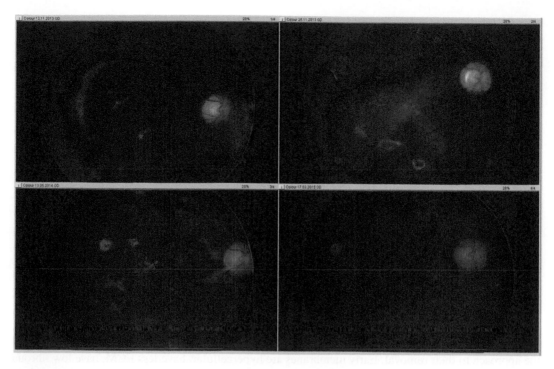

FIGURE 10.2 Preoperative and postoperative fundus images following surgery for diabetic tractional retinal detachment.

10.2 PROLIFERATIVE VITREORETINOPATHY

Proliferative vitreoretinopathy [PVR] could be defined as cellular proliferation occurring within the vitreous cavity, on the surface of the retina, and beneath the retina, in response to retinal tear induced retinal detachment. It is considered to have elements of wound healing, but in a wrong place, as the traction forces lead to deleterious effects on the delicate retinal tissue. PVR differs from wound healing in having a long drawn course and being devoid of a vascular component. The prevalence and severity depend on the duration of detachment, age, type of retinal tear [e.g., dialysis, giant retinal tear], etiology of retinal detachment [e.g., penetrating trauma, complicated cataract surgery, post vitrectomy], and secondary associations [e.g., choroidal detachment, high myopia]. Although PVR could be evident preoperatively and add to the complexity of management, it also is the most common cause of late redetachment and poor outcome after retinal detachment surgery. This is because it can induce tissue contraction, reopen the primary break or retinotomy, create new breaks, produce macular distortion (macular pucker), and cause retinal tautness and shortening. Similar to wound healing, PVR evolves through a complex process of migration and proliferation of native and alien cells, synthesis of extracellular matrix proteins, remodelling of connective tissue, collagenization, and contraction. The stimulus for PVR is creation of a retinal tear with subsequent dispersion and exposure of retinal pigment epithelial cells and glial cells to an altered biological milieu. Under these conditions, both retinal pigment epithelium [RPE] cells and glial cells [astrocytes and Mueller cells] acquire some characteristics of fibroblasts and macrophages. PVR then begins to evolve at the sites of deposition of these altered cells under the effect of stimulatory and inhibitory factors. Stimulatory factors include epidermal growth factor [EGF], platelet-derived growth factor [PGDF], tumour necrosis factor [TNF-α], fibroblast growth factor [FGF], insulin-like growth factor [I and II], and interleukin-1. Inhibitory factors are fewer and include [TNF-β] and interferon-beta [INF-β]. These factors reach the vitreous cavity and subretinal space due to breakdown of the blood retinal barrier after the occurrence of a retinal tear and detachment. Cytokeratin positive cells are found in the majority of PVR membranes wherein they may form epithelium like layers or may present as focal aggregates of rounded fibroblastic cells. Their numbers dwindle with increasing duration of the membrane. Glial cells that contribute to PVR include astrocytes and Mueller cells [both glial fibrillary acid protein (GFAP) positive]. They are the predominant cell type in simple epiretinal and retrolental membranes. In addition, the other cellular components include fibroblast-like spindle-shaped cells [cytokeratin and GFAP negative] of indeterminate origin, vascular endothelial cells, and inflammatory cells [macrophages and T lymphocytes]. Contribution of inflammatory cells may predominate in patients with choroidal detachment and perforating injury. PVR is less severe in patients with high myopia and those with hypopigmented fundus [e.g., albinos] owing to a paucity of RPE cells.

The natural history of PVR has been arbitrarily classified into four overlapping phases: the phase of cellular proliferation, phase of extracellular matrix formation, phase of membrane formation and contraction, and phase of maturation and organization of fibrous tissue. In the phase of cellular proliferation, RPE and glial cells divide by mitosis, and this process may occur for several months [in contrast to the short wave of cell division in dermal wound healing]. Growth usually occurs in the form of membranes that have contractile tendency. In the phase of extracellular matrix (ECM) formation, synthesis of collagen types I, III, and IV and glycoproteins such as fibronectin and vitronectin is seen. Membrane contraction is thought to occur secondary to a process termed *reel in*, a process in which cells drag components of ECM, such as collagen, towards themselves. In the later phase, the membrane appears hypocellular. It is important to know that membranes in the early phase of PVR differ from those in the later phases, and this difference has a bearing on the timing of surgery and the approach to their removal. Early membranes are hypercellular, have less ECM, have low fibrous elements [hence low mass with which to grasp the membrane], are fragile, are flimsy, and are stickily adherent to the retina. Late membranes, on the other hand, are hypocellular, have well-formed ECM and fibrous tissue and adhere to the retina in the form of a 'dry' single sheet or focally. These characteristics explain why membranes in the later phases of PVR are relatively easier to peel and are less likely to recur compared to removal of membranes in the earlier phases. In addition, it also explains why drugs targeting PVR are likely to be most effective in the earlier phases.

Based on the extent and severity of the proliferation, PVR has been classified in a slightly different manner by the three most widely used classification systems, the Retina Society classification, Silicone Oil Study Group classification, and updated Retina Society classification. Some of the terms used in these systems are self-explanatory. For clinical purposes, the Retina Society classification seems most appropriate. The updated classification made no changes to features of grade A and B PVR but made significant descriptive changes to grade C PVR and completely abolished grade D PVR. These modifications have importance because they assist in better preoperative surgical planning and seem to have better prognostic value. Clinically, however, the original classification system is simpler to convey the severity of PVR. Grade A is characterized by vitreous haze and pigment clumps in the vitreous and surface of the retina (usually inferior). In grade B PVR, there are wrinkling of inner retinal surface, vessel tortuosity, rolled and irregular edges of the tear, and reduced mobility of vitreous. The presence of fixed folds in the retina is the sine qua non of grade C and D PVR (in the Retina Society classification). It is termed C1, C2, and C3, implying the presence of fixed retinal folds in one, two, or three quadrants, respectively. In grade D, fixed folds are present in all four quadrants [D1 if the entire retinal surface is still seen clearly (open funnel), D2 if there is constricted view of the retina and optic disc (narrow funnel), and D3 when optic disc is not visible (closed funnel)] [Figure 10.3a-c]. In the updated Retina Society classification, grade D has been eliminated, and grade C has been assigned two subtypes, anterior and posterior, in relation to the vitreous base and into clock hours (1–12 clock hours). Specific diagrammatic 'codes' have also been assigned to depict focal contraction (solitary or few fixed folds less than 4DD), diffusion contraction (multiple fixed folds, more than 4DD), subretinal band, anterior displacement, and so on. It also introduces features such as circumferential contraction [characterized by posterior radial folds and 'purse stringing' of the equatorial retina], anterior loop traction [forward and often severe

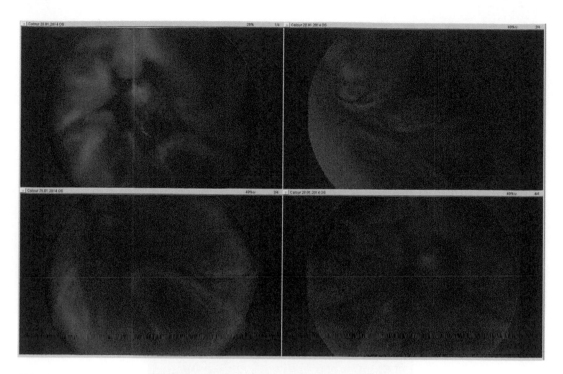

FIGURE 10.3A Fundus photograph of patient with total retinal detachment and narrow funnel [PVR D2].

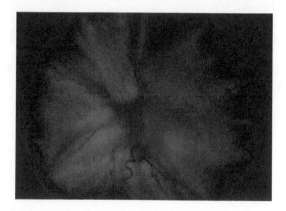

FIGURE 10.3B Fundus photograph of patient with total retinal detachment and closed funnel [PVR D3].

displacement of the retina due to contraction of the vitreous base and retro-iridial tissue], and ante-rior displacement [stretched peripheral retina]. Based on the morphology, subretinal PVR could be sheet like, napkin ring, moth-eaten, or clothesline like [Figure 10.4a-b]. From these classifications, it is evident that in managing grade C PVR, one needs to consider the contribution from three components: the vitreous component, epiretinal component, and retro-retinal or subretinal compo-nent. Despite the detailed preoperative grading, the status of the posterior vitreous detachment and intraoperative hyaloidal–retinal relationship (HRR) could be difficult to fathom. In view of this, the author and his colleagues reported on their observations between preoperative PVR, intraopera-tive HRR, and anatomical outcomes after triamcinolone-assisted small-gauge vitreoretinal surgery. We perceive that triamcinolone-assisted intraoperative visualization is probably the most sensitive method to accurately identify, define, and classify PVR.

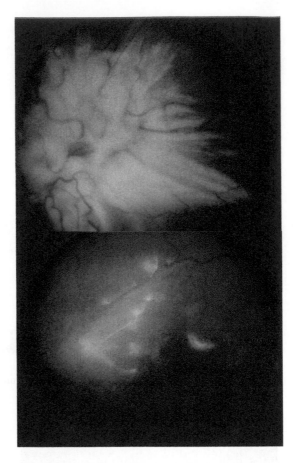

FIGURE 10.3C Preoperative and postoperative fundus photographs following vitreoretinal surgery for proliferative vitreoretinopathy [PVR D3].

Currently, the choice of surgery in phakic patients with retinal detachment and mild to medium PVR [below C1] and break localized to the area of the equator and beyond remains scleral buckle. Scleral buckle may be successful even in the presence of multiple breaks [Figure 10.5]. In pseudophakic patients, the trend is towards primary vitrectomy, irrespective of PVR grade. More than one surgery may become necessary in some cases with advanced PVR to achieve anatomical success. The principle in conventional retinal detachment surgery is to search all retinal breaks and seal them by external buckling and retinopexy [see section on surgical approaches and steps]. In vitreoretinal surgery, in addition, the surgeon identifies internal forces that could prevent the success of conventional surgery, and having done so, eliminates these forces (vitreous, epiretinal, subretinal) and replaces the lost vitreous using substitutes such as silicone oil and long-acting gases.

The current standard for managing retinal detachment with PVR is small-gauge vitreoretinal surgery. In the presence of concurrent choroidal detachment, ocular hypotony, and severe anterior PVR, the risk of subretinal or choroidal location of the small-gauge infusion cannula is more likely. So, the surgeon must be more cautious to rule out this concern before switching on the infusion. The surgeon should also be prepared to insert a 6-mm 20G infusion cannula in the event of subretinal location of the small-gauge cannula. In this situation, one could also perform surgery with the infusion cannula located adjacent to either of the superior ports. Irrespective of the statistics, it is the author's belief that a scleral band (with or without buckle) always acts as a 'friend' in improving the long-term success of vitreoretinal surgery in patients with anterior and circumferential PVR. Rather than blindly placing these supportive buckles from the ora serrata, it would sometimes be useful to

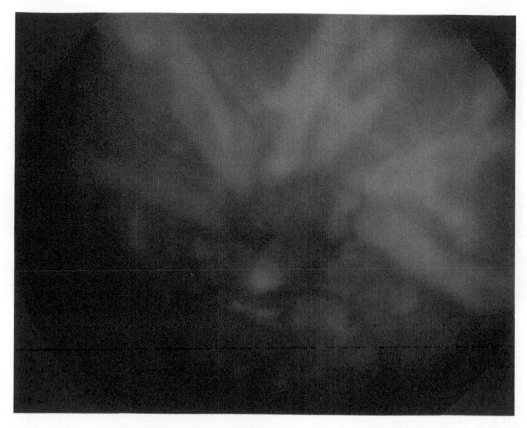

FIGURE 10.4A Proliferative vitreoretinopathy with subretinal bands [double napkin ring].

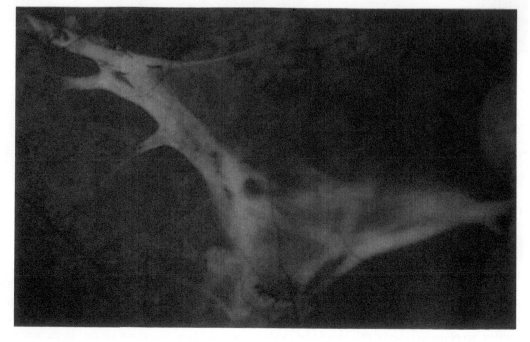

FIGURE 10.4B Proliferative vitreoretinopathy with broad sheet of subretinal proliferation.

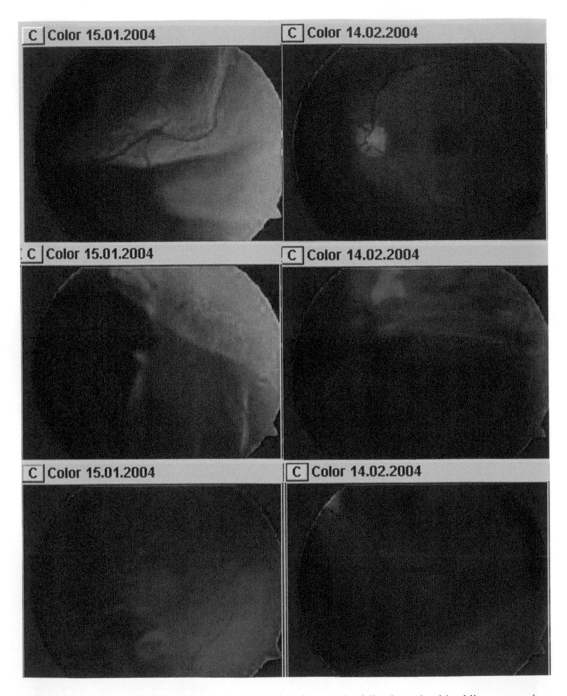

FIGURE 10.5 Preoperative and postoperative fundus photographs following scleral buckling surgery in a young phakic patient with multiple retinal tears and bullous retinal detachment.

first mark the location of the break and align the sutures accordingly. In general, crystalline lens and a stable intraocular implant does not need removal even in the presence of giant retinal tear [GRT] and most anterior PVR. This is because of improvements in illumination, wide-angle viewing, and safety of vitreous cutters. An exception is the presence of iris-fixated lenses; these may tend to tilt or retroflex, so plans to counter this should be made beforehand [e.g., retention sutures in the anterior chamber]. In the presence of a breach in the posterior capsule [following capsular rent or yttrium aluminum garnet (YAG)capsulotomy], there is likelihood of air entering into the anterior chamber during air fluid exchange [also read section on complications], and this, too, must be anticipated and measures planned to overcome the ensuing difficulty in visualization [injecting suitable viscoelastic into the anterior chamber].

In the initial steps of vitreous surgery, first clear the pupillary plane and central vitreous. Then it may be useful to manage anterior and peripheral PVR before managing posterior PVR. This is because posterior PVR maintains a stretch on anterior PVR, and this stretch aids the dissection efforts. Peripheral indentation by the assistant in a controlled manner is very helpful in this situation. While dissecting posteriorly located membranes, move from the thicker posterior retina to the thinner anterior retina [i.e., centrifugal dissection]. This approach reduces the risk of iatrogenic break formation. The epiretinal component in PVR is best managed by membrane peeling using end-opening forceps (apply tangential force and peel centrifugally). Peeling of star folds is started from their epicentre. Segmentation using vertical scissors may be useful when membranes are more adherent. With the cutter opening of small-gauge vitreous cutters being close to the tip, the need for pick- and bent needle–assisted removal of membranes has significantly reduced. Rarely, one may have to resort to bimanual surgery to remove membranes located close to the vitreous base and beyond [e.g., anterior loop traction]. Subretinal bands rarely prevent reattachment, so their removal must be considered only in the presence of napkin ring or if they are found to tent the macula. In the presence of early and immature membranes, gentle massage of the retinal surface over the affected area using DDMS, finesse loop, or silicone tip helps to loosen and remove the fine membrane.

Once the retina seems adequately mobile, attempt internal drainage via one of two routes, preexisting break or posterior retinotomy (1–2DD). In the presence of bullous detachment, it would be useful to make an early posterior retinotomy and undertake fluid-fluid exchange before trying to remove peripheral vitreous. This would convert a bullous detachment into a shallow detachment intraoperatively, thus making further removal of the vitreous safer [Figure 10.6]. During fluid-fluid exchange, subretinal fluid can be evacuated by active suction or passively using a silicone-tipped

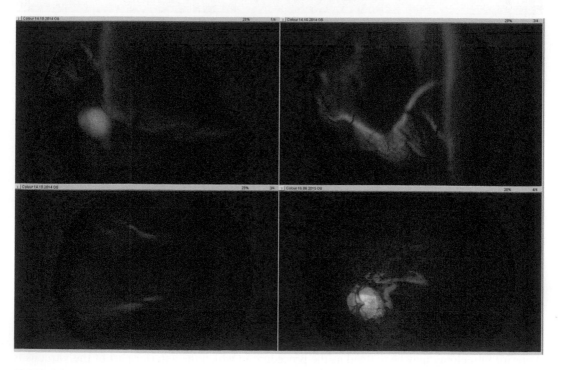

FIGURE 10.6 Preoperative and postoperative fundus photograph following vitreoretinal surgery for bullous retinal detachment.

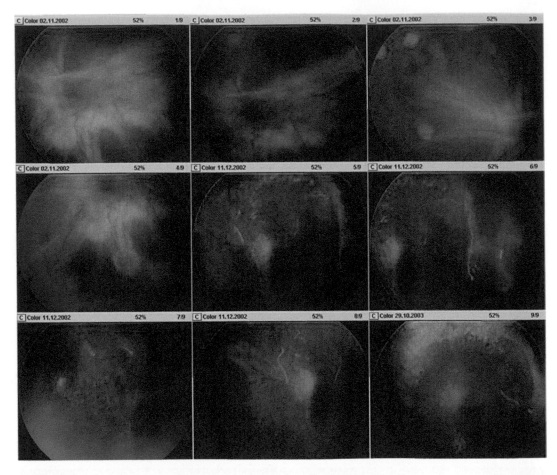

FIGURE 10.7 Preoperative and postoperative sequential fundus images following vitreoretinal surgery with retinectomy in a patient with proliferative vitreoretinopathy [PVR D3].

flute needle. Once vitrectomy is completed safely [assisted by injection of triamcinolone into the vitreous cavity one or more times], further evacuation of subretinal fluid and retinal reattachment is assisted by fluid-air exchange. This process has to be gradual to prevent dramatic extension of tears in areas of unrelieved traction and dissection of air into the subretinal space. Retinectomy may be necessary in a small group of patients [Figure 10.7]. Once the retina has flattened, retinotomy and any other breaks should be treated by endolaser photocoagulation. Marking all the retinal tears using internal diathermy before air-fluid is very helpful in not missing them out later on. Delimitation all around (360 degrees) was also recommended by most vitreoretinal surgeons in the past, but there is less emphasis now on its utility in reducing the risk of redetachment. [Very high laser energy should be avoided because it can lead not only to necrotic break formation but also impede venous drainage from peripheral retina and increase the risk of choroidal detachment and postoperative inflammation.] Following completion of laser, silicone oil or long-acting gas is injected for adequate long-term internal tamponade. During this step, a vent is needed to allow egress of fluid across a valved cannula.

10.3 ANTERIOR VITRECTOMY

Anterior vitrectomy may be defined as the procedure in which the anterior part of the vitreous is removed by means of efficient aspiration and cutting. There is no clear delineation of vitreous as anterior and posterior, but for practical purposes, it may be considered as the vitreous lying just behind the crystalline lens and posterior surface of the iris. In the natural state, it is limited by the anterior hyaloid face and merges imperceptibly into the rest of the core vitreous. Intraoperatively, it could be considered as that part of the vitreous that prolapses into the anterior chamber following a breach in the posterior capsule. Anterior vitrectomy, in addition to the situation of complicated cataract surgery, is also utilized in a planned manner while performing lens aspiration with primary posterior capsulorrhexis in very young children with congenital cataract and during lensectomy with anterior vitrectomy in children with complicated cataract secondary to juvenile idiopathic arthritis. As with posterior segment surgery, technological advances in phaco machinery have significantly enhanced the safety and outcomes of the surgical intervention. Loss of vitreous during cataract surgery was almost the norm during the days of intracapsular surgery, was less common during manual extracapsular cataract surgery, and is very infrequent with phacoemulsification. Nevertheless, the final outcome of phacoemulsification, in the event of rupture of the posterior capsule and vitreous loss, is impacted strongly by the efficiency with which the surgeon handles the prolapsed vitreous. It is best, however, to prevent this eventuality by being aware of high-risk associations during the preoperative workup and recognizing indicators of its possibility during early steps of the surgery. But the most important attribute is to perform each step of phacoemulsification meticulously and be able to pick up subtle features, such as the ring sign or spider leg sign, that are indicative of imminent risk of posterior capsular rupture and take immediate reversal or corrective measures. If a rent does occur, it must be noted at its smallest dimensions and further enlargement prevented. Immediate measures to prevent risk of posterior capsular rent from enlarging would be to stop the aspiration or phacoemulsification, reduce infusion pressure [lowering bottle height in gravity-dependent systems], inject viscoelastic into the anterior chamber to tamponade the rent, consider dry aspiration of epinuclear or cortical remnants, and viscoexpression of nuclear fragments. Abrupt withdrawal of the phaco probe must be avoided. These measures are likely to reduce the amount of vitreous prolapsing into the anterior chamber across the posterior capsular defect. The anterior chamber must be freed of vitreous by thorough and careful anterior vitrectomy.

Anterior vitrectomy is best performed in a closed chamber, so the cataract incision must be sutured if it had been enlarged for delivery of a large nuclear fragment. The objectives of vitrectomy are to remove the herniated vitreous from the anterior chamber and for a short depth behind the pupillary zone but without causing further prolapse of the posterior vitreous; ensuring no damage to the pupillary margin, the iris, both lens capsules, and the retina; and preventing hypotony. Two approaches can be used, combined pars plana–limbal route [irrigation through limbal incision and vitreous cutting through pars plana] or entirely limbal route. The former has the advantage of allowing more efficient clearing of vitreous from the retrolental space and reducing the risk of vitreous hydration; its disadvantage is that it may be difficult to make a trocar cannula entry once the scleral rigidity is lost [due to the cataract incision and loss of vitreous]. The advantage of the latter is that it is easier to perform, but there is an increased risk of vitreous hydration and further prolapse. During vitrectomy, the important variables that the surgeon must pay attention to are amount of irrigation, direction of irrigation, amount of aspiration force, wound stability, wound leak, iris prolapse, and vitreous upthrust. The cut rate selected must be the maximum setting on the available machine [2500 for White star, 4000 for Centurion, and 5000 for Stellaris and Constellation]. Low-flow, low-vacuum, high-cut-rate surgery is the preferred approach. The direction of fluid flow through the irrigation handpiece plays an important role in the procedure and must always be directed away from the pupillary opening [usually directed towards the anterior chamber angle]. If the irrigating fluid is allowed to flow into the vitreous cavity through the pupil, it would hydrate the core vitreous and lead to its further prolapse into the anterior chamber. The end point of anterior vitrectomy is when the iris falls back and there is no distortion of the pupillary margin [due to adherent vitreous strands]. At the same time, the eye must not be allowed to become hypotonus. Injecting a small amount of triamcinolone into the anterior chamber may help in better visualization and cutting of the vitreous fibrils. It is again emphasized that direct damage to the pupillary margin, iris, and lens capsule must be avoided during anterior vitrectomy.

Premium machines that allow both phacoemulsification and vitrectomy to be performed have preset wet vitrectomy [WetAnt] and dry vitrectomy [VitDry] modes. In **wet vitrectomy**, irrigation and cut rate are fixed, while vacuum can be controlled linearly. The foot pedal has two ranges: the first range actuates irrigation at a fixed rate, while the second range [pressing down the foot pedal farther] actuates cutting at fixed cut rate as well as linearly controlled vacuum. [Irrigation continues to flow in the second range.] In **dry vitrectomy**, the cut rate is fixed, and the vacuum increases linearly through the entire range of the foot pedal. As there is no machine-controlled irrigation, a separate irrigation line with desired flow is necessary to maintain anterior chamber stability.

10.4   POSTERIORLY DISLOCATED [DROPPED] CRYSTALLINE LENS

The crystalline lens is an important optical element of the eye as it molds itself, under the influence of accommodation, to enable focused rays of light to fall on the neurosensory retina when viewing objects, both far and near. Although avascular and seemingly metabolically inert, it undergoes constant structural changes throughout life. Structural changes include changes in lens dimensions during early childhood, changes in capsular 'elasticity' during the mid-years of life, and changes in lens transparency (sclerosis) during later life. In situ, the crystalline lens resides within the patellar fossa, suspended by three sets of zonular fibres. Dislocation of the lens could also occur into the anterior chamber. However, it is relatively less complicated to manage and can usually be removed by visco-expression and, if warranted, limited anterior vitrectomy.

Crystalline lens may drop into the vitreous cavity owing to small dimensions of lens (microspherophakia), large dimensions of the eyeball (e.g., in buphthalmos), or from weak or broken zonules (e.g., Marfan's syndrome, Ehlers-Danlos syndrome, pseudo-exfoliation, syphilis, trauma). In these situations, it is usually the entire lens that is dislocated. Sometimes, however, part of the crystalline lens—nucleus, epinucleus, or both—without the lens capsule, drops into the vitreous cavity. This situation is usually secondary to complicated cataract surgery [phacoemulsification, small-incision manual surgery, extracapsular cataract surgery] but may also result from trauma to the lens capsule following injury or as a rare adverse event of intraocular injections, implants, or pars plana vitreoretinal surgery. Posterior dislocation of the lens requires more complex management approaches.

Several factors need to be considered to decide if surgery is indeed necessary, including the method of surgical removal and the plan for optical rehabilitation. These factors include visual potential, age of the patient, etiology of the dislocation, duration of dislocation, intactness or otherwise of the dislocated lens, mobility and size of the dislocated lens, presence of concurrent sequelae like cystoid macular edema [CME], elevated IOP, or endophthalmitis, status of the corneal endothelium, and presence of other concurrent pathology like retinal detachment. Rare situations include subretinal location of the crystalline lens and presence of a dropped intraocular lens (IOL) in addition to the crystalline lens.

Preoperative evaluation must also pay attention to the status of the corneal endothelium [endothelial cell count and other indices by specular microscopy]; depth of the anterior chamber; presence of vitreous in the anterior chamber and pupillary margin; extent of pupillary dilatation; damage to the iris, ciliary body, or trabecular meshwork; and presence of retinal tears. Taking note of the amount of capsular remnant, available, if any, would aid in planning the type of IOL that could be implanted. In addition, in case of dislocation following open globe trauma or cataract surgery, integrity of the open wound must be doubly confirmed. Any form of pressure on the globe must be avoided during local anaesthesia to prevent sudden wound dehiscence, vitreous loss, or even expulsive haemorrhage.

The only indication when one would avoid any form of surgical intervention is in the presence of a dislocated lens that is fixed [indicative of its long-standing nature]. Watchful observation and deferral of surgery could be considered when the amount of lens matter is less than 25% and there is no intraocular inflammation or elevated IOP. However, it may be difficult to determine exact dimensions of the dislocated lens fragments owing to their hydration.

The age of the patient has a significant bearing on the surgical approach. Dislocated lens in the younger age [younger than 30 years] can usually be removed by lensectomy and lens aspiration of the whole dislocated lens or its fragments using a vitrectomy cutter within the posterior chamber. The smaller the gauge of the vitreous cutter, the greater the time taken for removal; 23G may be preferable to 25G/27G. In the presence of an intact capsule, it would be first necessary to remove the capsule in the cutting mode. Once the capsule is removed, the reminder of the lens can be removed in the aspiration mode using moderate vacuum of about 400 mmHg. Dislocation at a young age when this approach can fail include those in patients with coloboma [nuclear sclerosis can be significant even at this age]. In patients older than age 40 years, there is invariably some degree of nuclear sclerosis, so phacofragmentation using an ultrasonic fragmentor [23G] should be the preferred choice. The fragmentor could be introduced into the vitreous cavity through a separate scleral port [preferable] or by enlarging the active port. When the entire crystalline lens has dislocated into the vitreous cavity, it is again important to realize that the fragmentor should be used only after removing the lens capsule [with the vitreous cutter]. The author's preferred mode for removing dropped lens nucleus and fragments in the momentary mode [Figure 10.8a-b].

In earlier times when access to phacofragmentation was not available, several other approaches were attempted during surgery for dislocated lens. These methods included impalement, aspiration or cutting with the vitreous cutter and simultaneous crushing with the light pipe (endoilluminator), levitation using PFCL followed by delivery through the limbus, and rarely, posterior segment phacoemulsification [after removal of the irrigation sleeve]. Of these, levitation using PFCL and delivery through a limbal incision could be preferred over phacofragmentation in the presence of a grade 4

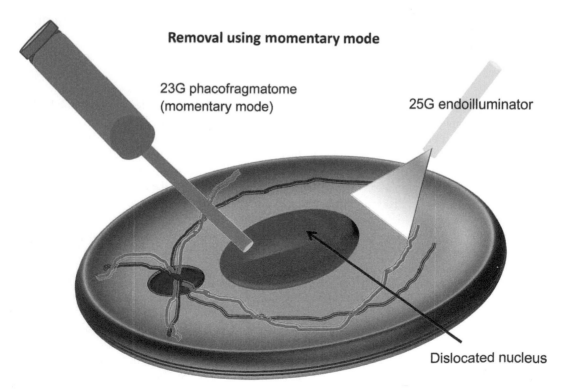

Removal using momentary mode

23G phacofragmatome
(momentary mode)

25G endoilluminator

Dislocated nucleus

FIGURE 10.8A   Removal of dislocated crystalline lens using fragmatome in momentary mode allows better precision and control than linear mode.

Final removal of lens fragments

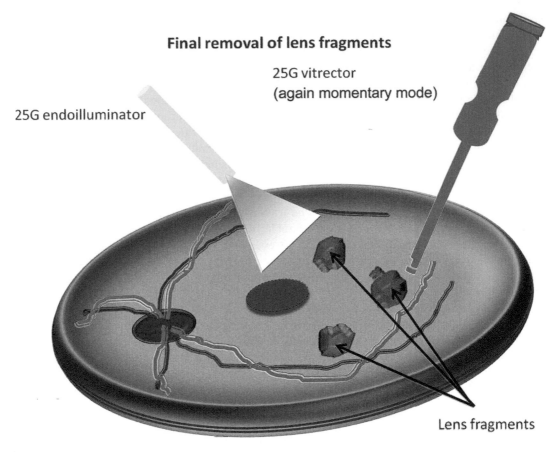

25G vitrector
(again momentary mode)

25G endoilluminator

Lens fragments

FIGURE 10.8B   Removal of dislocated crystalline lens using fragmatome in momentary mode allows better precision and control than linear mode.

dislocated nucleus or lens. If PFCL levitation and removal of the dislocated lens through the limbus is chosen, it is important to protect the corneal endothelium using adequate layering of viscoelastics.

Routine use of PFCL is not necessary during the removal of dislocated crystalline lens but is mandatory if there is concurrent retinal detachment. If there is a large tear, PFCL injection in the routine manner may inadvertently push the levitating nucleus or lens into the subretinal space. So, caution and constant manipulation of the lens away from the tear [using the light pipe] could become necessary. Sometimes the dislocated nucleus is already in the subretinal space at presentation, and this is quite challenging to overcome. In this situation, blind injection of PFCL into the vitreous cavity may further trap the lens within the subretinal space. A bimanual four-port approach [using two aspiration tips] may be useful to first move the lens out of the subretinal space and into the vitreous cavity. In this approach, one aspiration tip is used to move the retina away from the lens lying within the subretinal space, while the other is used to simultaneously move the lens into the vitreous cavity. The former can be achieved using passive aspiration while the latter would need high vacuum delivered from the vitreous machine.

Irrespective of the approach used, it is important to remove as much of the vitreous as is safely possible [which is facilitated by PVD induction]; ensure that there is no vitreous remnant along the pupillary surface, anterior chamber, and cataract wound; retain as much of the peripheral capsular rim [to facilitate secondary sulcus implantation of IOL]; meticulously examine the retinal periphery for breaks [port site, equator, vitreous base] and manage these using endolaser and cryopexy; and finally ensure proper wound closure [at the limbus or scleral ports].

10.5   POSTERIORLY DISLOCATED [DROPPED] INTRAOCULAR IMPLANT

Up until the late 1980s, there continued to be raging debates on the safety of implanting IOLs after cataract surgery. Currently, cataract surgery occupies the very pinnacle of all surgeries in its ability to improve the quality of vision and quality of life. Hence, an eye without an intraocular implant after a planned cataract surgery is considered abnormal. To avoid this situation, all cataract surgeons endeavor to somehow implant an IOL into the eye. In more than 99% of the surgeries, IOL implantation is carried off successfully, either into the capsular bag or within the ciliary sulcus. In fewer than 1% of cases, however, an implanted IOL gets dislocated posteriorly, into the vitreous cavity. Surgical intervention is imperative in such situations because no visual rehabilitation would be possible otherwise.

Risk factors for intraoperative and early postoperative dropped IOL include failure to recognize a posterior capsule [PC] rent [during the early learning curve], recognizing but underestimating the size of the rent and hence opting for 'in-the-bag' implantation, overestimating the available capsular support at the ciliary sulcus, or choosing the wrong IOL [size and type] in the presence of a posterior capsular rent and traumatic IOL insertion [faulty instrument or technique]. Late postoperative dislocations are generally secondary to ocular trauma but may be rarely seen in eyes with pseudoexfoliation or following vitreoretinal surgery with extensive dissection of tissues in the vitreous base region.

The timing of surgery and the surgical plan would depend on several variables. These include the time of detection of IOL dislocation, which can be immediate [intraoperative] or during the early postoperative period or late postoperative period, presence of collateral tissue damage [e.g., corneal edema, vitreous haemorrhage, retinal detachment], location of the IOL [retrocapsular, anterior vitreous, mid-vitreous, posterior vitreous or on the retinal surface], type of IOL [plate haptic, loop haptic, hydrophilic or hydrophobic], amount of capsular remnant available, corneal endothelial count, integrity of the anterior chamber angle, presence of double [rarely, even triple] IOL syndrome, status of zonules or presence of diseases associated with zonular weakness [e.g., pseudoexfoliation, Marfan's disease, homocystinuria], presence of predisposing lesions in the retinal periphery or retinal tears. Rare surprises include the concurrent presence of dislocated capsular tension ring [Figure 10.9], more than one dislocated IOL, or subretinal location of the dropped IOL. The extent and severity of dislocation indicate the causative factor behind the dislocation: if only the IOL is dislocated, it is usually secondary to loss of the capsular support, but if the entire capsular bag is located, then it indicates loss of zonular support.

The primary objective of surgery is to restore visual recovery in such a manner that it resembles an uneventful cataract surgery. While this can be achieved in a majority of patients, a significant number would have suboptimal recovery owing to a higher risk of cystoid macular edema, secondary glaucoma, corneal decompensation, and retinal detachment. Optical rehabilitation could be achieved by IOL repositioning, primary IOL exchange, or secondary IOL implantation. Prerequisites for being able to reposition a dropped IOL include the extent and nature of capsular support that is still available and the type and dimensions of the dislocated IOL.

Preoperative evaluation must pay attention to best corrected visual acuity, presence of relative afferent pupillary defect [RAPD], integrity of the corneal wound, corneal clarity and endothelial count, depth of anterior chamber and angle, vitreous herniation into the anterior chamber, pupil shape and ability to dilate [indirect evidence of vitreous adherent to the pupil or iris trauma], location of IOL [partial visibility in the capsular area/ retrolental space or complete aphakia], media clarity [USG may be necessary in the presence of vitreous haemorrhage to confirm the dislocated IOL and to rule out retinal or choroidal detachment], retinal periphery, and retinal detachment.

In early postsurgery IOL dislocation, it is highly probable for the cataract wound to have been left sutureless or with a solitary suture. When this is encountered, it is safe to first secure the wound by passing additional sutures under topical anaesthesia and only then administer peribulbar or retrobulbar block. Application of super-pinkie or digital massage is absolutely contraindicated.

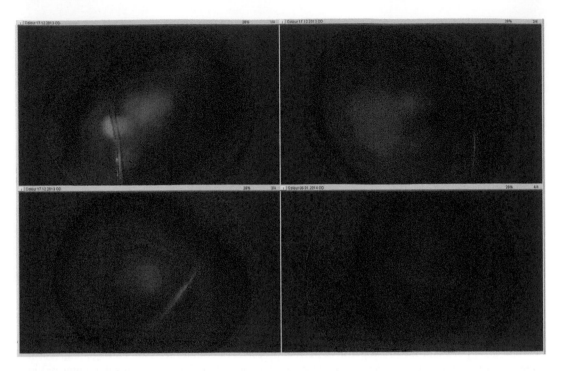

FIGURE 10.9 Preoperative and postoperative images following surgery for removal of dropped capsular tension ring and intraocular implant.

In patients in whom no corneal wound is visible, one must look for the presence of a scleral wound under the conjunctiva. This is a likelihood when the demographics and circumstances indicate the possible surgery as being manual small incision cataract surgery rather than phacoemulsification.

Standard precautions recommended for port construction and initial steps of pars plana vitreous surgery must be adhered to. Scleral ports are to be made with a trocar and cannula from a freshly opened pack so as to keep the force of scleral entry to a minimum, reducing the IOP elevation and/ or distortion of the cataract wound, and hence averting the risk of iris prolapse. If the IOL is still situated in the patellar fossa, a minimally invasive approach can be attempted. In this approach, the IOL should be held at the optic–haptic junction and stabilized using an intravitreal forceps, either through a small-gauge limbal incision or through the pars plana. No pull–push forces must be transmitted to the IOL before stabilizing it with a forceps and removing vitreous all around. With the infusion in low flow, vitreous all around the IOL and pupillary margin is removed using a high-speed cutter. Once the IOL is free of vitreous, it should be carefully manipulated into the anterior chamber under a cushion of viscoelastic. After the IOL has been retrieved into the anterior chamber, further decisions on IOL replacement or removal or exchange may be implemented. Despite minimal vitrectomy, retinal periphery still needs to be meticulously examined using wide-angle lenses and endoillumination. Scleral indentation to view the retinal periphery and ora must be gentle.

When the IOL is dislocated and lying on the retinal surface, complete pars plana vitrectomy is mandatory and the sequence of 4Ps—port site, posterior, PVD induction, and peripheral vitreous removal—must be followed. Then two methods have been described to lift up [levitate] and bring it into the anterior chamber. The first approach, to directly hold the IOL at the optic–haptic junction and manipulate it into the anterior chamber, is one single step. Although not mandatory, it would be prudent to layer the macula with a bubble of PFCL while using this approach. In the second approach, the IOL is first lifted away from the retinal surface into the vitreous cavity using high, active, steady suction with the extrusion cannula. The IOL is then gripped in this safe zone at the optic–haptic junction using an intravitreal forceps and then manipulated into the anterior chamber. In both approaches, the intravitreal forceps could be introduced either through the limbus [combined approach] or through the pars plana scleral port. The author's experience suggests that it is easier to manipulate the dropped IOL into the anterior chamber using the combined limbal–pars plana approach. The combined approach allows placement of the chandelier illumination through the non-dominant scleral port [i.e., no fourth scleral port is necessary]. While using the pars plana approach, it is often necessary to use the endoilluminator to support and then gently move the IOL from the pupillary plane into the anterior chamber. Use of serrated 23G forceps rather than 25G forceps is preferred because of its sturdiness, firmness, and fixity of hold over the IOL. Having an extra forceps of the same kind is helpful. In a new approach being evaluated by the author, the retractable finesse loop is used to grasp the haptic of the IOL. This approach reduces the risk of injury to the retina that may rarely occur while grasping the IOL lying on the retina, using an intravitreal forceps. Moreover, the finesse loop allows a firm grasp and prevents slippage of the IOL.

Having the cataract tray alongside the vitreoretinal tray allows quick access to instruments such as a 3.2 blade, Sinskey hook, and MacPherson's forceps that would allow a seamless completion of the procedure. If IOL removal has been planned, it is important to complete the process by rotating the IOL out of the wound, along the curvature of the haptic, and not directly pull out the lens. This allows atraumatic delivery of the IOL, prevents breakage of the haptic, and minimizes the risk of wound distortion and iris prolapse. During manipulation of the IOL into and out of the anterior chamber, it is crucial to maintain the anterior chamber using protective viscoelastic. Failure to do so would increase endothelial cell loss and risk evolution of corneal decompensation. Plate haptics are usually more difficult to grip than loop haptics, and one may have to choose an intravitreal end grasping forceps accordingly. In some situations, as the jaws of the forceps may have to be slightly widened mechanically to enable purchase on a plate haptic, it would be useful to undertake this step using a resterilized forceps and avoid the use of a fresh forceps for IOL removal.

10.6   MYOPIC SCHISIS AND TRACTION MACULOPATHY

Unique and characteristic changes on ophthalmoscopic evaluation within the macula of patients with high myopia have included macular edema, choroidal neovascular membranes, Foster-Fuch's spot, lacquer cracks, posterior staphyloma, macular hole, and posterior pole detachment [Figure 10.10]. Now, with the availability of OCT, it has become evident that many of these pathologies may be related to hyaloidal traction on the macula and may be a continuum. Myopic traction maculopathy [MTM] is an umbrella term encompassing all macular lesions secondary to evident macular traction in patients with moderate to high myopia. Its most identifying features [on OCT] include vitreomacular traction [VMT], multi-layer schisis, macular hole, and posterior pole detachment. The earliest feature, sometimes even in the absence of prominent VMT, is separation of the internal limiting membrane (ILM) from the nerve fibre layer and splitting of inner layers of the neurosensory retina. With time, these changes progress to involve a wider area as well as deeper layers of the retina. Subsequently there is subfoveal detachment, and in the final stages, there are macular hole formation and detachment of the posterior pole. Macular hole may initially be lamellar. Staphyloma may or may not be in evidence. While progression is the rule, the rate of progression is quite varied. The disease is reported to occur in 10% to 30% of patients with high myopia, tends to have a female predilection, and usually presents between the fourth and seventh decades of life. Some factors that could be responsible for the evolution of MTM include early vitreous liquefaction, reduced vitreous mass, slow progression of vitreoretinal separation [PVD in slow motion], anomalous posterior vitreous detachment, persistent hyaloidal traction on the macula, dehiscence of the internal limiting membrane, metaplasia of glial elements, weakening of intercellular attachments and then obvious separation, and splitting of cellular layers. Rare reports of spontaneous resolution do exist, however. The presence of concurrent staphyloma may augment the tractional force vectors and result in more severe and more rapid evolution of the pathological

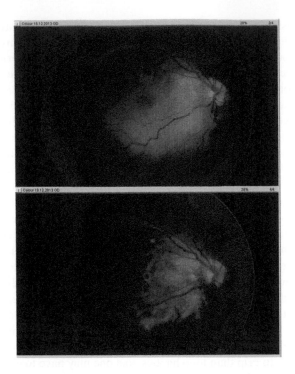

FIGURE 10.10   Preoperative and postoperative fundus images of a patient with high myopia after vitreoretinal surgery for macular hole and retinal detachment.

changes. Contrarily, dome-shaped macula is said to retard the progression of MTM by its natural 'buckling' effect. VMT in emmetropic eyes is a comparable entity, but herein the traction tends to be relatively stable and slowly progressive.

MTM has only recently become well characterized, so authors have used their own means of classifying the condition. As there is yet no consensus classification, study design, management approaches, and outcome measures would be variable. Classifications are evidently dependent on OCT characteristics and have three essential components: changes on the surface of the retina [vitreomacular attachment, VMT, epimacular membrane (EMM)], intraretinal changes [inner retinal layers, outer retinal layers, involving all layers], and status of the foveal contour [unchanged, lamellar hole, full thickness hole and macular detachment]. Other associated findings include those of dome-shaped macula, posterior staphyloma, and macular atrophy or scar [secondary to neovascular membrane]. The area of schisis too could be focal [involving fovea, perifovea, or peripapillary region] or diffuse [involving a larger area of the macula]. These possibly represent stages in the evolution of MTM. While the detection of MTM is straightforward, the treatment is very challenging as there are no international guidelines on how frequently these patients must be followed, at what visual acuity or symptoms surgical intervention must be considered, what the most appropriate intervention is, and how long could observation be considered without jeopardizing final outcome. In addition, information on the risk-to-benefit ratio of early versus delayed intervention, based on multicentric trials, is lacking. Options available for managing patients with MTM include observation, small-gauge vitreoretinal surgery, and macular buckle. Patients with MTM detected incidentally and with good visual acuity could be observed closely in the initial period, and then the follow-up interval could be gradually increased. Patients should also be encouraged to check the gross visual acuity [near and distance with spectacles] in each eye at 4-week intervals and to report immediately on noting an appreciable difference. The role of monitoring with an Amsler grid is not known. Risk factors for early progression include higher axial length, presence of posterior staphyloma, status of fellow eye, female gender, and persisting papillovitreal traction. The effect of cataract surgery on MTM remains unexplored.

Challenges during vitreoretinal surgery are similar to those encountered during surgery for retinal detachment in patients with high myopia: poor contrast owing to thinned retina and atrophic choriocapillaris, vitreoschisis, difficult access owing to increased axial length, and risk of suboptimal retinopexy. Careful study of preoperative OCT may help in planning and implementing surgical dissection meticulously. Taking appropriate measures to improve visualization of the vitreous (triamcinolone suspension) and membranous structures such as EMM and ILM (dyes such as indocyanine green or brilliant blue) add to the safety of the surgery. ILM peeling, even in the absence of macular hole, is considered important to the success of surgery. Use of a flat contact lens provides the best resolution, so one must resist dissection of membranes at the macula using a wide-field lens. Instruments (forceps and cannula) with longer shafts, when available, must be requisitioned from the inventory or surgical store prior to surgery. Surgery assisted by intraoperative OCT, 3D viewing, and digital filters may be helpful. Long-term tamponade is probably not indicated if there was no pre-existing macular hole and if the surgery was uneventful. Controversy on choice of tamponade and duration of prone positioning persists owing to conflicting reports on the rapidity of MTM resolution, incidence of post-surgery macular hole, and final visual recovery. Fovea-sparing ILM peeling is considered to be a safer approach in these patients owing to the high risk of deroofing a thinned-out, central foveal schitic cavity. Despite ILM peeling, tractional forces on the fovea may not be completely eliminated in patients with macular hole and posterior pole detachment. This has been linked to straightened and stretched retinal vessels running from the optic disc to the temporal retina and to scleral vector forces from the posterior staphyloma. Non-compliant Bruch's membrane could also be a contributive factor.

Macular buckling, first described by Schepens, is now being resurrected as an effective procedure to treat patients with complications of MTM. Silicone is the dominant material used, and several shapes have been marketed [L, T, quadrangular, circular]. Some of these have wires to allow the buckles to be molded into a desirable curvature [Ando-stainless steel], while others have optical fibres to facilitate visualization of buckle location [AJL Ophthalmic, Spain]. Surgical steps are identical to that during scleral buckling surgery using a segmental buckle [with limited peritomy]. The most important steps during surgery include safe passage of posterior scleral suture and precise localization. The latter is commonly detected using an indirect ophthalmoscope; however, internal illumination using a chandelier light [similar to EASB] and wide-angle viewing may be more effective. Macular buckles with inbuilt illuminated optical fibre also improve the outcome of surgery by allowing precise localization. In addition to complications similar to those that could occur during scleral buckle surgery [particularly with drainage], macular buckle surgery has added risks like compression of the optic nerve and damage to vortex veins. A third approach claimed in some small case series has having higher success is pars plana surgery combined with macular buckling. Owing to lack of appropriate guidelines, the surgeon must individualize each case and discuss the objectives, anticipated intraoperative challenges, risks, and unpredictable and delayed positive impact on visual recovery and stability.

10.7 GIANT RETINAL TEAR

When the circumferential extent of a retinal tear extends beyond 3 clock hours [90 degrees], it is designated as GRT. These tears are unique in multiple ways, including their etiopathogenesis, systemic associations, clinical features, natural history, surgical approach, and outcomes, so they need consideration as a separate entity from all other forms of rhegmatogenous retinal detachment. GRT tends to occur at an earlier age; has an increased risk of retinal detachment developing in the fellow eye; and is likely to be associated with systemic conditions like Marfan's syndrome, Ehlers-Danlos syndrome, Stickler's syndrome, or ocular conditions like pathological myopia or Wagner's syndrome. Like other retinal detachments, trauma and intraocular surgery are also risk factors for GRT formation. In predisposed eyes, it could result from minor trauma. GRT-associated retinal detachment tends to progress rapidly into more severe and complex forms and must hence be considered as an emergency. Precursor clinical features are said to include white with pressure and white without pressure, both probably indicative of abnormal vitreous collagen and vitreoretinal relation. In the normal course, senile PVD takes 6 or more weeks for completion. In patients who develop GRT, it is possible that PVD evolves in a hyperdynamic manner [hyperdynamic PVD]. Hyperdynamic PVD in the presence of abnormal, strong vitreoretinal attachment due to some peripheral pathology or early-onset hyperdynamic PVD in the presence of normal vitreoretinal attachment for that age is a possible pathomechanism. The circumferential extent of the tear may range from 90 to 360 degrees, and as a rule, the larger the tear, the more rapid the evolution. Classic GRT has radial extensions at its terminating ends. The more posterior the radial ends extend, the more severe is the rolling in [in-folding] of the detached neurosensory retina towards the centre of the vitreous cavity [due to the inherent mass of the detached retina and gravitational effect]. At the same time, the anterior 'flap' of the torn retina rolls out towards the ora serrata and ciliary body, owing to pull from the vitreous base [resulting ultimately in anterior loop traction, severe anterior PVR, ciliary body dysfunction, and hypotony]. In addition, PVR evolves rapidly in these eyes due to abundant release of RPE cells into the vitreous cavity at the time of tear formation and the continued presence of a large area of bare RPE. It is important to remember that patients may also harbour other tears and predisposing lesions in parts of the retina not involved by the GRT. For management purposes, GRT could be classified into three grades of severity: in-rolling of the posterior retina is absent; in-rolling of the posterior retina is present, but the flap is free; and in-rolling of the posterior retina with fixed flap. PVR in GRT may involve only the posterior retina, only the anterior retina, or both the anterior and posterior retina. Retinal slippage is an intraoperative complication unique to GRT surgery. Postoperative peculiarities include risk of inadvertent retinal rotation and foveal displacement, high risk of PVR [and hence the need for additional surgeries], and high risk of hypotony [from anterior PVR and ciliary body traction].

It can thus be seen that management of GRT entails addressing multiple components of the complex pathology. These components include detached posterior vitreous, posterior in-rolled flap of retina, anterior vitreous, anterior flap, PVR involving other parts of the retina, vitreous base in parts of attached retina, and other concurrent lesions [independent breaks and predisposing lesions]. What makes GRT surgery different from surgery for other forms retinal detachment is management of the in-rolled flap, anterior vitreous, and anterior flap. In addition, there is also a need to aggressively suppress the high risk of postoperative PVR, but no successful strategies for this have been developed so far.

The problem of stabilization of the rolled-in posterior flap has been solved with the introduction and widespread use of PFCL. However, use of PFCL could itself lead to some intraoperative and postoperative situations. These include incomplete removal of the posterior hyaloid [from premature injection of PFCL], failure to achieve a single PFCL bubble [and risk of migration into the subretinal space] and obscuration of the surgical field, precipitous raise of IOP [due to lack simultaneous egress of fluid from the vitreous cavity], anterior ballooning of the detached retina [more likely when GRT is limited; occurs due to displacement of subretinal fluid anteriorly], and rarely incarceration of the unfolding flap into the scleral ports. Unless the GRT has folded in completely over the optic nerve head, a small amount of triamcinolone should be injected cautiously over the region of the optic disc and efforts made to identify an attached posterior hyaloid [while moving and supporting the inverted flap away using the endoilluminator]. This step must be undertaken before PFCL injection. Failure to do so could result in the residual posterior hyaloid going undetected under the weight of the PFCL and worsening the chances of early redetachment. Some of the other situations related to PFCL injection can be reduced by lowering the infusion pressure before the start of injection and by taking measures to allow fluid to egress while PFCL is being injected. Various methods used to allow egress of fluid within the vitreous cavity include the use of a double-bore cannula for PFCL injection, use of non-valved cannulas at the active port and injecting with a soft tip of a smaller gauge [e.g., 25–23G mismatch], and intermittently exiting the instrument from one of the ports and letting some fluid egress or using chandelier assisted illumination to undertake simultaneous passive extrusion of [with flute needle] fluid or actively using the bimanual mode. In the absence of a double-bored cannula, the last approach is likely to maintain the most optimal stability. Although rare, anterior ballooning of the detached retina is a possibility in eyes with limited GRT and can be avoided by intermittently aspirating the subretinal fluid through the GRT. Completion of peripheral vitrectomy, debulking of the vitreous base, and excision of the anterior flap are carried out after stabilization of the posterior retina with PFCL. Margins of the GRT [anterior and posterior] will have abruptly terminating small and large blood vessels, and these could bleed while the margin [if it remains curled up] of the posterior flap is being trimmed or anterior flap is being excised. So, it is helpful to diathermy the larger vessels beforehand. Bleeding is venous or arterial, from the anterior flap and posterior flap, respectively. If severe, this can quickly flow into the subretinal space and so must be avoided. Once the retina is attached, four or five rows of laser photocoagulation are placed along the posterior margin and as far into the periphery as possible. In phakic patients, the anterior extent of the tear may have to be treated with cryopexy. Retinal slippage and formation of a fold [Figure 10.11] is a potential risk when PFCL is being replaced with long-term tamponade. The risk can be minimized by undertaking direct PFCL–silicone oil exchange in comparison with PFCL–air exchange followed by silicone oil injection [see section on surgical approaches and steps]. Additional aspects that need to be discussed and considered during preoperative planning and during surgery include the ideal site for placement of the infusion line, need for scleral buckle or encircling band, cautious injection of just adequate amount of triamcinolone or dye [to avoid subretinal injection or/ migration of triamcinolone or vital dye], only laser or combined with cryo of the peripheral ends of the tear, and the type of tamponade. It is likely that prophylactic placement of dexamethasone implant at the end of surgery may help to reduce the risk of postoperative PVR, but

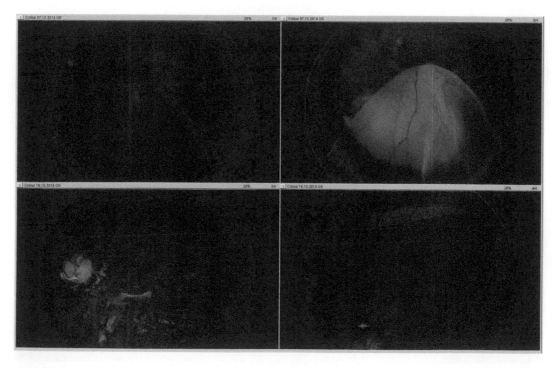

FIGURE 10.11   Preoperative and postoperative fundus photographs of a patient following surgery for retinal detachment secondary to a large giant retinal tear and retinal inversion [note the fold in the superior retina secondary to slippage].

studies addressing this are yet to come by. Postoperative positioning would be more critical in these patients and must be discussed during preoperative counselling. In addition, one must not neglect to follow recommended guidelines for screening and follow-up of patients with diseases like Marfan's syndrome.

10.8   IDIOPATHIC EPIMACULAR MEMBRANE

Epiretinal membrane is a contractile membrane on the surface of the retina that results from proliferation of either glial elements or metaplastic retinal pigment epithelial cells. When the membrane is located in the macular region it is termed EMM. EMM that develops without any evident predisposing condition is termed idiopathic, while those that develop as a response to retinal detachment (proliferative vitreoretinopathy) and other conditions such as retinal vascular occlusions, diabetes mellitus, or intraocular inflammation are termed secondary EMM. Unlike secondary membranes, it is unusual for idiopathic membranes to be vascularized. Idiopathic EMM may be a reactive tissue response to micro-dehiscence of the ILM as a result of ageing or hyaloidal traction or separation during the evolution of PVD. These membranes are most commonly seen in older adults, but they may also occur in the young and rarely as a congenital abnormality [must be distinguished from combined hamartoma of the retina and retinal pigment epithelium]. Depending on the severity of contraction, idiopathic EMMs have been graded into cellophane maculopathy (grade 0), membrane distorting partial thickness of the retina (grade 1), and membrane distorting full thickness of the retina (grade 2, also called macular pucker) [Figure 10.12]. Examination with red-free light may be useful in very early cases. Microaneurysms, axoplasmic stasis (and appearance of cotton-wool spots), and punctate retinal haemorrhages are infrequent associated findings. Sometimes, dehiscence of the epiretinal membrane may give an appearance of a macular hole (pseudohole). Most patients with primary or idiopathic EMM have good vision [the only symptom may be metamorphopsia or

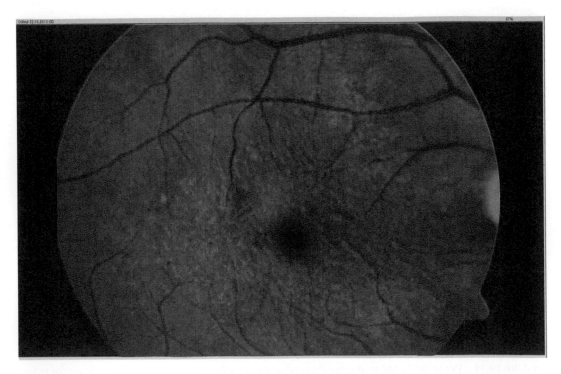

FIGURE 10.12   Fundus image of a patient with epimacular membrane. Note the crinkling of the retinal surface.

macropsia], and the membrane itself remains stationary over many years or may evolve very slowly. Hence, the decision to remove the membrane by surgery must be taken only after detailed discussion [and consent] with the patient about her or his symptoms, expectations from the surgery, and understanding of the risks. It may be safer to avoid surgery in a patient with 6/9 vision and insignificant metamorphopsia.

Distinguishing EMM from VMT is very important because they have different clinical courses, management strategies, and prognoses. Unlike EMM, VMT may not always be evident on clinical examination but gets detected on OCT. This is because VMT causes absent to minimal distortion of the retinal surface and vasculature, and the hyaloid is relatively translucent. Unlike this, EMM is generally thicker and more opaque and invariably causes retinal distortion, varying from subtle wrinkling of the ILM to obvious distortion of the retinal surface and foveal blood vessels. On following the membrane outwards, the edge of an EMM can be identified but not so in cases of VMT [Figure 10.13]. PVD is almost always absent in VMT, and contrarily, is often seen in patients with EMM. On OCT, EMM has variable thickness and may reveal focal attachment pegs and crowding with distortion of inner retinal layers [rarely all layers] and absence of inner retinal cystoid spaces and neurosensory detachment. In VMT, the membrane or hyaloid has a relatively uniform thickness, no focal pegs are seen, and inner retinal layer cystoid spaces and neurosensory detachment are common rather than distortion or thickening of the retinal layers. While most patients with EMM have stable vision over many years without intervention, those with VMT invariably deteriorate. As a result, patients with EMM with good visual acuity may be observed periodically until progressive decline in vision is documented, while early surgical intervention should be considered in patients with VMT. Following surgery, visual recovery and outcomes are more satisfactory in patients with EMM than with VMT.

In the preoperative period, it is important to screen these patients for potential predisposing lesions like PVD-induced tear and lattice degeneration. When present, these should be treated

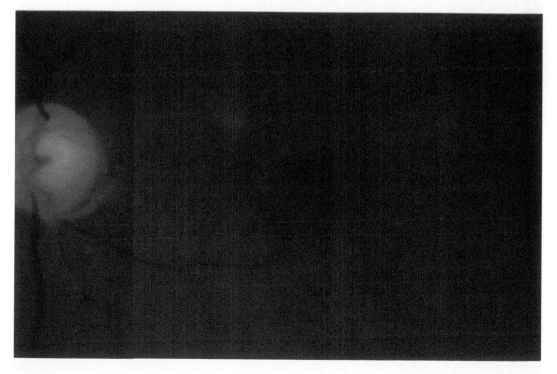

FIGURE 10.13 Fundus image of a patient with vitreomacular traction syndrome [VMT and epimacular membrane].

using prophylactic laser or cryopexy and surgery scheduled about 4 weeks later. Surgery for EMM involves standard three-port pars plana vitrectomy with removal of vitreous from the port, posteriorly and periphery. Triamcinolone-assisted surgery improves visualization of the vitreous body and hyaloid and hence makes the surgery safer. If absent, PVD induction must be undertaken [see section on induction of PVD; infrequently, EMM may also separate during PVD induction] and carefully extended to the equator. Forceful extension of PVD to the vitreous base and aggressive debulking of the vitreous base may increase the risk of traction-induced iatrogenic retinal tears, so caution is advised. Following PVD induction, EMM removal should be performed using standard plano-concave contact lenses because they provide the best clarity and stereopsis [see section on lenses for visualization]. As most of these membranes are thick and opaque, staining with a dye is not as important. It is better to use an end grasping forceps rather than an ILM forceps for removal of EMM. This is because the latter provides a wider surface area of grasp and hence reduces the likelihood of membrane fragmentation. With the advent of small-gauge surgery, only rarely is there a need for bent MVR or special picks to initiate the peel. As a general rule, it is useful to avoid initiation of the peel in the temporal macula [as retina is thinner], over the foveal centre, near large blood vessels, and where the membrane is very opaque [as underlying anatomy is masked]. Two approaches can be used to peel the membrane, 'pinch and peel' or 'lift and peel'. In the former, the membrane is directly grasped on its surface and carefully elevated, while in the latter, the edge of the membrane is grasped first, carefully elevated and then gradually extended. The applied force initially, in the former, is more anteroposterior, while in the latter, is tangential. The latter approach is a safer approach and is recommended. During the peel, it is important to release and regrasp the membrane [more proximally towards the attached margin] on multiple occasions [Figure 10.14, Video 10.1]. Failure to do so may increase the risk of retinal tear formation adjacent to the EMM

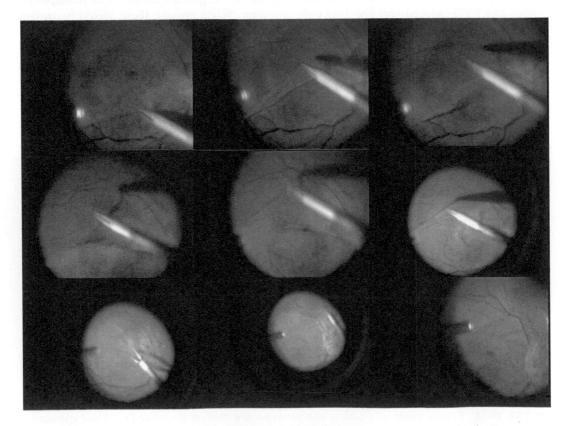

FIGURE 10.14   Snapshot of sequential steps during surgery for removal of epimacular membrane.

attachment or direct trauma to the retina from the tip of the forceps [as it is moved peripherally, the narrow field of view of the contact lens restricts visualization and hence the leading edge of the forceps may strike against the retina if the direction of pull does not follow the curvature of the globe]. Rarely, one may encounter a vascularized membrane or a focal and tight attachment of the EMM to the retina [more likely in secondary membranes]. Diathermy of vascularized membranes before continuation of the peel is necessary to prevent the possibility of an unexpected severe intraocular bleeding [and loss of anatomical details]. Sometimes it is observed that the presumedly tight attachment becomes amenable to peeling on changing the direction of traction applied by the forceps. If this fails, then, it may be prudent to trim the tightly adherent EMM with the vitreous cutter. Unless histopathological or other laboratory studies are being planned, the surgically detached EMM must be removed using the vitreous cutter. Attempts to remove the EMM with a forceps, through small-gauge cannulas, is usually unsuccessful and often leads to entrapment of the membrane in the peripheral vitreous and so must be avoided. Staining with a dye may be considered after this step in order to identify any residual EMM or for ILM peeling. [Although ILM peeling reduces the rate of EMM recurrence, visual acuity outcomes with and without ILM peeling have been found comparable.] As for every vitreous surgery, the peripheral retina must be screened for iatrogenic breaks [with scleral indentation] before fluid-air exchange. Routine 360-degree laser of the retinal periphery may reduce the risk of post-surgery retinal detachment. Long-term tamponade is not necessary, and the surgery can be closed under air tamponade. Prone position for 12–24 hours may suffice [supine position must be avoided to prevent prolonged contact of air or gas with the crystalline lens and to reduce the risk of anterior chamber shallowing].

10.9 VITREOMACULAR TRACTION AND SYNDROME

Posterior vitreous detachment is a natural outcome of the senescent changes occurring with the vitreous humor. It is characterized by a clean, complete, and uncomplicated separation of the posterior hyaloid face of the vitreous from the ILM. Complications at the periphery of the retina such as retinal haemorrhage and retinal tear following complicated PVD are well recognized. These complications result from the strong attachment of the vitreous to the retina at the vitreous base. Posteriorly, the hyaloid is firmly attached to the margins of the optic disc, fovea, and blood vessels. VMT is also a form of complicated PVD in which the posterior hyaloid fails to separate from attachments at the foveal region, causing subtle tractional changes. Unlike EMM, in which retinal distortion results from static forces, VMT causes retinal changes owing to dynamic traction. Hence, the clinical course, characteristics, management approach, outcomes, and prognosis are different [see section on idiopathic EMM]. VMT is usually a diagnosis that is confirmed only after OCT imaging and has been classified as primary [without other pathology] and concurrent [with other pathology like vascular occlusion]. Based on the size of attachment on 2D OCT scan, it is termed focal and diffuse, when less than and greater than 1500 μm, respectively. It is termed vitreomacular traction syndrome [VMTS] when there is also associated ERM. Ultramicroscopic imaging of the vitreomacular cone resected at surgery has revealed the uniform presence of fibrocellular proliferation along the surface of the inner retina and posterior surface of the hyaloid. This proliferation is also thought to contribute to the strong adherence between the fovea and hyaloid in patients with VMT. Tractional CME, tractional DME, and myopic foveoschisis [see section on MTM] are considered as variants of VMT. It is important to note that fluorescein angiographic leakage is absent in tractional CME. Unlike in classic VMT, wherein the area of attachment is broad based, in tractional CME, it is very focal and narrow. Tractional CME has two further subtypes, one with shallow neurosensory separation and one without. Spontaneous separation of vitreomacular adhesion [VMA, or mere attachment of partially separated hyaloid to the fovea without any structural and functional changes in the retina] during follow-up has been observed in about one third of patients and so these patients need only follow-up. On the other hand, spontaneous release of VMT is considered infrequent.

Several interventions have been evaluated in patients with symptomatic VMT; these include intravitreal injection of air, long-acting gas, ocriplasmin [Jetrea; see section on enzymatic vitreolysis], and vitreoretinal surgery. Release of VMT with intravitreal air and gas injection, though simple as a procedure, can lead to macular hole formation in a high number of patients, either immediately after the procedure or as a delayed adverse effect. Hence, it is to be considered only by trained vitreoretinal surgeons after adequate patient counselling. Although ocriplasmin was found to be effective and had received Food and Drug Administration approval for managing patients with VMT, it did not gain widespread acceptance due to the high cost of the injection, poorly understood natural history of VMT, and lack of precise guidelines on when to intervene surgically in these patients. The company stopped production of Jetrea in 2020 as a business decision, and hence it is no longer commercially available. Small-gauge vitrectomy remains the most effective option and can achieve resolution of VMT in all patients. The primary objectives of surgery are relief of symptoms, stabilization of visual acuity, and arrest of the progression to more prognostically poorer conditions [e.g., macular hole formation]. The procedure involves safe removal of vitreous from the port site, core, and periphery using standard three port surgery followed by triamcinolone-assisted cautious separation of the posterior hyaloid. Unlike PVD induction in most other situations, application of very high vacuum must be avoided. It is recommended to inject only a gentle layering of triamcinolone particles on the posterior hyaloid. Injection of concentrated triamcinolone suspension or injection of diluted triamcinolone in large amounts over the posterior pole must be avoided. This is because the particles may get strongly enmeshed into the posterior cortical fibres and seriously impede visualization of the underlying, delicate vitreoretinal anatomy that needs to be released. A combination of forceps peel and sharp dissection may become necessary. In very tightly adherent hyaloid, it may be safer to truncate the cone of vitreous and hyaloid overlying the fovea, with the vitreous cutter. ILM peeling is not recommended as it could increase the risk of deroofing of the foveal cysts and increase the risk of creating a macular hole. If ILM peeling is contemplated, foveal sparing is advisable. Dissection of concurrent EMM also needs more caution. Before air-fluid exchange, the periphery must be evaluated for breaks. Air tamponade is adequate in uncomplicated surgery. Long-term gas tamponade is necessary in the event of complications like macular hole formation or peripheral retinal tear. Strict prone positioning in the postoperative period is not warranted. Postoperative visual recovery is gradual and only modest in most patients. Whether preoperative injection of air or gas, followed a week or two later by vitrectomy, improves the ease and safety of the surgery remains unexplored.

10.10 MACULAR HOLE

Like a retinal hole, a macular hole is also a full-thickness breach in the neurosensory retina albeit located at the foveal centre. However, the term *full-thickness macular dehiscence* may be better suited to describe this condition rather than *macular hole*. The reasons for this are that other than the fact that it is a full-thickness defect in the retina, there are many features dissimilar to a retinal hole. These include the documentation of precursor stages, the ability to close spontaneously, the rarity with which it results in retinal detachment, and the ability to close completely following removal of the hyaloid and ILM. None of these are features of a retinal hole elsewhere in the retina.

The ILM is considered to be the basal lamina of the Mueller cells and measures about 2 μ. It delineates the neurosensory retina from the vitreous cavity, but its exact function remains poorly defined. It is possible that it has a role in modulating ocular growth during development and in the orderly cellular layering of the various layers of the retina within the confines of the retinal pigment epithelium and itself. The ILM probably acts like a tight easy wrap covering the entire inner retinal surface. With age, some degree of micro-dehiscence of the ILM could set in. As this dehiscence progresses, forces are also transmitted to the other retinal layers within the vicinity and finally results in full-thickness separation of the inner retinal layers. These progressive changes may correspond to the recognized clinical stages in the evolution of a macular hole. In some situations, concurrent existence of VMT, EMM, and cystoid changes may be in evidence. Separation of such overlying tissue from the neurosensory retina may result in the formation of a pseudo-operculum.

Based on the etiology, macular holes are broadly categorized as idiopathic or secondary. Idiopathic macular holes are seen in older adults, affect women more often than men, and could develop in the fellow eye in about 10% of patients. Some causes of secondary macular hole include ocular trauma, solar burn, laser induced, and as a sequela to other macular diseases like cystoid macular edema, macular schisis, and parafoveal telangiectasis. Macular hole could also be an adverse event following vitreous surgery for diabetic macular edema, epiretinal membrane, VMT, optic disc maculopathy, myopic foveoschisis, and submacular surgery.

Until the first reports on vitreous surgery for macular hole and the positive outcomes by Kelly and Wendel in 1991, there was no respite for these patients. Steadily however the procedure gained acceptance and is now considered a regular part of vitreous surgery. Nevertheless, several components of the surgical approach and postoperative care continue to be debated, even to this day. Macular hole, along with optic disc pit maculopathy, seems to be the two conditions on which the majority of surgeons seem to be 'experimenting' in order to improve safety, patient comfort, and outcomes. The lack of consensus about the most suitable approach could see young surgeons gaining expertise in one or two standard approaches to macular hole surgery.

About a decade ago, one criterion that was considered an obstacle to satisfactory visual recovery was duration of macular hole beyond 12 months. In most recent times, however, some surgeons advocate repair of all idiopathic macular holes, Irrespective of the duration, size, and status of the fellow eye. Until there are systematic reviews, meta-analyses, quality of life studies, and cost-effective analysis of this approach, it is recommended that macular hole surgery be approached with some rationale and individual patient considerations. In addition to this is the increasing trend of undertaking combined phacoemulsification–macular hole surgery, even when the lens opacity is negligible and minimal. This approach also needs detailed analysis before being accepted universally.

Anatomical closure rates following surgery are reported to be way in excess of 95% in the majority of cases, even in those with prior failed attempts. However, it is the functional outcome that should be taken into consideration before offering surgery. It is important to remember that most macular holes are detected incidentally during routine evaluation, and even after several years, they retain useful vision without any intervention. In addition, these are older adult patients with other comorbidities and social and financial dependency. Also, the risk of having a major complication still remains between 2% to 5%, and it may not be acceptable to accept this risk when dealing with a condition that is relatively stable and whose functional gains are unpredictable and modest and may not be contributing to the patient's quality of life. So, the only macular holes that should be advised surgery are those that are of a short duration (6–12 months) and less than 600 microns at their narrowest region. If there is already complete posterior vitreous detachment in the fellow eye, surgery could even be avoided in incidentally detected [and likely long-standing] macular holes.

The surgical approach to macular hole surgery is a standard three-port pars plana vitrectomy, PVD induction, and ILM peeling. Details on how to proceed with wound (port) construction, induction of posterior vitreous detachment, and removal of ILM are provided in the chapter on surgical steps. To determine the outcome of surgery, innumerable factors have been described in literature. These include minimum linear dimension, hole form factor, macular hole index, and tractional hole index. Although there is some agreement on designating macular hole as being chronic when they have been present for more than 1 year, there is yet no consensus on what constitutes a large macular hole; some define it as anything larger than 400 μ, others as 600 μ, and still others as more than 800 μ. The range 400–800 μ has been termed *intermediate-size macular hole*.

Standard ILM peeling has a high rate of efficacy in patients with hole sizes of about 400 microns. As the hole size increases, standard peeling has a lower chance of anatomical success, and so one could adopt one of a dozen approaches that have now been described, mostly in small case series. These approaches include inverted flap, multilayered flap, autologous serum, transplantation

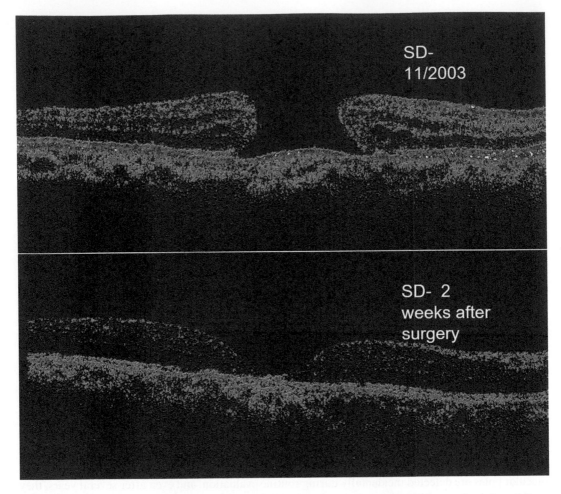

FIGURE 10.15 Preoperative and postoperative optical coherence tomography images of a patient following successful closure of macular hole after surgery. Note the time domain image and loss of the pigment epithelial layer.

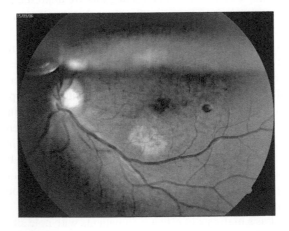

FIGURE 10.16 Postoperative fundus photograph showing development of iatrogenic eccentric macular hole following macular hole surgery.

of autologous ILM, autologous full-thickness retinal tissue, amniotic membrane, and lens capsule. While these approaches may achieve mechanical anatomical closure, claims of significant recovery of visual function and functional integration of the transplant with the recipient's retinal layers defies the long-established observations on the limitations of photoreceptor recovery. Any improvement in visual recovery can only be explained by some narrowing of the visual angle. Contraction of the transplanted tissue [like any scar tissue] could draw in the margins of the large macular hole closer, resulting in narrowing of the visual angle [hill of vision]. Commonly reported complications after macular hole surgery include cataract, raised IOP, peripheral break formation, retinal detachment, RPE alterations [Figure 10.15], endophthalmitis, cystoid macular edema, and late reopening of the macular hole. Rarely, iatrogenic hole could also occur within the area of ILM peeling [Figure 10.16].

10.11 PAEDIATRIC RETINAL DETACHMENT

Rhegmatogenous retinal detachment in infants and children presents different challenges in terms of pathogenesis, diagnosis, and treatment. In the paediatric age group (birth to 18 years of age), rhegmatogenous retinal detachment accounts for 3.2% to 5.6% of all retinal detachments (approximately 0.38–0.69 per 100,000 individuals). Paediatric retinal detachments tend to present late with the macula detached in most of the cases at presentation. As a result, management is relatively more difficult, and the final result in often suboptimal. Children with rhegmatogenous retinal detachment have one or more risk factors such as trauma (open and closed globe), peripheral retinal degenerations (with and without myopia), iridofundal coloboma [see section on rare surgeries], regressed retinopathy of prematurity, aniridia, buphthalmos, persistent foetal vasculature, and past history of surgery for congenital cataract or glaucoma. They are also associated with syndromic conditions like Marfan's syndrome, Stickler's syndrome, Wagner's syndrome, and hereditary vitreoretinopathies like familial exudative vitreoretinopathy. Retinal detachment in childhood may also be associated with systemic disorders such as Patau's syndrome, Norrie's disease, incontentia pigmenti, and Walker-Warburg syndrome. Other challenges include difficulty in evaluating visual acuity and conducting a complete evaluation of the retinal and overall ocular condition, need for general anaesthesia, lack of compliance to postoperative positioning and incompleteness of postoperative evaluation without re-examination under anaesthesia. Since most retinal pathology in this age group is bilateral, one must make a detailed documentation of the fellow eye and promptly treat any predisposing conditions at the first opportunity. Intraoperatively, it is essential that attention be paid to the smaller dimensions of the eyeball and the differing surgical landmarks during the newborn period, infancy, and the toddler years [see section on surgical anatomy].

Proliferative vitreoretinopathy is one of the major causes of failure in retinal detachment surgery and occurs at a rate higher than in adults. The finding of more advanced PVR in children has been generally ascribed to late presentations and greater intraocular cellular activity. The anterior form of PVR has a uniformly worse prognosis than the posterior form, and its treatment requires more complex surgical procedures. Buckling surgeries are preferred to vitreoretinal surgery whenever possible because vitrectomy is more complex and has a greater complication rate. Moreover, the infant cortical vitreous is usually firmly adherent to the retina and difficult to separate from it in a risk-free manner. In very young children, compliance with prone positioning is also difficult to achieve, as indicated earlier. In paediatric patients, as single surgery anatomical success tends to be lower compared with adults, there may be a need for multiple surgeries. Even if vitreoretinal surgery is planned, it is useful to place a band-buckle at the first surgery. This is because vitreous is more adherent, and being phakic, removal of the peripheral vitreous and peripheral membranes would be difficult without risking lens touch. Multiple factors account for poor visual outcome in these patients, including delay in diagnosis, development of severe PVR, difficulty in proper positioning in the postoperative period, difficult visual rehabilitation by contact lenses or glasses, and development of amblyopia. There is a need for continued efforts to improve treatment strategies for children with retinal detachments. Regular screening of the retina during early childhood in high-risk cases may be a useful approach to initiate prophylactic measures and for early detection. Children who have been diagnosed with retinopathy of prematurity, have undergone surgery for congenital cataract or glaucoma, and have a past history of significant ocular trauma should regularly undergo screening of the retinal periphery until adulthood. In addition, legal and social efforts to reduce the availability of toys with a high potential to injure the eye would be a necessary preventive measure. It must also be made mandatory, for children involved in active sports, to wear high-impact-resistant, protective eye wear.

SUGGESTED READING

1. Stewart MW, Browning DJ, Landers MB [2018]. Current management of diabetic tractional retinal detachments. *Indian J Ophthalmol.* 66(12): 1751–1762.
2. Oshima Y, Shima C, Wakabayashi T, Kusaka S, Shiraga F et al [2009]. Microincision vitrectomy surgery and intravitreal bevacizumab as a surgical adjunct to treat diabetic traction retinal detachment. *Ophthalmol.* 116(5): 927–938.
3. Sundar D, Takkar B, Venkatesh P, Chawla R, Temkar S et al. Evaluation of hyaloid-retinal relationship during triamcinolone-assisted vitrectomy for primary rhegmatogenous retinal detachment. *Eur J Ophthalmol.* 28(5): 607–613.
4. Mancino R, Aiello F, Ciuffoletti E, Di Carlo E, Cerulli A, Nucci C [2015]. Inferior retinotomy and silicone oil tamponade for recurrent inferior retinal detachment and grade C PVR in eyes previously treated with pars plana vitrectomy or scleral buckle. *BMC Ophthalmol.* 15: 173.
5. Tabandeh H [2017]. A surgical technique for the management of retinal detachment associated with severe proliferative vitreoretinopathy. *Retina.* 37(7): 1407–1410.
6. Shroff D, Saha I, Bhatia G, Dutta R, Gupta C, Shroff CM [2020]. Tug of war: A bimanual technique for anterior circumferential proliferative vitreoretinopathy in recurrent retinal detachment. *Indian J Ophthalmol.* 68(10): 2155–2158.
7. Vajpayee RB, Sharma N, Dada T, Gupta V, Kumar A, Dada VK [2001]. Management of posterior capsule tears. *Surv Ophthalmol.* 45(6): 473–488.
8. Chakrabarti A, Nazm N [2017]. Posterior capsular rent: Prevention and management. *Indian J Ophthalmol.* 65(12): 1359–1369.
9. Hong AR, Sheybani A, Huang AJ [2015]. Intraoperative management of posterior capsular rupture. *Curr Opin Ophthalmol.* 26(1): 16–21.
10. You TT, Arroyo JG [1999]. Surgical approaches for the removal of posteriorly dislocated crystalline lenses. *Int Ophthalmol Clin.* 39(1): 249–259.
11. Yao K, Shentu X, Jiang J, Du X [2002]. Phacofragmentation without perfluorocarbon liquid for dislocated crystalline lenses or lens fragments after phacoemulsification. *Eur J Ophthalmol.* 12(3): 200–204.
12. Stenkula S, Byhr E, Crafoord S, Carlsson JO, Jemt M et al [1998]. Tackling the "dropped nucleus". *Acta Ophthalmol Scand.* 76(2): 220–223.
13. Sella S, Rubowitz A, Sheen-Ophir S, Ferencz JR, Assia EI, Ton Y [2021]. Pars plana vitrectomy for posteriorly dislocated intraocular lenses: Risk factors and surgical approach. *Int Ophthalmol.* 41(1): 221–229.
14. Chan CK, Agarwal A, Agarwal S, Agarwal A [2001]. Management of dislocated intraocular implants. *Ophthalmol Clin North Am.* 14(4): 681–693.
15. Bajgai P, Tigari B, Singh R [2018]. Outcomes of 23- and 25-gauge transconjunctival sutureless vitrectomies for dislocated intraocular lenses. *Int Ophthalmol.* 38(6): 2295–2301.
16. Parolini B, Palmieri M, Finzi A, Frisina R [2020]. Proposal for the management of myopic traction maculopathy based on the new MTM staging system. *Eur J Ophthalmol.* Dec 20. 1120672120980943.
17. Shiraki N, Wakabayashi T, Ikuno Y, Matsumura N, Sato S et al [2020]. Fovea-sparing versus standard internal limiting membrane peeling for myopic traction maculopathy: A study of 102 consecutive cases. *Ophthalmol Retina.* 4(12): 1170–1180.
18. Gómez-Resa M, Burés-Jelstrup A, Mateo C [2021]. Myopic traction maculopathy. *Dev Ophthalmol.* 54: 204–212.
19. Lee KS, Lee JS, Koh HJ [2020]. Surgical outcomes of myopic traction maculopathy according to the international photographic classification for myopic maculopathy. *Retina.* 40(8): 1492–1499.

20. Berrocal MH, Chenworth ML, Acaba LA [2017]. Management of giant retinal tear detachments. *J Ophthalmic Vis Res.* 12(1): 93–97.
21. Ghosh YK, Banerjee S, Savant V, Kotamarthi V, Benson MT, Schott RAH et al [2004]. Surgical treatment and outcome of patients with giant retinal tears. *Eye.* 18: 996–1000.
22. Ambresin A, Wolfensberger TJ, Bovey EH [2003]. Management of giant retinal tears with vitrectomy, internal tamponade, and peripheral 360 degrees retinal photocoagulation. *Retina.* 23(5): 622–628.
23. Dabour SA [2014]. The outcomes of surgical management for giant retinal tear more than 180. *BMC Ophthalmol.* 27(14): 86.
24. Schechet SA, DeVience E, Thompson JT [2017]. The effect of internal limiting membrane peeling on idiopathic epiretinal membrane surgery, with a review of the literature. *Retina.* 37(5): 873–880.
25. Huang Q, Li J [2021]. With or without internal limiting membrane peeling during idiopathic epiretinal membrane surgery: A meta-analysis. *pLoS One.* 16(1): e0245459.
26. Fang XL, Tong Y, Zhou YL, Zhao PQ, Wang ZY [2017]. Internal limiting membrane peeling or not: A systematic review and meta-analysis of idiopathic macular pucker surgery. *Br J Ophthalmol.* 101(11): 1535–1541.
27. Flaxel CJ, Adelman RA, Bailey ST, Fawzi A, Lim JI et al [2020]. Idiopathic epiretinal membrane and vitreomacular traction preferred practice pattern®. *Ophthalmol.* 127(2): 145–183.
28. Steel DH, Lotery AJ [2013]. Idiopathic vitreomacular traction and macular hole: A comprehensive review of pathophysiology, diagnosis, and treatment. *Eye.* 27(Suppl. 1): S1–S21.
29. Reid GA, McDonagh N, Wright DM, Yek JTO, Essex RW, Lois N [2020]. First failed macular hole surgery or reopening of a previously closed hole: Do we gain by reoperating? -A systematic review and meta-analysis. *Retina.* 40(1):1–15.
30. Viana KÍS, Gordilho CT, Almeida FPP, Esperandio MM, Lucena DR et al [2021]. Combined pars plana vitrectomy (PPV) and phacoemulsification (phaco) versus PPV and deferred phaco for phakic patients with full-thickness macular hole (FTMH) and no significant cataract at baseline: 1-year outcomes of a randomized trial combined PPV/phaco vs PPV/deferred phaco for MH. *Graefes Arch Clin Exp Ophthalmol.* 259(1): 29–36.
31. Parravano M, Giansanti F, Eandi CM, Yap YC, Rizzo S, Virgili G [2015]. Vitrectomy for idiopathic macular hole. *Cochrane Database Syst Rev.* 12(5): CD009080.
32. Read SP, Aziz HA, Kuriyan A, Kothari N, Davis JL et al [2018]. Retinal detachment surgery in a pediatric population: Visual and anatomic outcomes. *Retina.* 38(7): 1393–1402.
33. Scott IU, Flynn HW Jr, Azen SP, Lai MY, Schwartz S, Trese MT [1999]. Silicone oil in the repair of pediatric complex retinal detachments: A prospective, observational, multicenter study. *Ophthalmol.* 106(7): 1399–1407.
34. Raman R, Kalluri Bharat RP, Bhende P, Sharma T [2021]. Managing paediatric giant retinal tears. *Eye.* 35(11): 2913–2914.
35. Rejdak R, Nowakowska D, Wrona K, Maciejewski R, Junemann AG, Nowomiejska K [2017]. Outcomes of vitrectomy in pediatric retinal detachment with proliferative vitreoretinopathy. *J Ophthalmol.* 8109390.
36. Ghoraba HH, Mansour HO, Abdelhafez MA, El Gouhary SM, Zaky AG et al [2020]. Comparison between pars plana vitrectomy with and without encircling band in the treatment of pediatric traumatic rhegmatogenous retinal detachment. *Clin Ophthalmol.* 14: 3271–3277.
37. Kelly NE, Wendel RT [1991 May]. Vitreous surgery for idiopathic macular holes. Results of a pilot study. *Arch Ophthalmol.* 109(5): 654–659.

11 Vitreoretinal Surgery in Rare Conditions

11.1 IRIDOFUNDAL COLOBOMA

Choroidal coloboma is characterized by poor development of chorioretinal structures within a focal area representative of the embryonic fusion line of the developing optic cup. It is of varying extent and severity and is often associated with absence of the iris and ciliary body at the fusion line, along with a corresponding lens notch [Figure 11.1a]. Failure of fusion of the fetal cleft, the reason behind development of iridofundal coloboma, is said to occur from defective evolution of epiblasts, mesoderm, or crystalline lens. Histopathology studies of choroidal coloboma and optical coherence tomography (OCT) reveal poor differentiation of both retinal pigment epithelium (RPE) as well as neurosensory retina. While outer sensory layers cannot be discerned in the region of the coloboma, inner retinal layers are said to continue as a bridging membrane across the margins of the coloboma [intercalary membrane]. Fundus coloboma is sometimes associated with other anomalies of the eyeball such as microphthalmos and microcornea. It could also be associated with a myriad of systemic conditions such as coloboma, heart defects, choanal atresia, growth retardation, genital defects, and ear abormalities [CHARGE] syndrome. Colobomas have been classified into various clinical types based on the superior extent of the defect in relation to the optic nerve head [Ida Mann classification]. These types are coloboma extending beyond the anatomic disk [type 1], abutting the superior margin of the disc [type 2], reaching just below the inferior disc margin [type 3], significantly away from the optic disc but extending to the periphery [type 4], an island of defect along the line of fusion but surrounded by healthy retina and choroid all around [type 5], peripheral pigmentation along the line of fusion [type 6], and defect confined to the periphery along the fusion line [type 7]. Based on the type and involvement of the foveal region, visual acuity [VA] may range from very poor with accompanying nystagmus to almost normal. In patients with subnormal vision, fixation as well as point of highest VA may reside along the temporal margin of the coloboma within the evident or presumptive temporal arcade. Hence, it may be unwise to laser this segment of the coloboma margin, either as a prophylactic measure or at the conclusion of surgery for associated retinal detachment.

Rhegmatogenous retinal detachment in patients with fundus coloboma [Figure 11.1b] usually presents in childhood or during the early adult years. The majority of cases with iridofundal coloboma require primary vitreoretinal surgery as the breaks are located posteriorly, either within the intercalary membrane, or at the margins of the coloboma. This should not, however, be presumed as universal, as rare cases with peripheral retinal tears have been seen by the author, and these are better managed by scleral buckling. Owing to poor contrast from lack of RPE and poorly developed choroidal vasculature, causative breaks may be difficult to identify preoperatively, as well as intraoperatively. At surgery, dye-assisted localization of breaks, by injecting diluted trypan blue into the subretinal space, may be useful in some patients. Creating adequate chorioretinal adhesion around breaks located at this region is also challenging due to the absence of RPE. In addition, there is a host of other concerns while undertaking vitreoretinal surgery in these patients. These include abnormal shape and size of the eyeball and cornea [making intravitreal instrumentation and placement of viewing contact lens challenging], poorly defined surface anatomy [which makes measurements less accurate], absence of zonules at the region of lens notch [owing to which air, gas, or silicone oil can migrate into the anterior chamber], presence of dense nuclear sclerosis even at a young age, presence of hyaloid remnant in some cases, absence of a landmark from where to

DOI: 10.1201/9781003179320-12

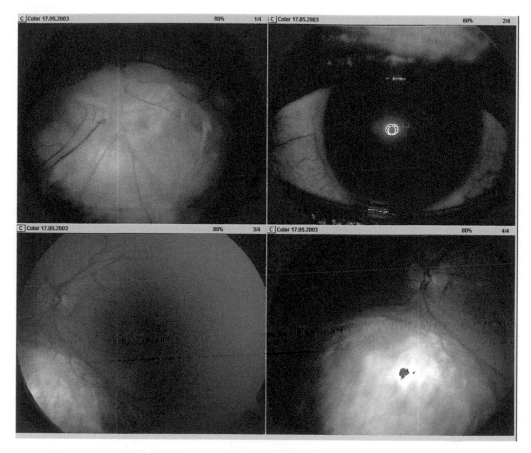

FIGURE 11.1A Fundus photographs of a patient with bilateral iridofundal coloboma [type 2 RE, type 4 LE]. Also shown is lens notch in the left eye [anterior image].

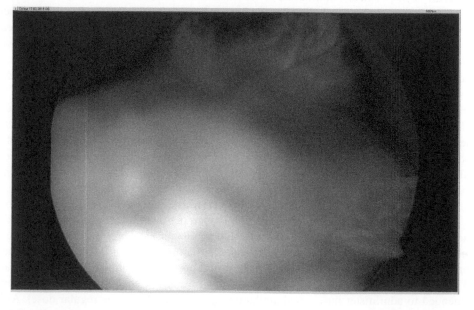

FIGURE 11.1B Fundus photograph of a patient with fundus coloboma and retinal detachment.

induce posterior vitreous detachment [PVD], relatively tighter adherence of hyaloid to the retina, and in some cases the existence of only a small region of normal retina. Whether placement of a scleral buckle-band during vitreoretinal surgery improves long-term results is not clear. Presence of nystagmus is a poor prognostic feature. The objective of surgery in most cases is to provide at least long-term ambulatory vision. Owing to significantly higher risk of redetachment, it is advisable to prefer silicone oil as a long-term vitreous substitute.

11.2   ENDOPHTHALMITIS

Endophthalmitis is an inflammation of the internal layers of the eye resulting from intraocular colonization of infectious agents and manifesting with an exudation into the vitreous cavity. This is an entity that can rapidly destroy vision, and despite the best available therapeutic efforts, even today, the prognosis remains extremely unpredictable. Based on the type, severity, etiology, and drug sensitivity of the etiological organisms, vitrectomy is used as a treatment approach in its management. The timing 'when to do vitrectomy' in endophthalmitis is difficult to decide and a controversial issue because choosing a time that is neither too late nor too early is subjective, usually based on the surgeon's past experiences and because the benefit versus safety window for this procedure is very narrow. The advantages of vitrectomy are that it decreases infectious, toxic, and inflammatory load; provides adequate undiluted specimen for culture, next generation sequencing, and drug sensitivity studies; and enables more rapid visual recovery by removing vitreous opacification. In reality, however, the functional outcome may be less than that theoretically possible because of a surgical bias in undertaking vitrectomy only in the more severe and advanced cases. As a result of this bias, not only does the surgery become more difficult, but also the risk of complications like retinal detachment increases and so also the possibility of a relapse. With advances in technology allowing access to the vitreous with minimal tissue trauma, precise control of fluidics and intraocular pressure [IOP], and vitrectomy probes with high cut rates, there is an increasing trend towards earlier vitrectomy. This is certainly advantageous when there is a high suspicion of infection with gram-negative organisms, as such patients tend to develop worsening corneal edema and corneal abscess rapidly [which may completely preclude any chances of performing vitrectomy]. The indications recommended in literature for undertaking immediate vitrectomy are severe cases, cases in which gram-negative organisms are seen on smear examination of the vitreous aspirate, and in cases showing no response to medical treatment (intravitreal injection). Severe case has been defined as one in which there is a total absence of red reflex, inaccurate projection of light [PL], afferent pupillary defect, corneal ring infiltrate, and worsening 24–48 hours after an intravitreal injection. Although the Endophthalmitis Vitrectomy Study [EVS; see section on studies in vitreoretina] was not designed to address when to undertake vitrectomy, indirectly it concluded that immediate vitrectomy must be considered if vision at presentation is only light perception.

Vitrectomy for endophthalmitis might be required either in the acute stage or in the resolved stage. In the resolved stage, vitreous surgery is less complex in the absence of retinal detachment, and the surgery may be facilitated by the presence of total PVD. However, in the presence of active infection (acute stage), vitreous surgery is prone to a high risk of surgical complications. Problems generally encountered include significant lid edema, boggy conjunctiva, wound dehiscence [in exogenous cases], corneal haze, edema, folds and abscess, exudates in the anterior chamber, pupillary membrane, perilenticular membrane [on the anterior and posterior surface of implant or crystalline lens], choroidal thickening and congestion [hence the need for a 6-mm cannula], adherent and sticky vitreous without PVD, and a necrotic and friable retina. Three cardinal principles to be remembered while undertaking vitrectomy for endophthalmitis are use the maximal cut rate, use minimal suction, and do not attempt to induce posterior vitreous separation forcefully. Also, attempt should be made not to work very close to the necrotic retina. At the end of vitrectomy, it is generally recommended to administer intravitreal antibiotic injection [1/10th of the regular dose]. Although vitrectomy is not the procedure of choice in all endophthalmitis cases, it is generally required if the patient fails to respond to intravitreal antibiotic injection, in severe cases which have initial VA of PL only, fungal endophthalmitis, bleb-related endophthalmitis, and posttraumatic endophthalmitis with retained intraocular foreign body [IOFB] [Figure 11.2]. Small-gauge vitrectomy would be the procedure of choice as it minimizes the risk of conjunctival trauma as well as port site complications. In the presence of pre-existing hypotony, however, it may be safer to create a 20G scleral port for infusion using a microvitreoretinal [MVR] blade and inserting a 6-mm cannula [with proper attention to direction of the cannula, this can be safely used even in phakic patients].

Proportional pars plana vitrectomy [PPV] has been described by Morris and colleagues wherein the extent of vitrectomy was advised to be proportional to safe visibility, expertise of the surgeon and the retinal condition. It could vary from minimum diagnostic vitrectomy to total PPV with cleaning of the posterior retinal surface. In complete and early vitrectomy for endophthalmitis [CEVE], a vertical well is dug within the opaque vitreous in the nasal part. The posterior vitreous face is then identified by its opaqueness or by the deposits of infective colonies over it [as yellowish or white dots]. A drop of triamcinolone may also be used to delineate the posterior vitreous clearly. PVD is then induced using suction of the cutter. Induction of PVD is avoided over necrotic retina; hyaloid is shaved over these areas as there is a high chance of retinal break or retinal detachment. In other areas, PVD is induced, and vitreous is removed to decrease the infective load optimally. However, detachment of vitreous anterior to the equator is not 'aggressively pursued', and peripheral vitreous must be trimmed carefully. Thus, in CEVE posterior hyaloid is removed contrary to the recommendation of the EVS, though they retain same treatment philosophy regarding peripheral vitrectomy. The primary goal of CEVE is to cure the infection, and vacuuming of the macular surface was always performed using a silicone tip extrusion cannula (flute needle) with passive suction. Aspiration by vitrectomy probe was done once the sticky material was mobilized from the retinal surface. European Society of Cataract and Refractive Surgeons [ESCRS] recommends that in acute endophthalmitis, induction of PVD (in cases without a pre-existing PVD) should be reserved for experienced vitreoretinal surgeons.

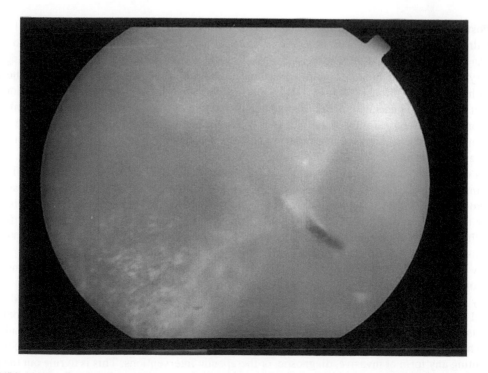

FIGURE 11.2A Fundus photograph of endophthalmitis following trauma with a broom stick.

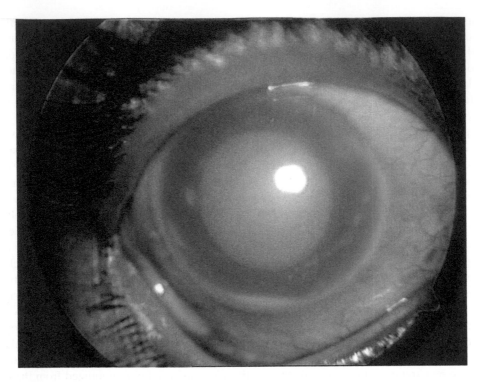

FIGURE 11.2B   Anterior segment photograph of a child with pseudo-hypopyon and pseudo-exudates in the anterior chamber secondary to retinoblastoma and not metastatic endophthalmitis [masquerade syndrome]. Retinoblastoma was also seen in the fellow eye on fundus examination.

Postoperative endophthalmitis. In the majority of patients with postsurgical bacterial endophthalmitis, the clinical presentation is very classical and causes few problems in diagnosis. In the early follow-up period after surgery, if there is doubt about the unexpected reaction being secondary to sterile inflammation or infectious endophthalmitis, diligent observation over the next 6–24 hours is very critical to make a definitive diagnosis. During this period of observation, the patient is started on adequate doses of topical and systemic anti-inflammatory agents (mainly corticosteroids). Endophthalmitis of an infectious origin usually progresses significantly, while sterile inflammation either remains stable or shows some improvement. When uncertainty still prevails, it is better to err on the side of infectious endophthalmitis and start appropriate treatment. Three forms of bacterial endophthalmitis are recognized after surgery based on the clinical profile. The fulminant variety occurs within about 4 days and is usually caused by gram-negative bacteria, streptococci, or *Staphylococcus aureus*. The acute form develops between 5–7 days and is most likely to be caused by *Staphylococcus epidermides* or coagulase-negative cocci (rarely by fungi). The chronic type of endophthalmitis usually develops 1 to several months after the surgery, and organisms involved are fungi, *Propionibacterium acnes*, or *S. epidermides*.

VA and grade of media clarity are the two most important considerations in decision making. Loss of light projection is an absolute indicator of infectious endophthalmitis. In the EVS, media clarity was graded into 5 grades: more than 20/40 (6/12) view of the retina [grade 1], second-order retinal vessels visible [grade 2], some vessels visible but not second order [grade 3], no retinal vessels visible [grade 4], and no fundus glow [grade 5]. In any patient with suspected endophthalmitis and when retinal details are not visible, it is mandatory to undertake ultrasonography (USG) before instituting any form of invasive, diagnostic, or therapeutic interventions. This is to rule out the possibility of conditions that may mimic endophthalmitis such as dislocated nucleus and to detect the presence of concurrent pathology like choroidal detachment or retinal detachment and to note the degree of vitreous exudation and PVD. Ultrasonography is a useful aid in planning and safe execution of surgical steps.

Gram-positive organisms are the predominant bacteria and are responsible for 90%–95% of all postsurgical endophthalmitis cases. Despite the lower prevalence of gram-negative infection, they are important to recognize early as these organisms are highly virulent, produce endotoxins, and rapidly begin to colonize the vitreous cavity. They need a more vigorous management approach, and early vitrectomy may also become necessary. Fungal endophthalmitis following intraocular surgery is seen in about 3% of patients.

EVS was the first randomized, multicentric study on postoperative endophthalmitis and concluded that if initial vision is hand motions or better, then there is no difference in outcome between immediate vitrectomy or intravitreal antibiotics. However, if initial vision is only light perception, then final VA and media clarity are substantially better in patients undergoing vitrectomy and intravitreal injection rather than intravitreal injection alone [see section on studies in vitreoretinal surgery].

Special forms of exogenous endophthalmitis include cluster endophthalmitis, *P. acnes* endophthalmitis, post-intravitreal injection endophthalmitis, bleb-associated endophthalmitis, posttraumatic endophthalmitis, and paediatric endophthalmitis. *P. acnes* is an anaerobic, gram-positive bacillus that is normally present in the conjunctival sac as a commensal and is reported as a common isolate in patients with chronic postsurgical endophthalmitis. A few cases of endophthalmitis by *Propionibacterium granulosum* have also been reported. Rare cases of acute infection have also been reported, but these respond well to treatment and are not associated with relapses. *P. acnes* endophthalmitis presents as a low-grade, smouldering type of intraocular inflammation following cataract surgery. Because of this pattern of inflammation, it tends to be missed in its early stages. The inflammation may show an initial response to steroids, but subsequent relapses appear. On clinical evaluation, it is characterized by the presence of whitish plaques [composed of bacterial colonies and inflammatory cells] in the capsular bag. A history of unexpected inflammation after yttrium aluminum garnet [YAG] capsulotomy should also raise the suspicion of this infection. Laboratory confirmation of the diagnosis is difficult and often delayed because the organism has a low replication rate and begins to show up on culture only after about 2 weeks. Hence, for laboratory confirmation of *P. acnes* infection, the aspirate must be cultured on anaerobic media and observed for at least 14 days. Management of endophthalmitis caused by *P. acnes* infection poses a peculiar challenge. Being sequestered within the spaces of the capsular bag and intraocular implant, they are difficult to eradicate [antibiotics fail to reach these spaces and achieve the needed minimum inhibitory concentration]. Treatment approaches include intravitreal antibiotics alone [injected into the capsular bag] in mild cases, to vitrectomy, total capsulectomy and intraocular lens [IOL] explantation along with intraocular and systemic antibiotics in very severe cases. The objective of total capsulectomy and IOL explantation is to eradicate colonies of *P. acnes* sequestered within the confines of the capsular bag. Surgical measures like partial capsulectomy and retaining of the IOL may provide only transient respite. The antibiotic of choice in treating endophthalmitis caused by *P. acnes* is vancomycin in the same dose recommended for other forms of bacterial endophthalmitis. Small-gauge vitreoretinal surgery is ideally suited for this form of endophthalmitis. Unlike in other types of endophthalmitis, induction of posterior vitreous separation and more extensive removal of vitreous are considered to be relatively safe. In addition, the need for long-term vitreous tamponade is also unlikely to be necessary. An important consideration is the need for removal of the IOL through the limbal route or scleral tunnel. This step is likely to induce significant endothelial cell loss if adequate care is not taken to protect the corneal endothelium using viscoelastics. Although it is infrequent to encounter significant posterior synechiae, the surgeon must be prepared to use iris hooks to retract an undilated pupil in order to gain access to the entire capsular bag. Gentle traction on the capsular bag using an intravitreal forceps with one hand may add safety during this step. It would be useful to inject intravitreal vancomycin at the end of the surgery [with no need for ceftazidime]. The surgeon must send samples of the aspirate and capsular extract as well as the explanted IOL to the laboratory for reconfirmation of *P. acnes* infection.

In metastatic endophthalmitis caused by fungi, there is an associated fungaemia and involvement of extraocular sites, and hence systemic anti-fungal therapy is necessary. Following intraocular surgery, however, fungal colonization is restricted only to the intraocular cavity. In addition, most anti-fungal drugs have the potential to cause significant systemic adverse effects and have very limited ocular penetration. Hence, exact management guidelines for the management of exogenous fungal endophthalmitis are not available in literature. The relative paucity of controlled studies on the treatment approach in this form of endophthalmitis is related to the infrequent occurrence of fungal endophthalmitis in comparison with bacterial endophthalmitis after intraocular surgery. Unlike in postoperative bacterial endophthalmitis, in which the mainstay of treatment is intravitreal administration, in fungal endophthalmitis, this mode of drug administration seems to have only a limited role. This is because fungi multiply less rapidly than bacteria, and correspondingly, treatment of fungal endophthalmitis requires a prolonged duration of drug action within the vitreous cavity. This objective cannot be achieved effectively with intravitreal administration. Development of sustained-release intraocular devices may be useful, but tissue toxicity may remain a concern. The method of injection and the precautions while administering an intravitreal injection are the same as for postoperative bacterial endophthalmitis. However, the follow-up guidelines (e.g., when to repeat the injection, how long to wait before vitrectomy.) following this injection are not clearly defined. Steroids are absolutely contraindicated.

In fungal endophthalmitis, it is generally recommended that vitrectomy be performed early and an antifungal injection [usually amphotericin B] be injected at the end of the surgery. Here again, small-gauge surgery has advantages over 20G vitreous surgery.

Endophthalmitis in patients with a filtering bleb following glaucoma surgery is usually considered separately because of differences in pathogenesis, bacteriological isolates, and treatment. It occurs infrequently and is usually a late complication. Although the occurrence is late, the symptoms are acute as the disease is related to a delayed entry of the pathogenic organism into the intraocular cavities and not a delayed manifestation. Whether thinness of a bleb contributes to an increased risk of endophthalmitis has been a matter of considerable debate. Filtering procedures with anti-mitotic agents like mitomycin C and 5-fluouracil are known to increase the risk of late-onset endophthalmitis. The reported incidence is 2% with mitomycin C [0.04% concentration] and about 6% with 5-fluorouracil. Filtering blebs made along the inferior limbus are considered to be at a higher risk of developing endophthalmitis. Bleb-associated endophthalmitis is frequently caused by streptococci and *Haemophilus* spp. [probably related to the ability of these organisms to penetrate intact conjunctiva], and since these are relatively more virulent, bleb-related endophthalmitis carries a poorer prognosis. It is important to distinguish 'blebitis' from bleb-associated endophthalmitis. In the former the infection is still confined to the bleb and the anterior chamber, and the prognosis is good when diagnosed and managed early. Failure to initiate early treatment can allow blebitis to develop into frank endophthalmitis. Blebitis must be promptly evaluated for the etiological organism and drug sensitivity [by sending a swab from the area of the bleb]. In the presence of severe blebitis at presentation, it is necessary to send vitreous samples for culture as they still remain the best source from which to obtain positive growth and because organisms cultured from the conjunctival sac and even from the surface of the bleb may be frequently different from growth obtained from intraocular specimens. Initial treatment revolves around the use of concentrated topical drops of ceftazidime and tobramycin. Efforts must be made to maintain pupillary dilatation with regular instillation of a parasympatholytic and sympathomimetic drops. Simultaneous administration of broad-spectrum systemic antibiotics is needed. Use of topical steroids and systemic steroids must be delayed until the effects of topical and systemic antibiotics have set in. When intravitreal samples are collected, it should be combined with injection of intravitreal broad-spectrum antibiotics [combination of vancomycin and ceftazidime]. As cases treated with intravitreal antibiotics alone fare poorly, early vitrectomy is necessary. Despite early vitrectomy, the prognosis in terms of visual and anatomical outcomes remains unsatisfactory. Patients with bleb-related endophthalmitis are particularly suited to surgery using small-gauge vitrectomy instrumentation owing to the scarred conjunctiva and presence of a bleb. As most blebs are located in the superonasal region, one may have to use a temporal approach vitrectomy [with infusion line placed in the inferonasal pars plana and the active ports in the inferotemporal and superotemporal pars plana]. The Collaborative Bleb-related Infection Incidence and Treatment study group used a staging of bleb-related infections: confined to bleb with mild anterior chamber inflammation [stage 1], with significant involvement of the anterior chamber and no vitreous involvement [stage 2], with mild vitreous involvement [stage 3a], and advanced vitreous involvement [stage 3b]. Stage IIIb cases received immediate vitrectomy with intravitreal antibiotics along with topical and systemic antibiotics. Early PPV with intravitreal antibiotics has been shown to reduce risk of final vision of no PL and improve final VA in culture positive bleb associated endophthalmitis.

Posttraumatic endophthalmitis. Open globe injury is associated with an increased risk of endophthalmitis because most objects [e.g., vegetable matter, stones, broom sticks (Figure 11.2a), needles, metal fragments] are contaminated. The reported mean intervals from injury to the onset of endophthalmitis are about 1–2 days in fulminant cases [bacillus, *Clostridium* spp., and streptococcus], 3–4 days in acute cases [*S. epidermides* and gram-negative organisms], and about 2 months for endophthalmitis caused by fungi. Most posttraumatic intraocular fungal infections are caused by filamentous fungi with greater virulence, and infection with yeast like fungi does not occur.

Endophthalmitis following ocular trauma is different from other forms of endophthalmitis because of several reasons. First, disorganization of the normal anatomy may cause difficulty in assessing the clinical features and in making an accurate diagnosis of endophthalmitis in its early stages; second, the organisms producing the infection are more virulent and have a high degree of pathogenicity; and third, the protocol for management remains ill-defined. Collection of intraocular samples for laboratory investigations is necessary as in cases of postsurgical endophthalmitis. However, it is more difficult to collect the sample because of the distorted anatomy and associated clinical features (e.g., extreme hypotony). The procedures adopted are again paracentesis, vitreous aspiration, and vitreous biopsy. Whenever a foreign body is removed, it should also be sent to the laboratory for culture. Treatment should not be delayed for want of diagnostic specimens. Similar to that in postsurgical endophthalmitis, *S. epidermides* is the commonest isolate in posttraumatic endophthalmitis. Unlike postsurgical cases, *Bacillus cereus*–related endophthalmitis occurs in a large number of cases (22%) following trauma. Infection caused by *B. cereus* has certain characteristic features: in the presence of retained IOFB, the patient develops severe orbital pain within 24 hours of the injury, associated with significant proptosis, chemosis, and periorbital inflammation. Corneal ring infiltrate and ring abscess occur frequently. Most patients become febrile and have moderate polymorphonuclear leucocytosis. The only other endophthalmitis-producing organism capable of causing similar constitutional symptoms is *Clostridium*.

If *B. cereus* infection is suspected, then treatment measures have to be instituted urgently. The preferred drug combinations for intravitreal injection are as recommended for postsurgical endophthalmitis. It is important to remember that *B. cereus* is resistant to cephalosporins. Vancomycin, clindamycin, and gentamicin (amikacin) are effective against this organism and are given in combination. Intravitreal antibiotics alone have limited efficacy in posttraumatic endophthalmitis, so many such patients need early vitrectomy followed by intravitreal injection of antibiotics. Early vitrectomy has been advocated in all cases with a retained IOFB. However, there are several considerations that need to be addressed before performing vitrectomy, such as the choice of anaesthesia; corneal clarity; status of the crystalline lens; pupillary dilatation; IOP; integrity of the ocular coats and need for strengthening before making the scleral ports; location of the scleral ports; risk of choroidal haemorrhage; size, shape, and chemical composition of the foreign body; presence of cilioretinochoroidal detachment; and vitreous haemorrhage [preoperative USG is mandatory].

Whether prophylaxis with antibiotics helps in preventing or decreasing the risk of posttraumatic endophthalmitis is not known with certainty. Nevertheless, the practice of prescribing systemic antibiotics for at least 5 days after trauma is widespread. The role of prophylactic intravitreal antibiotics is also favoured by most surgeons, particularly if vitreous involvement is present or a retained IOFB exists.

Endogenous endophthalmitis. Colonization of the vitreous cavity by bacterial or fungal organisms by hematogenous dissemination is known as endogenous or metastatic endophthalmitis. Its two forms are bacterial and fungal endogenous endophthalmitis. The source of organism is usually from a foci elsewhere in the body such as the gastrointestinal tract (hepatic abscess, appendicitis), heart (endocarditis), ear (suppurative otitis media), skin (pyoderma), pelvic inflammatory disease, lung, or urinary tract. Common to most cases of metastatic endophthalmitis are the presence of an immunocompromised status, prolonged alimentation, complicated systemic surgery, indwelling catheters, prolonged systemic antibiotics, complicated major surgery, malignancies (leukaemia, lymphoma), diabetes mellitus, chronic alcoholism, chronic malnutrition, liver disease, organ transplantation, prolonged corticosteroid therapy, premature infants, and puerperal sepsis.

In metastatic endophthalmitis, the presentation is usually delayed because of the indolent course of the infection and because most cases have a systemic illness of greater concern. Clinically, in patients with metastatic endophthalmitis, anterior segment inflammation typically lags behind the posterior segment inflammation. The involvement also tends to be bilateral. The commonest fungal isolate in metastatic endophthalmitis is *Candida albicans*, followed by *Aspergillus fumigatus*. Early stages in the evolution of *Candida* endophthalmitis are characterized by a focal inner choroidal lesion with a variable intensity of inflammation of the overlying retina and vitreous. The lesion is round to oval, usually multifocal, and about 1/8–1/4 disc diameter in size. With further growth (usually over days to weeks), it breaks into the vitreous with budding extensions. This is accompanied by focal perivascular inflammatory deposits, strand-like collection of inflammatory cells, and increasing vitreous reaction. Focal small intraretinal haemorrhages and retinal necrosis may also occur. The latter, along with the formation of vitreoretinal membranes and contraction, are the usual causes of visual loss. Most patients with *Aspergillus* endophthalmitis have other foci such as endocarditis, allergic bronchopulmonary aspergillosis, or invasive pulmonary aspergillosis. Unlike in endogenous *Candida* endophthalmitis, the symptoms can be quite marked in patients with *Aspergillus* endophthalmitis. These include, pain, redness, blurred vision, chemosis, and periocular swelling. Signs of inflammation are clearly evident in both the anterior chamber and vitreous. A hypopyon may also be present. The chorioretinal inflammation appears as depigmented lesions with a pale yellow or fluffy appearance. Occlusion of the choroidal and retinal vessels by invasion of fungal hyphae is also known to occur. The mainstay in the management of metastatic endophthalmitis is early diagnosis and appropriate treatment. As most cases of metastatic endophthalmitis have non-ocular foci of fungal colonization, the preferred route of drug administration is systemic. Most patients need treatment for a prolonged period of several weeks to months. It takes a minimum of 1 week to detect any appreciable response to treatment unlike in patients with bacterial endophthalmitis. It is again important to remember that corticosteroids by any route is contraindicated in the management of metastatic endophthalmitis as it tends to encourage further fungal colonization. The most effective drug remains amphotericin B, but it has the potential to cause severe side effects, including nephrotoxicity. Hence, azole derivatives are generally preferred by some. With azole derivatives, the effect is, however, fungistatic, and drug resistance may develop. Drug combination of amphotericin B and azoles is not recommended as they may have antagonistic effects. Endogenous endophthalmitis should ideally be managed in consultation with an internist because of the disseminated nature of the disease and the need for an intensive drug therapy. No invasive procedures are advisable in endogenous fugal endophthalmitis in the initial stages of management, including diagnostic vitrectomy and intravitreal injection. Unlike in exogenous endophthalmitis, vitrectomy and intravitreal injection are reserved only for patients not responding to intensive medical treatment.

Endogenous bacterial endophthalmitis is a rare form of endophthalmitis. Nevertheless, it is important to be aware of this entity because the infection is often very severe, progression extremely rapid, and visual prognosis dismal. Several organisms have been reported to cause this form of endophthalmitis, including *Klebsiella*, *Pseudomonas*, *Neisseria*, *Streptococcus*, *Escherichia*, *Proteus*, and *Bacillus* spp. Predisposing factors are the same as those seen in endogenous fungal endophthalmitis. *Listeria monocytogenes*, *Neisseria meningitides*, and *Hemophilus influenzae* have been reported to cause endogenous endophthalmitis even in the absence of any risk factors. Greenwald and colleagues have classified endogenous bacterial endophthalmitis into posterior focal, posterior diffuse, anterior focal, and anterior diffuse. The focal nature of the infection can rapidly evolve into a diffuse form if it is not recognized and managed early. In the posterior diffuse group, vision may deteriorate to no light perception within hours, and occlusion of the central retinal artery is a usual occurrence. With further delay in treatment, the condition may progress into a fulminant and life-threatening panophthalmitis. Endogenous bacterial endophthalmitis has to be managed as a medical emergency, and as in postsurgical endophthalmitis, time elapsed between the onset and institution of appropriate treatment is the critical factor in determining the final outcome. Unlike in exogenous endophthalmitis, however, the route of choice for drug administration is parenteral. Therapy has to be intensive and prolonged. The recommended doses of antibiotics are about the same as those given in cases of bacterial meningitis. The role of intravitreal injection of antibiotics is debatable. While it definitely has no role in the anterior focal and diffuse form of infection, it may be of benefit in the posterior focal group if no bacterial isolate has been cultured. In the posterior diffuse group, intravitreal injection of broad-spectrum antibiotics has to be given early. The recommended doses of intravitreal antibiotics is the same as that indicated under postoperative bacterial endophthalmitis. Corticosteroids should be considered [under cover of systemic antibiotics and in consultation with an internist] in the posterior form of infection to counter the effect of endotoxins and cytokine-mediated damage. Other topical and periocular medications (antibiotics, corticosteroids, and cycloplegics) are prescribed as in postsurgical endophthalmitis. The frequency of administration is determined by the severity of anterior chamber infection or inflammation. The role of vitrectomy is controversial with very few reports available in literature. It is definitely indicated in posterior diffuse form of endogenous bacterial endophthalmitis whenever there is a lack of prompt response to intensive systemic treatment. It has no role in the anterior focal, anterior diffuse, and posterior focal group of endophthalmitis. The principles of vitrectomy are similar to postsurgical endophthalmitis; however, the risk of complications in the form of retinal tear and detachment are uniformly higher owing to absence of prior PVD, subretinal location of the septic focus, and more severe retinal necrosis.

Endophthalmitis in children. The commonest forms of endophthalmitis in children, unlike in adults, is probably posttraumatic endophthalmitis followed by endogenous endophthalmitis and endophthalmitis secondary to spread from contiguous structures (e.g., corneal ulcer). Postsurgical endophthalmitis is relatively rare. Another cause is sclerosing endophthalmitis secondary to parasitic infestation with *Toxocara canis* and *Cysticercus cellulosae*. *Toxocara* endophthalmitis in some series has contributed to 16% of the cases of leukocoria in children.

The organisms causing endophthalmitis in children also tend to be different compared to that in adults. Streptococcal species has been reported as the commonest isolate in paediatric posttraumatic endophthalmitis (unlike *S. epidermides* in adults). In children with endophthalmitis, there are several diagnostic problems. The nature of trauma may not be easy to ascertain, the presentation may be delayed, clinical examination may be difficult, the complete extent and nature of the trauma may become evident only during examination under anaesthesia, and this may have to be switched to full anaesthesia if immediate surgery is mandated. Masquerade syndromes like retinoblastoma [hypopyon may be present] need to be ruled out by USG and fellow eye examination [Figure 11.2b]. As repeated and frequent anaesthetic exposure is not desirable, one may have to consider examination under a sedative during follow-up. In addition to concerns about visual outcome, in children, there is the added concern of anatomical outcome. All efforts should be made to retain the anatomical integrity of the globe, as the effect of an empty socket in children is a cause of great psychological trauma to the child and parents, and it also retards further development of the orbital bones, leading to a facial asymmetry. Hence, vitrectomy, although more challenging than in adults, should be considered in all children with endophthalmitis following surgery or trauma. For complex cases, silicone oil should be the preferred vitreous substitute. Evisceration should be avoided except as a desperate last resort to contain panophthalmitis.

11.3   INTRAOCULAR CYSTICERCOSIS

Cysticercosis is the extraintestinal lodgement and development into cystic form of oocysts of either the pork (*Taenia solium*) or cattle (*Taenia saginata*) tapeworm. The tapeworm usually enters the body through the oro-fecal route and develops within the intestines to produce the condition, taeniasis. Some oocysts may migrate across the gut and extrahepatic pathways into any of the tissues within the body, resulting in cysticercosis of that organ [e.g., neurocysticercosis]. In relation to the eye, cysticercosis may involve intraocular structures [except crystalline lens], extraocular muscles, orbital tissue, and ocular adnexa. While it is common to find neurocysticercosis in a patient with intraocular cysticercosis, it is rare to find concurrent involvement of the extraocular tissues. The former observation makes it mandatory for all patients with intraocular cysticercosis to undergo neuroimaging to rule out neurocysticercosis and for patients with neurocysticercosis to be screened for intraocular cysticercosis. Neurocysticercosis may manifest as abrupt onset of seizures and other neurological symptoms. In many developing countries, cysticercosis is the most common parasitic infestation, and its prevalence is often considered as an indicator of social hygiene.

Manifestations of intraocular cysticercosis include sense of foreign body within the visual field, either fixed or floating, defective visual function, and sometimes features of ocular inflammation [pain, redness]. It is infrequent to find more than one cyst and bilateral cysts. The most frequent intraocular location is within the posterior chamber [vitreous cavity and subretinal space]. Concurrent findings include signs of anterior chamber inflammation or panuveitis, inflamed iris vessels, posterior synechiae, cataract, cyclitic membrane, dense vitreous inflammatory membranes [that may be vascularized and hence mistaken for the retina], inflammatory deposits over the hyaloid, focal area of dense scarring [site through which the cyst has entered the subretinal space or vitreous cavity], and retinal detachment. The natural history of eyes with intraocular cysticercosis is eventual phthisis, and hence there is a need for early diagnosis and management. In doubtful cases wherein the cyst and its scolex cannot be discerned on ophthalmoscopic evaluation, USG of the eyeball is an immensely helpful and mandatory investigation.

Intraocular cysticercosis may be classified based on its location, on being alive or dead, on the presence or absence of mild to severe structural damage, and on the existence or otherwise of cysticerci elsewhere [e.g., neurocysticercosis]. Unlike cysticercosis elsewhere in the body [including extraocular], medical therapy has no role in the management of intraocular cysticercosis. Surgical removal of the cyst is the sole option. Removal of cysts from the anterior chamber is usually without hurdles. In contrast, removal of cysts from within the vitreous cavity and subretinal space can be associated with significant difficulties like resection of a vascularized inflammatory or cyclitic membrane, induction of PVD, incising the capsule surrounding the cyst and teasing out the cyst from within the subretinal space, and reattaching an often taut retinal detachment. In addition, there are unique differences noticed during surgery for a cyst that is still alive and one that is dead. When the cyst is alive, it tends to move away from the light source, and the cyst wall is also more elastic. This makes it necessary to use higher vacuum to aspirate the cyst from its location and into the cutter port. Contrarily, when the cyst is dead, it tends to get encapsulated, and one may have to first incise this capsule before being able to successfully aspirate and remove the cyst [Video 11.1]. Unlike in the past, there is no role for removing the cyst in toto. This is associated not only with increased surgical time but also with increased ocular morbidity. The current recommendation is to undertake cystectomy using relatively high suction and moderate cut rates. Small-gauge instruments, including 25G, are efficient in achieving this objective, and there is no need to use 20G cutter. Once the intraocular cysts have been removed surgically, it is safe to initiate medical therapy

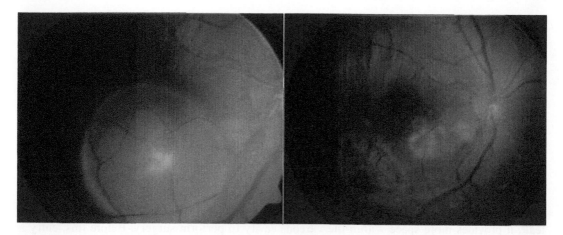

FIGURE 11.3 Preoperative and postoperative images of a patient following PPV for subretinal cysticercosis.

with antiparasitic drugs for cysts elsewhere, like the brain. Even in the early postoperative period, the eye remains relatively quiet, with no undue inflammation after cystectomy, and systemic corticosteroids are not routinely recommended [Figure 11.3]. Visual recovery may not be gratifying in cases where in the cyst is located within the submacular region, when the presentation is delayed, or when there is concurrent structural damage. Even when visual prognosis is poor, removal of the cyst may reduce the risk of phthisis.

11.4 RETINOPATHY OF PREMATURITY

Retinopathy of prematurity [ROP] is a proliferative vascular vitreoretinopathy that occurs in babies born prematurely. The incidence of ROP has an inverse relationship with the gestational age at birth [more than 70% when less than 23 weeks and less than 10% when 32 weeks] and birth weight [60% when below 750 gm and about 10% if above 1500 gm]. The risk increases in the event of protracted intensive care, unmonitored oxygen administration, sepsis, and hypoxia. Protective measures against the development of ROP include use of surfactant, antenatal corticosteroids, monitored oxygen supplementation, prevention of hospital-acquired infections, and healthy nourishment. Owing to improved and meticulous neonatal care, ROP has shown a decline in developed countries [despite improving survival rate of very low birth weight babies and gestational age] but continues to worsen in low-middle income countries. The natural history of the disease progresses rapidly through five stages: demarcation line, ridge, retinal neovascularization, retinal detachment without retrolental proliferation, and retinal detachment with retrolental proliferation. Large majority of ROP undergoes spontaneous regression from stage 1/2. If progression is documented at follow-up screening, it can be arrested in a significant majority by laser ablation of the avascular retina [according to guidelines developed by the early treatment of ROP Study Group and other international experts]. Cryotherapy is no longer a recommended treatment alternative for retinal ablation. In newborns who progress despite treatment and in those who have stage 4 at presentation, prompt vitreous surgery is effective in preventing evolution to stage 5 ROP. Visual outcomes of vitreous surgery in stage 5 disease have been very varied and generally unsatisfactory, so the enthusiasm for intervention at this stage has waned. Currently, treatment of high-risk eyes with intravitreal anti-VEGF injection has resulted in improved revascularization of the retina and a significant decline in the occurrence of retinal detachment. However, these eyes need a more prolonged follow up as a delayed recurrence of proliferation and its sequelae is known to develop.

The objectives of surgery in stage 4 ROP are to remove the contracting vitreous scaffold, retain the crystalline lens, and not create any retinal tear at surgery. Challenges at surgery include a high prevalence of systemic comorbidities, unstable homeostasis, need of experts in neonatal anaes-thesia, and provision for specialized postoperative care in a high-dependency unit. In addition, there could be bilateral disease for which a plan of simultaneous or sequential surgery needs to be discussed with the team and parents beforehand. It is important to suppress any plus disease before surgery by intravitreal injection of anti–vascular endothelial growth factor [anti-VEGF] about 1 week prior to surgery. This significantly reduces the chances of intraocular bleed during surgery. Surgical steps may be difficult in view of narrow pupillary aperture and limited exposure of the surgical field, lack of clear anatomical landmarks, boggy conjunctiva, small globe and vitreous cavity with a disproportionately large crystalline lens, low scleral rigidity, and risk of intraopera-tive haemorrhaging from new vessels. Unlike in the past, placement of scleral explant is only rarely recommended. Owing to smaller globe dimensions, it may be beneficial to prefer 27G instrumen-tation over 25G instruments for managing stage 4 ROP. Some surgeons prefer to use small-gauge cutter and endoilluminator without the cannula. While this could increase the chances of wound leak, it provides more space within the vitreous cavity to perform surgery. Before this, entry is gained into the vitreous cavity using corresponding 25–27G trocar but without the cannula. During vitrectomy, care is taken to specifically identify and remove several forms of traction, including ridge to ridge, ridge to peripheral retina, ridge to lens, and ridge to optic nerve. Performing the pinch test [momentarily lowering the IOP by pinching the infusion tubing] helps to identify and effectively diathermize any intraoperative bleeders. No attempt must be made to drain subretinal fluid. After this, partial air fluid exchange at 25–30 mmHg infusion pressure is performed, and then the ports are closed with absorbable sutures [preferable 9-0 Vicryl]. Optical rehabilitation of the child through periodic refraction is as important as undertaking the surgery and must not be neglected.

11.5 FAMILIAL EXUDATIVE VITREORETINOPATHY

Familial exudative vitreoretinopathy [FEVR] is a bilateral and often symmetrical disorder of peripheral retinal vascular development. Systemic features are generally absent, although a rare association with Turner syndrome has been reported. ROP is an important differential diagno-sis. The condition was first described by Criswick and Schepens and is most commonly inherited as an autosomal dominant trait. There is a high degree of penetrance but variable expressivity. History of prematurity is absent. The disease can manifest at birth in some and remain quiescent in others until adulthood. The severity of manifestations ranges from mild and stable to severe and progressive. Clinical features include zone of avascular retina in the retinal periphery [usually temporal], straightening of temporal vessels, abrupt termination of blood vessels at the avascular zone in a brush border pattern, sclerosis of terminal vessels, peripheral exudation, and neovascu-larization [Figure 11.4]. Severe cases are characterized by congenital retinal fold, macular ectopia, and tractional and combined tractional–rhegmatogenous detachment. The benefit of prophylactic laser treatment or cryotherapy to the avascular area is a matter of debate because many reports sug-gest non-progression and regression of new vessels. In bilateral cases however, prophylactic laser ablation of avascular retina may be useful in the worse eye. Regular follow up of these children, if necessary, by examination under anaesthesia [EUA], is important to note signs of progression and to consider treatment options. In patients with progressive traction involving the macula and in those with combined traction–rhegmatogenous detachment, vitreoretinal surgery is helpful in maintain-ing vision. Since these patients are young and phakic and vitreoretinal attachments are strong, placing a band-buckle would improve the outcomes of vitreoretinal surgery. Aggressive attempts at inducing PVD are discouraged, but this must be compensated by careful debulking and shaving of the vitreous around regions of vitreous traction. As long-term vitreous tamponade is inevitable, silicone oil [preferably 5000 cs] should be preferred. In the event of silicone oil emulsification, it may be prudent to plan silicone oil exchange instead of silicone oil removal [owing to the higher risk of redetachment].

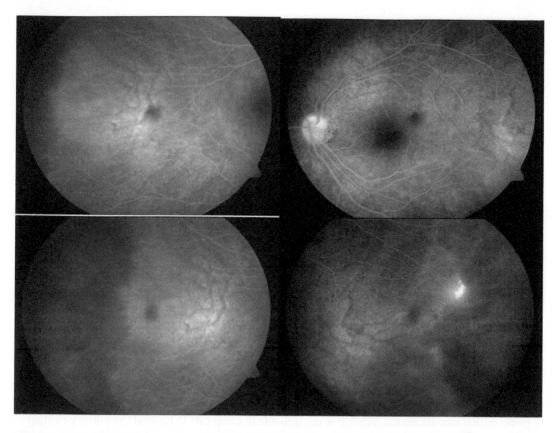

FIGURE 11.4   Fundus fluorescein angiographic images of the right and left eye of a patient with familial exudative vitreoretinopathy. Note the straightening of the vessels, peripheral avascular retina, and early neovascularization in the left eye.

11.6   RETINAL ANGIOMATOSIS

Retinal angiomas are rare tumours [hamartoma] that develop within the vascular bed of the retina. It may be sporadic or a part of the multisystem disorder, von Hippel Lindau [VHL] syndrome. VHL is inherited as an autosomal dominant disease with high penetrance and variable expressivity; the genetic defect being in the *VHL* gene located on the short arm of chromosome 3. These tumours express brachyury, FlK-1, and Scl, and so are thought to develop from embryologically arrested mesodermal cells programmed to develop into hemangioblasts. Tie-2 and CD31 endothelial markers have also been detected in these tumours. Other than retinal angiomas, VHL is associated with hemangioblastomas of the central nervous system (mainly infratentorial); renal cell carcinoma; pancreatic carcinoma; pheochromocytoma; and adrenal, pancreatic, and epidydimal cysts. Extraocular lesions could develop over a variable time frame, as late as the fifth decade of life, so periodic screening is recommended in all patients diagnosed with retinal angiomas.

Retinal angiomas are the earliest and most frequent manifestation of VHL. They evolve as small aneurysmal dilatations and inexorably progress to vision-threatening retinal complications like macular exudation, exudative retinal detachment, tractional detachment, and combined tractional–rhegmatogenous detachment. Before the stage of retinal detachment develops, several methods of treatment for retinal angiomas have been reported like thermal laser, cryotherapy, transpupillary thermotherapy, photodynamic therapy, plaque radiotherapy, and external-beam radiotherapy. In the

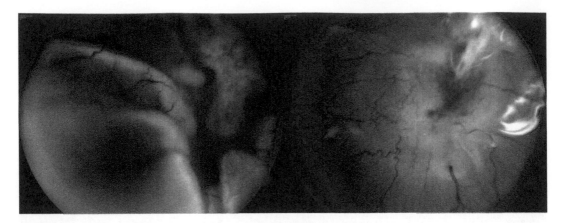

FIGURE 11.5   Preoperative and postoperative fundus photographs of a patient with optic disc hemangioblastoma and exudative retinal detachment.

presence of retinal detachment, vitreoretinal intervention becomes imperative. Exudative retinal detachment resulting from an angioma is best managed by external drainage followed by cryotherapy or thermal laser of the tumour. Standard three port small-gauge vitreous surgery is necessary to manage tractional and combined tractional–rhegmatogenous retinal detachment [Figure 11.5]. It is prudent to place a buckle and band during vitreoretinal surgery as most patients are young and phakic, and the majority of the tumours are in the periphery [zone 3] and have tight adherence to the vitreous, along with some degree of fibrovascular proliferation. This makes it difficult to completely eliminate vitreous traction without increasing the risks of lens touch, intraocular bleeding, and iatrogenic retinal tear formation. Also, it is not possible to extend PVD beyond the posterior extent of the angioma(s). In regions of tight vitreous attachment, vitreous shaving is the safest approach. To eliminate the traction completely and prevent recurrent development of traction and its complications, some surgeons routinely recommend excision of the entire tumour at surgery. However, this aggressive approach is also associated with a higher risk of intraocular haemorrhage, proliferative retinopathy, retinal shortening, and recurrence of detachment. Treatment of the feeder vessels using intravitreal diathermy before tumour excision is said to make surgery safer. Performing surgery at the earliest detection of macular traction may be safer and more beneficial than intervening after the establishment of more severe and extensive tractional changes. In patients with peripheral angiomas and limited traction and or macular exudation, combining ablative treatment [cryotherapy, thermal laser] with scleral buckle and band may delay the progression of the retinal detachment in comparison with undertaking ablative treatment alone. Formation of a retinal fold is a possible counter side to placement of an external buckle.

Visual morbidity from retinal angiomas is high, and many patients have visual loss in one eye at presentation due to complex retinal detachment. Preventing vision loss seems most likely when the lesions are detected and treated in early stages, and continued monitoring is undertaken for several decades for early detection and management of new lesions.

11.7   OPTIC DISC PIT MACULOPATHY

Optic disc pit maculopathy is an exceedingly rare developmental pathology of the optic nerve with secondary changes at the macula leading to progressive diminution of vision. Ninety percent of the cases are unilateral. The presence of macular pathology as a result of optic disc pit is also called Kranenberg syndrome. Macular changes are reported to develop in 30% to 40% of patients with optic disc pit. Risk factors for the occurrence of maculopathy include the size of the pit, location of the pit [along the temporal margin], advancing age, evolving vitreous traction, and unsubstantiated

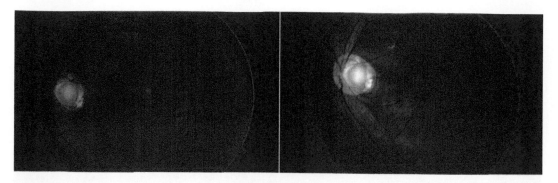

FIGURE 11.6 Preoperative and postoperative images following surgery for a large optic disc pit and maculopathy. Note the development of macular hole in the postoperative photograph.

acts like eye rubbing, Valsalva maneuver, and elevated IOP. Typical macular changes noted in optic disc maculopathy include intraretinal schisis and neurosensory detachment. Based on the structural changes noted on OCT, a classification system has been proposed. Long-term [more than 5 years] natural history observations have shown that about 80% of patients with optic disc maculopathy tend to develop progressive vision loss [down to 6/60 and even lower]. To arrest this decline, laser photocoagulation along the margins of the temporal disc margin was advocated until the past decade. Gradual flattening of the macular schisis and detachment over several months does occur following this intervention; however, visual recovery is infrequent. With advances in vitreous technology and presumably increased safety, more surgeons now advocate vitreous surgery to manage optic disc maculopathy. Several factors must be borne in the decision-making process: most patients are young and phakic, vitreous attachments are firm, the rate of vision decline is variable, and there is no consensus on the vision range at which to intervene. In addition, there are additional and unusual intraoperative and postoperative risks like deroofing of the schisis and conversion to a macular hole [Figure 11.6] as well as migration of air during air-fluid exchange or intraocular gas and silicone oil tamponade, through the optic pit into the subarachnoid space. These additional risks must clearly be explained to the patient or legally authorized representative/guardian and consent obtained accordingly.

Surgical steps include those of standard small-gauge vitrectomy. Special care is, however, needed during PVD induction, and undue traction over the macular schisis must be strictly avoided to prevent deroofing. For the same reason, a complete peel of the internal limiting membrane [ILM] over and above the schitic macula is best avoided. ILM peeling, if planned, must spare the macula. There is lack of clarity on the safety and efficacy of steps performed by some surgeons to 'close' the pit. These maneuvers include ILM flap rotation to cover the pit, ILM 'stuffing' into the pit, and closure with allogenic grafts like amniotic membrane, free ILM flap, autologous sclera, etc. Vitrectomy is also combined in the majority of cases with photocoagulation along the temporal margin of the pit. Other rare methods described in literature include macular buckle and pharmacologic interventions like acetazolamide.

11.8 REMOVAL OF RETAINED METALLIC IOFB

Magnets have played an important role in the extraction of posterior segment intraocular foreign bodies. Advances in vitreoretinal techniques have led to a change in the management of magnetic metallic IOFB from being an external approach to that of an internal one [Figure 11.7]. The use of an external magnet can be complicated by impaction of the foreign body or collateral damage to surrounding ocular structures due to an unpredictable trajectory. An intraocular approach not only avoids these complications but also enables removal of the vitreous gel along with any vitreous

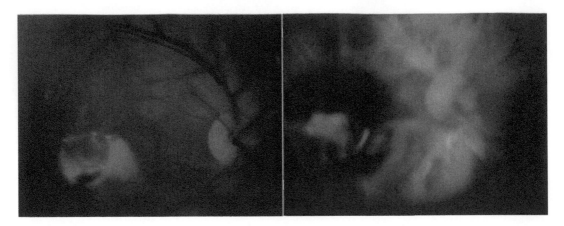

FIGURE 11.7 Preoperative and postoperative photographs following removal of retained metallic IOFB impacted at the fovea.

haemorrhage. This reduces the incidence of postoperative tractional and rhegmatogenous retinal detachment. Removal of a foreign body that is impacted and encapsulated within the retina can be particularly challenging. In such cases, the surgeon has to first incise the capsule and gently free the foreign body before attempting to extract it from the eye. Most such foreign bodies are large in size, so removal through a small-gauge sclerotomy is not possible. The options available are to enlarge one of the original sclerotomy ports, make a separate fourth sclerotomy of a size appropriate for the dimensions of the foreign body, or remove it through the limbus [in surgery combined with removal of a cataractous lens]. The 20G MVR blade seems best suited to make the fourth sclerotomy [after passing preplaced sutures] and to incise the dense encapsulation. Subsequent steps involve the use of an intraocular magnet to bring the foreign body anteriorly and finally remove it through the sclerotomy using a foreign body forceps. In our modified approach, the strong magnetic property of an external magnet to magnetize the MVR blade itself [by applying it over the shaft of the myringotome] could be a useful alternate means of removing an iron IOFB. The magnetized MVR knife allows the foreign body to be safely lifted away from the underlying retinal surface in a controlled manner, without causing any damage to the retina. The stronger magnetic field of an external magnet compared with an internal magnet also precludes the need for using a foreign body forceps. Also, because the MVR knife is magnetized only after it is in contact with the foreign body, sudden release of the foreign body is avoided. Since the MVR knife helps in releasing fibrous adhesions around the foreign body, the need for repeated intraocular manipulation is also reduced.

11.9 PERSISTENT FETAL VASCULATURE

Intraocular fetal vasculature is a complex network of blood vessels that supply and nourish the developing anterior, intermediate, and posterior regions of the eye during intrauterine growth. Components of the fetal vasculature include the hyaloid artery, tunica vasculosa lentis, and a pupillary network [iridohyaloid and capsulopupillary artery]. These vessels develop by the process of vasculogenesis and, in the large majority of cases, undergo spontaneous dissolution at specific time intervals, long before the newborn is delivered. In some, however, their remnants could be discernible as Mittendroff's dot and Bergmeister's papillae on the posterior capsule of the lens and optic nerve head, respectively. These are detected incidentally, minor in nature, and do not lead to any pathological sequelae. In rare instances, the fetal vasculature fails to dissolute and leads to major sequelae, jeopardizing postnatal development of the eyeball as well as VA. This condition is referred to as persistent fetal vasculature [PFA]. In the past, a commonly used terminology for this was persistent hyperplastic primary vitreous (PHPV). In almost 90% of infants, the condition is unilateral and may be associated with persistent pupillary membrane, congenital cataract, macular ectopia, retinal drag, retinal fold, vitreous opacification, coloboma, optic disc hypoplasia, retinal detachment, and retinal disorganization. Some genetic anomalies [trisomies 13, 15, and 18] and systemic associations [neurofibromatosis] may be present in bilateral cases but not in typical unilateral PHPV. In bilateral cases, a rare variant called MPPC syndrome [microcornea, posterior megalolenticonus, PFA, and coloboma] must be considered. In this syndrome, the posterior lenticonus is sometimes said to be so large as to occupy the majority of the vitreous cavity. The usual presenting features are facial asymmetry [orbital], leukocoria, and microphthalmos. Important differential diagnoses to consider are ROP and FEVR. PFV has been classified into anterior, posterior, and combined forms, and recognizing this is important because it has a bearing on the long-term prognosis and in making management decisions. Each of these anatomical types has been further subdivided based on severity into mild and severe. Anterior PFV is characterized by an isolated dense retrolental plaque [cataract may or may not be present] and is termed mild when there is no involvement of the ciliary process and severe if there is. In posterior PFV, there is a stalk of hyaloid artery remnant running anteroposteriorly within the vitreous cavity and no attachment to the crystalline lens. It is mild when optic nerve traction and macular distortion are negligible and severe when it is significant. Combined anterior–posterior has features of both types and could again be either mild or severe. In some children, spontaneous vitreous haemorrhage and complex retinal detachment may be the presenting features.

Age is an important predictor of visual outcome and surgery; if its benefits are considered to outweigh the risks [based on severity of the condition], it must be planned before the critical time frame for postnatal visual development [6–10 weeks]. In anterior PHPV, both the mild and severe forms, lensectomy, removal of the plaque, and limited anterior vitrectomy [using small-gauge instruments] are important in early postnatal life to restore the visual axis. Most cases being unilateral, post-surgery optical rehabilitation remains challenging, and poor visual recovery due to amblyopia is high. As a result, every attempt is now made to place an intraocular implant in the capsular bag or sulcus at the initial surgery. In severe cases, surgery may prevent progression to phthisis bulbi. Posterior PHPV is normally detected beyond the amblyogenic period. If mild, the most prudent approach is periodic observation with a plan to intervene if further progression is noted. If severe, vitrectomy is advocated with the objective of reducing the risk of phthisis and glaucoma. The possibility of visual recovery is almost negligible. In combined PFV, it may be useful to first manage the anterior component surgically and then decide on a plan for the posterior component based on its severity. Preoperative USG may be a useful predictor of the posterior component. Nevertheless, the severity should be confirmed intraoperatively using an indirect ophthalmoscope or endoilluminator and wide-angle viewing of the posterior segment. Surgery for the posterior component should only proceed if it is likely to reduce the long-term risks of phthisis or glaucoma. In a one-stage surgery for combined PFV, it is helpful to insert the lens [non-foldable] through a superior scleral tunnel or postpone IOL implantation to a later date. Trocar and cannula entry site must be chosen [between 0.5 and 2.00 mm based on age, axial length, and lens status] carefully [see section on paediatric retinal detachment]. If single-stage surgery is planned, it is useful to place these before addressing the anterior component. However, infusion must be turned on only after the pupillary axis is cleared and the cannula opening is confirmed to be within the vitreous cavity. Removal of the vitreous, hyaloid, and abnormal attachments must be carried out cautiously, as in ROP surgery, and all efforts to prevent an iatrogenic break must be made. Creation of an iatrogenic break at surgery is an ominous event and enhances the risk and speed of progression to phthisis. No vitreous tamponade is generally recommended if the traction has been relieved uneventfully. The stalk and abnormal attachments are likely to be vascularized and so need to be adequately closed using diathermy before actual resection. Some surgeons recommend the use of endoscope-assisted vitrectomy to safely visualize and resect membranes close to the retinal periphery and ciliary processes. The need for ablation of the peripheral retina in the absence of a retinal tear is debatable.

11.10   POSTERIOR SEGMENT DRUG DELIVERY DEVICES

Chronic diseases of the retina and choroid such as age-related macular degeneration [ARMD], diabetic retinopathy, and chronic non-infectious uveitis are extremely challenging to manage in the long term. This is largely because delivery of drugs to the posterior segment of the eye has to overcome numerous anatomical and physiological barriers to achieve an effective and sustained concentration of the drug within the vitreous cavity, retina, and choroid. While intravitreal injections have been effective, repeated breach of the ocular coat increases the risk of endophthalmitis, traumatic cataract, increased IOP, intraocular haemorrhage, and retinal detachment. In addition, there are an added economic burden and time crunch with repeated intravitreal injections. In this background, the most appropriate solution seems to reside in the availability of safe and effective sustained drug delivery devices. These devices should be biologically and chemically inert, should be devoid of immediate and late procedure-related complications, must not impede optical clarity of the vitreous, must not obstruct the central visual field, must have an ease of surgical insertion and removal [or be biodegradable], and must be affordable. An ideal drug delivery device fulfilling all of these criteria is yet to become commercially available. An ideal solution for port-side sustained release drug delivery could be an inflatable drug reservoir [see section of port delivery system].

Drug delivery devices could be biodegradable or non-biodegradable, matrix or reservoir type, implantable or injectable type, and macro-implants or micro-implants. Non-biodegradable implants can provide more controlled and sustained drug release than the biodegradable implants but may be costlier to manufacture and may need removal in the event of a serious adverse event. Reservoir-type implants release the drug slowly [hence are used to treat chronic conditions], while matrix-type implants release the drug rapidly [hence are used to treat acute conditions]. Injectable implants may be delivered as an outpatient procedure, while implantable devices may need short-term admission as their placement into the vitreous cavity is more complex. Nonbiodegradable implants include Vitrasert, Retisert, and Iluvien; Posurdex is the only commercially available biodegradable implant for managing retinal disorders.

Vitrasert (Bausch & Lomb) was the first non-biodegradable sustained drug delivery device approved by the Food and Drug Administration [FDA] in 1996 for treatment of cytomegalovirus [CMV] retinitis in patients with AIDS. This implant contains 4.5 mg of ganciclovir [which inhibits viral DNA replication] in a 1-mm-thick, 2.5-mm-diameter tablet. The tablet is coated by polymers, polyvinyl alcohol [PVA] and ethylene vinyl acetate [EVA], which control the drug release. For implanting this device, an anchoring suture is first preplaced through a hole at one end of the base, and then the implant plate is inserted into the vitreous cavity through a 5- to 6-mm full-thickness pars plana incision. The two ends of the anchoring suture are then passed through the scleral lips of the incision and tied firmly in place. The scleral wound is closed using absorbable sutures followed by closure of the localized peritomy. Drug release occurs at a rate of 1.4 µg/hour over 9 months. Several complications are associated with implantation, including endophthalmitis, vitreous loss, intraocular haemorrhage, hypotony, cataract, retinal detachment, extrusion of the implant, and implant dislocation. In the pre–highly active antiretroviral therapy [HAART] era, Vitrasert doubled the time to disease progression compared to treatment with intravenous ganciclovir [214 days vs. 104 days] and was hence routinely implanted despite its known disadvantages and limitations [e.g., of being unable to prevent CMV retinitis in the fellow eye]. Subsequently, when HAART therapy was introduced, Vitrasert was found to be less effective than systemic therapy in reducing disease dissemination. This device is hence no longer commercially available.

Retisert [Bausch & Lomb] is the first FDA-approved non-biodegradable sustained-release fluocinolone acetonide implant for the treatment of chronic non-infectious uveitis. The implant consists of a pellet [carrying 0.59 mg of fluocinolone acetonide] enclosed in a silicone cup with a semipermeable release orifice. The silicone cup is attached to an anchoring suture strut with a silicone adhesive. It is placed into the vitreous cavity in a manner similar to that described for Vitrasert but with a smaller pars plana scleral incision size of small 3–4 mm [Video 11.1]. Flucinolone acetonide is released at a rate of 0.3–0.4 µg/day over a period of 2.5 years. Procedure-related complications include implant expulsion, migration of the implant, and wound dehiscence. Dissociation of the pellet during surgical implantation and late spontaneous dislocation of the implant have been observed by the author and have also been reported by others. Other complications observed by the author include hypotony, transient vitreous haemorrhage, and retinal detachment. Retisert was approved for treatment of non-infectious chronic uveitis but is sometimes used off label in patients with persistent diabetic macular edema [DME].

Iluvien [Alimera Sciences Products] is an elegant injectable, sustained-release device carrying fluocinolone acetonide as the active compound. The drug is compacted into a small cylindrical polyimide tube, 3.5 mm in length and 0.37 mm in diameter. A total of 0.19 mg of the drug gets released at the rate of 0.23–0.45 µg/day over 18 to 36 months. No major surgical incisions are needed, and the device can be injected directly into the eye across the pars plana using a prefilled, 25G needle injector. Post-injection, the implant may behave like a foreign body in the vitreous cavity, and this possibility has to be explained to the patient beforehand. For this reason, it may be preferable to inject this device in the inferotemporal quadrant. Although the device was approved by FDA for treatment of DME in 2014, it is yet to become available in several countries.

Posurdex is a sustained-release dexamethasone posterior segment drug delivery system [Allergan]. It is composed of biodegradable copolymer containing micronized 700-µg dexamethasone. The drug–copolymer complex gradually releases the total dose of dexamethasone over a period of 3–6 months after insertion into the vitreous. It has been approved by FDA for treatment of macular edema in retinal vascular occlusions [RVOs], non-infectious posterior uveitis, and DME. It is injected transconjunctivally via a 22-gauge preloaded applicator through the pars plana. The implant may create a sensation of a foreign body in the visual field, and the patient needs to be informed of this possibility before the injection. Owing to the larger gauge of the needle, some vitreous herniation is noted through the injection site in a significant number of patients. Care should hence be taken to displace the conjunctiva before injection to prevent a direct tract. Rare complications that could occur with this implant include displacement of a prior implant skeleton from the periphery into the central vitreous and impaction of the implant into the retina. The former can be prevented by avoiding the same site of injection whenever it is repeated. Impaction into the retina occurs due to a fault during the procedure wherein the 'stop stick' is removed after entry of the needle into the vitreous cavity and with pressure on the release button. This faulty method increases the velocity at which the implant is released from the injector.

11.11 SURGERY FOR NON-INFECTIOUS UVEITIS

Uveitis, particularly intermediate and posterior forms, have a propensity to result in secondary affliction of the vitreous and retina. This could vary from cystoid macular edema that can be managed by medical therapy to other pathologies like vitreous haemorrhage, vitreous opacification from inflammatory membranes, epiretinal membrane, macular hole, tractional retinal detachment, rhegmatogenous detachment, and combined traction–rhegmatogenous detachment. Anterior vitrectomy may have a useful role in certain patients with severe and chronic anterior uveitis, as in the uveitis of juvenile rheumatoid arthritis. Vitrectomy is also sometimes used for obtaining samples by the procedure of vitreous biopsy. No two uveitis cases behave similarly, so the approach must be rationalized, taking into consideration the benefits (in terms of vision potential) vis-à-vis the risks. The need for vitreous surgery in non-infective uveitis seems infrequent, as is highlighted by the fact that although there are several reports in literature, most have a small sample of patients. The indications for vitrectomy in uveitis include vitreous haemorrhage, disabling vitreous membranes, resistant vitritis, epiretinal membrane, macular hole, tractional retinal detachment, rhegmatogenous retinal detachment, combined tractional–rhegmatogenous detachment, lens-induced uveitis, dislocated posterior segment drug delivery devices, remove parasitic cysts [cysticercosis, subretinal worms in diffuse unilateral subacute neuroretinitis (DUSN), hydatid cyst], and to obtain vitreous sample

(Vitreous biopsy). Vitreous haemorrhage occurs in conditions like pars planitis and uveitic entities known to produce secondary vasculitis as in serpiginous choroidopathy and acute posterior multifocal placoid pigment epitheliopathy or neovacularization as in sarcoidosis and Behcet's disease. Vitreous haemorrhage is also a frequent presentation in patients with idiopathic retinal vasculitis and neuroretinitis [IRVAN] syndrome. Extensive vitreous membranes may be seen following severe attacks of intermediate uveitis, acute retinal necrosis, and Behcet's disease. Such membranes may also be the presenting feature in patients with intraocular lymphoma, a frequently underdiagnosed cause of masquerade syndrome.

The benefits of vitreous surgery in uveitis include restoration of media clarity, relief from vitreomacular distortions due to epimacular membranes as well as tractional detachment, reattachment of the retina, removal of an etiological agent [e.g., parasite], and identification of a pathology [e.g., intraocular lymphoma]. In some situations, it may be useful to perform vitreous surgery for uveitis under steroid cover, similar to that recommended for cataract surgery. Contrary to the prevailing thought, we believe that surgery for intraocular cysticercosis does not need any systemic preoperative and postoperative corticosteroids. In addition, it may be also important to perform surgery when there is no active systemic disease [e.g., in Behcet's disease] and ocular flare up. There are several factors that need to be taken into consideration before planning vitreous surgery in patients with uveitis. One must revisit the possibility of associated systemic conditions that can be treated medically before advising surgery. This is particularly so if the patient has been referred following workup elsewhere with a diagnosis of non-responsive uveitis. There have been situations in which patients with worsening inflammation, despite high doses of corticosteroids for presumed intermediate uveitis, have been referred for vitrectomy and repeat clinical examination revealed the cause of vitritis to be secondary syphilis. Also, surgery should be offered to patients with Behcet's disease only if the inflammation does not respond to biologic modifiers like infliximab. Before vitrectomy, one must exercise the option of treatment with sustained-release drug implants like Iluvien. Unless the inflammation is intractable and resistant to the best tolerated medical therapy, one must avoid vitreoretinal surgery in the very young. Intraocular surgeries in such eyes are known to affect ocular growth; optical rehabilitation and amblyopia management are needed, and treatment of secondary complications like cataract, glaucoma, and retinal detachment also needs consideration. These patients may also need frequent examination under anaesthesia. *Toxocara* infection can present as endophthalmitis, and often such children are misdiagnosed as presumed posttraumatic or metastatic endophthalmitis and subjected to surgery. This situation could be avoided by a good ultrasound evaluation and assessing initial response to corticosteroids.

Low IOP is a well-recognized sequela of various uveitis. The cause may be due to decreased cilary body secretion from severe inflammatory insult, ciliary body detachment due to formation of a cyclitic membrane or to ciliary body atrophy. Hypotony secondary to cyclitic membrane may respond well to vitreous surgery and resection of the membrane. Satisfactory improvements in VA and IOP have been reported after vitreous surgery [and silicone oil tamponade] in eyes with chronic hypotony. However, our observation is that such improvement is frequently transient. In the presence of severe hypotony, vitreous surgery demands more caution. As there could be difficulty in placing small gauge cannula, it would be preferable to use a 6-mm, 20G infusion cannula after making an entry with an MVR blade. After ascertaining that the tip of cannula is within the vitreous cavity, the IOP can be restored by switching on the infusion. The other two sclerotomies may be made in the usual manner once the IOP is normalized.

Patients with chronic uveitis are likely to have well-formed broad-based synechiae. Attempts to release such synechiae must be made only if the view under wide-angle lenses is inadequate for completion of vitreous surgery. If a decision to release the synechiae is made, it must be performed with small incision and instruments, avoiding intraoperative hypotony or pressure fluctuations. Blunt handling of the iris worsens postoperative inflammation. Gently passing a Healon cannula beneath the iris, injecting some viscoelastic, and then making gentle lateral movements may sometimes undo the posterior synechiae. Iris hooks may be helpful in selective cases, while microspincterec-tomies are infrequently necessary. It is common to find a very fine inflammatory membrane overly-ing the pupil in both phakic and pseudophakic eyes of patients with uveitis. Inflammatory debris on the anterior surface of the IOL may sometimes be cleared effectively by YAG sweeping before posterior segment surgery. Often, however, such membranes have to be removed or peeled to allow proper visualization. Membranes that are well formed need removal with microforceps. Often, it is noticed that beneath the pupillary membrane, the crystalline lens is devoid of significant opacities. This observation helps in avoiding needless removal of the crystalline lens. Inflammatory mem-branes are also frequently encountered in the anterior vitreous and behind the posterior capsule of the lens in patients with intermediate uveitis and sometimes in posterior uveitis. In pseudophakic eyes these membranes are easily removed with the vitreous cutter. In phakic eyes, however, there is a potential risk of lens touch and so removal of such membranes needs more caution. Gentle suction in the aspiration mode to create a 'safety zone' away from the crystalline lens followed by removal with actuation of the cutter is sometimes helpful. Hydrodissection of such membranes has also been reported, but its practical utility seems limited.

Complicated cataract is a frequent sequelae of uveitis and is likely to hamper visualization dur-ing vitreous surgery. The options that can be exercised are a two-stage surgery versus combined surgery. Small incision phacosurgery or microincisional surgery is again the preferred approach to remove the lens opacity. As early and significant opacification of the lens capsule develops in uveitic eyes, large anterior capsulotomy should be preferred, as well as good capsular polishing. In-the-bag placement of a foldable IOL (non-silicone) is recommended. IOL insertion is to be con-sidered in all cases as it helps maintain compartmentalization and reduces the risk of formation of iridocapsular adhesions. One must, however, avoid silicone IOLs. The superiority of heparin coated IOLs is not well established. It is prudent to prefer lensectomy and anterior vitrectomy over lens aspiration, IOL implantation, and capsulectomy in children with juvenile idiopathic arthritis-associated chronic uveitis. Patients with uveitis are also likely to have significant capsular opaci-fication following cataract surgery. YAG capsulotomy should be considered in milder grades of opacification. Often, however, the membrane is thick and needs removal by pars plana membra-nectomy using a vitrector. Excessive suction and repeated attempts at clearing peripheral opaci-fication must be avoided. Once adequate visualization in achieved in this manner, the posterior segment and ciliary zone must be reassessed intraoperatively with wide-angle lens visualization and scleral indentation. Decision on the benefits and risks of any further surgical steps must be calibrated accordingly.

A characteristic feature of intraocular inflammation is formation of inflammatory membranes. These membranes may be mistaken during preoperative evaluation (during fundus examination and by USG) as a detached posterior hyaloid. In addition, there is a higher prevalence of vitreoschisis in these situations. This pathoanatomy has to be well understood by surgeons lest they presume these to be indicators of complete PVD. If true PVD remains unachieved or undetected, significant poste-rior cortical vitreous is likely to remain resulting in persistence of CME and inflammatory media-tors. One must, however, avoid excessive use of suction in an attempt to induce PVD in patients with cystic changes at the fovea and in the presence of active retinal inflammation. Injection of intravit-real triamcinolone during vitreous surgery not only helps in visualization of the vitreous but may also aid in better control of postoperative inflammation. One must aim for vitreous removal that is 'safe' and avoid aggressive removal, particularly in the periphery. High cut rates must be used with just adequate suction. The periphery must be examined 360 degrees with indentation before per-forming air-fluid exchange. Although sutureless small-gauge surgery is very effective for vitreous surgery in patients with uveitis, it is preferable to suture all the ports. This is to reduce the increased risk of postoperative hypotony in these patients.

Outcomes of vitreous surgery in patients with uveitis is influenced significantly by the type of uveitis [e.g., patients with intermediate uveitis seem to have a better prognosis compared to patients with Behcet's disease]. Resolution of CME has been observed varying from 60% to 80% following vitrectomy, and the frequency of relapses and number of medications is also lowered. However, there is an increased risk of cataract progression, low IOP, elevated IOP, vitreous haemorrhage, and retinal detachment [rhegmatogenous, exudative] following surgery. Hence, the risk and benefits of surgery must be explained to the patient and informed consent obtained before vitrectomy is performed.

11.12   SURGERY FOR INFECTIOUS UVEITIS

Acute retinal necrosis syndrome is a rare disease caused by one of the neurotropic human herpes viruses: herpes simplex virus (type 1 or 2), varicella-zoster virus, or Epstein-Barr virus. The American Uveitis Society criteria for diagnosing acute retinal necrosis include focal, well-demarcated, peripheral areas of retinal necrosis; rapid circumferential progression; occlusive vasculopathy with arteriolar involvement; and a prominent inflammatory reaction in the vitreous and anterior chamber. The diagnosis of acute retinal necrosis syndrome is clinical, and the presence of optic neuropathy, scleritis, and pain supports the diagnosis. Immunological status of the patient [immunocompetent or immunodeficient] does not influence the clinical diagnosis of acute retinal necrosis syndrome. The fellow eye becomes involved in about 36% of patients with acute retinal necrosis, usually within 6 weeks of involvement of the first eye. Initial treatment is with intravenous acyclovir or oral valaciclovir, followed a few days later with addition of oral corticosteroids. Intravitreal anti-viral therapy may be helpful in arresting the disease earlier [but bilateral injection must be avoided]. Despite treatment, almost 75% of patients develop retinal detachment in the resolving phase [6–8 weeks]. Detachment results from the formation of multiple breaks at the junction of the necrotic and viable retina. Sieve-like breaks are characteristic and tend to coalesce at surgery. PVD is generally absent, but forceful attempts at creating one during surgery could result in iatrogenic complications. Prophylactic barrage laser was earlier believed to reduce the risk of developing vision-threatening retinal detachment. This has now been discontinued owing to the lack of evidence. The role of early vitrectomy, too, lacks clarity.

CMV is a double-stranded DNA virus belonging to the Herpesviridae family and is an obligatory intracellular organism. Most individuals are exposed to the virus in childhood or early adulthood, but innate immune response mechanism restricts the infection. Although the incidence of exposure increases with age, infection usually remains latent owing to defence mechanisms such as interferon and natural killer cells. CD4+ and CD8+ cells play an important role in virus infection and reactivation. There is positive correlation between CMV retinitis and CD4 lymphocyte count. Retinitis most commonly occurs when the CD4 cells are less than 50/µl. Unlike in HIV/AIDS, CMV retinitis in post organ transplant or in patients with malignancy treated with chemotherapy can occur with normal CD4+ cell counts. In adults, clinical disease most likely results from reactivation of latent infection but may also occur with newly acquired infection. CMV is a rare cause of disease, except in patients with severe immunosuppression because of either HIV/AIDS or pharmacologic immunosuppression following organ transplantation, autoimmune disease, or malignancy. In AIDS, CMV retinitis was a presenting feature in 2% of cases and was known to occur in 20%–30% cases in the pre-HAART era. This incidence has now significantly dwindled after the widespread availability of HAART therapy. Clinical presentation is quite varied, and VA at presentation depends on the zone of retinal involvement. Mild anterior uveitis with fine keratic precipitates may be seen, but there is no significant reaction in the vitreous. Fundus examination reveals areas of retinal whitening and haemorrhages in the affected zone. Some lesions are slowly progressive and indolent and reveal a granular 'demarcation' line between affected and normal retina; other lesions have an aggressive course with significant retinal haemorrhages [tomato ketchup or pizza-pie appearance]. Still others may have a white, mottled appearance. The risk of retinal detachment in CMV retinitis may be lower than that seen following acute retinal necrosis.

Small-gauge surgery is ideally suited to management of these detachments, and it may not be necessary to place an encirclage or scleral buckle. Removal of the hyaloid must be carried out gently and junction of affected and unaffected retina must be adequately lasered. Long-term tamponade with silicone oil is preferable.

Hydatid cysts may be encountered in almost every organ in the body. In humans, liver and lungs are the most common sites. While orbital echinococcosis is seen sporadically, reports of intraocular hydatid cysts are extremely rare. The condition is caused by infestation and lodgement of cysts of the parasite, *Echinococcus granulosis* and *Echinococcus multilocularis*. Two cases with intraocular infestation, both histopathologically confirmed, have been seen by the author. Both were of the paediatric age group, one with no light perception and the other with inaccurate light projection. No retinal details were discernible in both patients and USG revealed the presence of a uniformly anechoic vitreous cavity with the possibility of a thin cystic wall. In the second patient, USG also revealed multiple hyperechoic and freely moving 'bodies' within the posterior part of the vitreous cavity. In the first child, the diagnosis was confirmed on the enucleated specimen. In the second child, vitreous surgery was attempted to identify the diagnosis and salvage the eyeball. At surgery, fluid filling the presumed vitreous cavity was aspirated [and sent for histopathological examination] following which careful attempts were made to dissect the tissue overlying the entire inner surface of the eyeball. This turned out to be the capsule of the hydatid and was found to be tightly adherent and possibly invading the retinal layers. Attempts at dissection were encountered with significant haemorrhage from the underlying tissue and presumed optic nerve head. When further dissection was deemed futile, surgery was stopped after silicone oil tamponade. The confirmation of hydatid cyst was obtained only after study of the aspirated fluid [which revealed multiple scolex with characteristic hooklets].

DUSN is a zoonosis characterized by the presence of a nematode larva in the subretinal space. In the acute phase, there is optic disc edema, vitreous cells, and yellow-white crops of retinal edema at the location of the nematode. Untreated, there is progressive loss of RPE, arterial narrowing, and optic atrophy in the late stages. DUSN is said to occur most frequently in the second to third decades of life. The condition is usually unilateral, and there are no known systemic associations. The most characteristic feature of this disease is recognition of a subretinal helminth. A nematode, however, is visible in only about 25% of reported cases. Retinitis is the characteristic clinical feature and is seen as multiple, focal, yellow-white areas in the deep retina or RPE. They appear in clusters at sites wherein the subretinal nematode lodges and disappear within 7–10 days as the worm migrates elsewhere. Identification of these focal areas of retinitis is considered useful in detection of the worm. In late stages, there is significant visual loss, and fundus examination reveals optic disc pallor, retinal arteriolar narrowing, and focal areas of RPE atrophy. The latter occurs most typically in the paramacular region. The exact nature of the worm causing DUSN has been poorly defined. In endemic areas, two varieties of nematodes have been reported to produce this disease, *Ancylostoma canium* and *Baylisascaris procyonis*. *A. canium* is a frequent cause of cutaneous larva migrans and measures about 400–700 µm. This kind of small nematode has been identified as the cause of DUSN in reported cases from the southeastern United States, the Caribbean, Latin America, and Venezuela. *B. procyonis* is a rare cause of visceral and ocular cutaneous larva migrans and measures about 1000–2000 µm. The larger nematode has been observed as a cause of DUSN in cases reported from the north midwestern United States and Germany. Identification of the worm and direct laser photocoagulation is considered the treatment of choice. Following such treatment in the early stages of the disease, significant improvement in VA has been reported. Whenever the nematode remains undetected, a course of anthelmintics has been suggested, particularly in the presence of significant vitritis. The role of treatment with anthelmintics, however, remains controversial. Some authors have also reported surgical removal of the subretinal nematode, and this is said to enable proper identification of the subretinal nematode.

11.13   ENDORESECTION OF CHOROIDAL MELANOMA

Choroidal melanoma is the most common primary intraocular tumour in adults. They are usually classified as small, medium, and large based on their basal diameter and height [on USG]. These tumours have a low replication rate and so appear to remain dormant for many years. Choroidal melanomas most commonly metastasize to the lungs and liver, but the risk is much lower compared with extraocular melanomas and other malignancies in the body. Optimal therapy for uveal melanoma, however, still lacks consensus with current emphasis being primarily on preservation of globe and secondarily on preservation of vision. Depending on the size and location, choroidal melanomas are often managed using several options like periodic observation, transscleral resection, endovitreal resection, brachytherapy, proton-beam radiation, transpupillary thermotherapy, and enucleation. Endovitreal resection is usually reserved for the management of moderate to large tumours. Various advantages of the endovitreal surgery include complete removal of the tumour, photoablation of microscopic tumour elements under direct observation, preservation of globe integrity, and potential for retaining the vision in some patients. In addition, abundant tissue is available for histopathological and genetic analysis. Some reports have recently indicated comparable outcomes in plaque radiotherapy and endoresection for choroidal melanoma in terms of metastasis and VA, with fewer number of patients developing metastasis in the endoresection group.

Detailed informed consent explaining the objectives, short- and long-term risks, and benefits of the surgery is mandatory before undertaking an invasive procedure, including endovitreal resection, in patients with choroidal melanoma. In a small series of surgeries carried out by the surgeon using 25G small-gauge vitreous surgery, the surgical approach [Video 11.2] consisted of trocar–cannula insertion, tricort-assisted PVD induction and vitreous removal, creation of a drainage retinotomy, fluid and perfluorocarbon liquid [PFCL]–assisted drainage of exudative retinal detachment, laser ablation of the tumour surface, resection of the tumour to scleral base using 25G vitrector, endolaser of the resected area and 360 peripheral retina, and closure with PFCL tamponade for 7–10 days [with supine positioning]. After 7–10 days, delayed direct PFCL–silicone oil exchange was performed. Intraoperatively, choroidal bleeding was controlled by raising the IOP to 60 mmHg at the time of resection. Concurrent hypotensive anaesthesia with mean blood pressure of 80 mmHg was used when possible. The risk of tumour cell dissemination was reduced by using high suction of 600 mmHg and high flow rate. High suction was applied directly near the cutting edge of vitrector facing the tumour mass to aspirate all loose tumour cells. Tissue remnants at the scleral bed and 2 mm beyond the tumour margins were photocoagulated with high power (200–300 mW). Aspirated fluid from the vitrectomy cassettes was sent for histopathological diagnosis immediately after surgery. Intraoperatively, these tumours were surprisingly soft in consistency and the bulk of tumour resection and aspiration was possible without undue resistance. However, tight adherence of the tumour base to the lamina fusca was noted consistently in all patients. The lamina fusca could easily be elevated from the sclera beyond the margins of the visible tumour. This 'sign of adherence' could be used as an end point for base area resection of choroidal melanomas. With the advent of newer minimal-gauge vitrectomy systems, the entire surgery was performed in a close environment and at a very high suction and flow rate, thus minimizing spill-over of tumour cells. Moreover, software-controlled vented gas forced infusion [VGFI] in Constellation responds to any change in IOP within a few microseconds and thus is able to maintain high IOP despite high suction and helps to prevent significant intraocular bleeding and maintains haemostasis [Figure 11.8]. The chances of port site seeding are also minimized because of trocar cannula system compared with previous 20G vitrectomy systems. Postoperatively, these patients need lifelong follow-up for evidence of tumour relapse and distant metastasis using positron emission tomography scan, liver function tests, and chest radiography, in consultation with an oncology specialist. More recently, unexplained fatal air embolism has been reported following melanoma endoresection [even with no use of air during surgery].

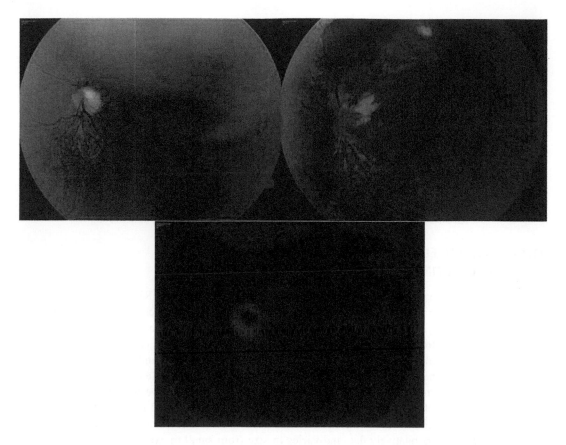

FIGURE 11.8 Preoperative and early postoperative images of a patients following 25G endoresection of a large choroidal melanoma.

11.14   ENDOILLUMINATION- [CHANDELIER-] ASSISTED BIOPSY [FINE-NEEDLE ASPIRATION BIOPSY]

Fine-needle aspiration biopsy [FNAB] is the most commonly used method of biopsy for obtaining tissue samples for histopathological studies. Obtaining tissue for diagnosis becomes necessary in the presence of atypical lesions and diagnostic uncertainty. A total of 2.4% to 10% of intraocular mass lesions diagnosed based on clinical judgement alone or in conjunction with non-invasive methods have a different and often benign histopathological diagnosis. The most widely described methods of FNAB for intraocular mass lesions, in the literature, have been transillumination and visualization with indirect ophthalmoscopy. These methods have a long learning curve and inherent limitations, with increased possibility of complications during the learning curve. One of the reasons for the limited use of intraocular biopsy has been attributed to concerns about serious eye complications. FNAB using chandelier-assisted endoillumination and wide-angle viewing was described by us as a safer and more accurate way of obtaining tissue samples from intraocular tumours. In this approach, two pars plana scleral ports are made using minimally invasive vitreosurgical trocar and cannula. Through one port, the chandelier light source [25G or 23G] is placed [Video 11.3]. A wide-angle contact lens system then provides excellent direct visualization of the choroidal mass under the operating microscope. FNAB of the mass is then obtained through a 24G, 1-inch needle inserted into the vitreous cavity through the second 23G cannula opening. Adequate tissue samples were obtained in all cases in which we have used this approach. As with other approaches, two potential side effects include bleeding from the surface of the retina or intraocular mass and hypotony. We were able to reduce these risks by immediately infusing air into the vitreous cavity through one of the ports [through an infusion line connected to VGFI of the constellation machine] at the conclusion of the procedure. As the aspirating needle passes through the cannula, there is no direct contact with the scleral tissue and the risk of tumour seeding is also reduced.

In the coming decade, FNAB of intraocular lesions is likely to become more widespread due to advances in management based on cytogenetic and molecular analysis of tissue specimens. There is hence a need to have an FNAB skill that is safe, precise, and easy to acquire. In contrast to the conventional techniques of transillumination and indirect ophthalmoscopy, FNAB using small-gauge two-port chandelier illumination and wide-angle viewing is likely to be better accepted, safer, and more precise for most surgeons and patients. This is because retinal surgeons are well trained in the use of microincision vitreous surgery and are unlikely to need any additional learning to perform FNAB.

11.15 COMBINED HAMARTOMA OF THE RETINA AND RETINAL PIGMENT EPITHELIUM

Combined hamartoma of the retina and retinal pigment epithelium [CHRRPE] is a rare, benign tumour formed by an overgrowth of several constituents of the retina such as the RPE cells, vascular elements, and glial components. [Hamartoma is a malformation that consists of a mass of disorganized tissue indigenous to the particular region.] It has a varied clinical appearance and may sometimes simulate intraocular malignancies like retinoblastoma and choroidal melanoma. Neurofibromatosis, incontinentia pigmenti, tuberous sclerosis, isolated café au lait spots, and facial hemangiomas are some of the reported systemic associations. Optic nerve head pit, drusen of the optic nerve, bilateral fundus coloboma, tractional retinoschisis, choroidal neovascular membrane, and full-thickness retinal break are known ocular associations. The tumour usually involves the posterior pole, appears relatively flat, and varies in size from small to extensive. As it involves all germinal layers of the retina, there is significant disorganization of the retinal anatomy. Varying degree of retinal disorganization and vascular tortuosity, in combination with hyperpigmentation of the adjacent RPE, is very characteristic. Intraretinal gliosis, epiretinal membranes, and condensation of the overlying vitreous may also be seen, with one type of tissue often predominating. In severe cases, OCT reveals marked disorganization of the retinal architecture, and individual retinal layers are often not delineated. Visual loss from intraretinal gliosis and epiretinal proliferation is common and may be slowly progressive. Patients in whom progression of visual loss has been documented at follow-up may benefit from vitreous surgery to remove the epiretinal membrane. Unlike idiopathic epimacular membrane, these membranes tend to be more extensive, thick, adherent, and vascular. It may also be more difficult to induce PVD as these are generally young patients. As full-thickness breaks have been reported earlier in association with this hamartoma, careful screening of the retina and prophylactic treatment of such lesions must be undertaken before surgery. Despite successful removal of the epiretinal proliferation, retinal layers remain disorganized at follow-up [Figure 11.9]. This accounts for the less than satisfactory improvement in VA in a large number of these patients.

11.16 INTRAOCULAR LYMPHOMA

Primary intraocular lymphoma [PIOL] is the most common ocular masquerade syndrome. It is a rare form of non-Hodgkin lymphoma and is considered a subtype of primary central nervous system (CNS) lymphoma. PIOL typically presents as a posterior uveitis with nonspecific findings of infiltrative vitritis, vitreous debris, optic nerve infiltration, subretinal infiltration, elevated chorioretinal lesions, and retinal detachment. It is usually bilateral, and the CNS is involved in 60% of cases. There are three main treatment options for PIOL—systemic high-dose methotrexate injection,

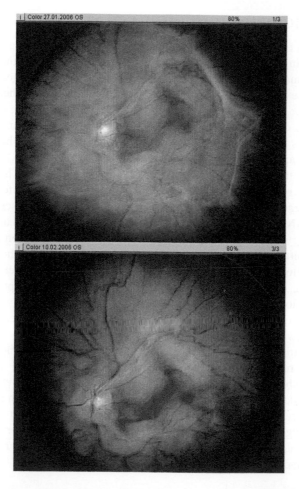

FIGURE 11.9 Preoperative and postoperative photographs of a young patient following surgical removal of the epiretinal component of combined hamartoma of the retina and retinal pigment epithelium.

orbital irradiation, and intravitreal chemotherapy with methotrexate. Therapeutic levels of methotrexate have been reported in the vitreous cavity for almost 5 days after an intravitreal injection compared with a few hours after systemic administration. Hence, repeated intravitreal injection of methotrexate seems to have become accepted as the first line of treatment in patients with primary intraocular lymphoma. Sometimes, however, the tumour cells develop resistance to methotrexate. As a result, there is persistent and worsening vitreous opacification from tumour infiltration into the vitreous cavity. In this situation, we believe that complete vitrectomy using small-gauge instruments is a safe and effective intervention. Diagnostic vitreous biopsy has been in use for several decades as part of the management algorithm of intraocular lymphomas, and no concerns of systemic spread as a result have been raised, unlike with retinoblastoma. In one such patient, we found no vitreal relapse 9 months after therapeutic vitrectomy [tragically, the patient succumbed to complications of CNS lymphoma thereafter]. As there was no PVD, it had to be induced in the standard manner. Other than early development of cataract, no other complications were noted after surgery. The prolonged remission seen in our patient following complete vitrectomy prompts us to wonder whether microincisional therapeutic vitrectomy should become the treatment of choice in patients with the vitreal form of PIOL. Observations from a larger number of patients comparing intravitreal methotrexate versus primary vitrectomy would be warranted to arrive at a firm conclusion.

11.17 IDIOPATHIC RETINAL VASCULITIS AND NEURORETINITIS

IRVAN is a rare form of retinal vasculitis of unknown aetiology that is characterized by the presence of multiple leaking aneurysmal dilatations along the arteriolar tree and over the optic nerve head. Rapid changes may be noted in the clinical picture in terms of emergence of new aneurysms and regression of pre-existing ones. The condition typically affects young, healthy individuals with a female predominance and is not associated with any systemic abnormalities. The presenting clinical symptom in these cases is diminution of vision either due to macular exudation or vitreous haemorrhage. Vitreous haemorrhage is a sequelae to proliferative changes that evolve secondary to extensive peripheral capillary non-perfusion. In contrast to Eales' disease, which forms the main differential diagnosis, the vasculitis in IRVAN is predominantly arterial. The presence of multiple aneurysms along the arteriolar tree and on optic nerve head, which are better appreciated on fluorescein angiogram, readily distinguishes IRVAN from other types of vasculitis. The aneurysms associated with IRVAN typically measure between 75μ and 300μ in diameter with a triangular or 'Y'-shaped morphology. A therapeutic protocol for IRVAN has not yet been established. Systemic corticosteroids have little effect on the progression of the condition and should be used, if at all, only for a short duration. The role of photocoagulation for treatment of peripheral capillary non-perfusion is uncertain. At present, the consensus is to follow up with asymptomatic patients and to initiate photocoagulation when retinal neovascularisation develops.

The disease is frequently bilateral and macular exudation is a consistent feature. In the presence of non-resolving vitreous haemorrhage, standard small-gauge vitreous surgery with endolaser is indicated. Proliferation is usually indolent, less extensive, and flat compared to patients with proliferative diabetic retinopathy. Hence, it is possible to safely separate the hyaloid at surgery [if complete PVD is absent preoperatively]. We have noted spontaneous but gradual resolution of macular exudation following vitrectomy [to clear vitreous haemorrhage] in a patient with IRVAN and non-resolving vitreous hemorrhage. Hence, aggressive treatment with intravitreal corticosteroids and anti-VEGF agents may not be necessary in these patients, after vitrectomy. In some cases, we have also documented significant vitreomacular traction and epimacular membrane formation, necessitating their removal by vitreous surgery.

11.18 VITREOUS AMYLOIDOSIS

Familial amyloidosis polyneuropathy (FAP) is an autosomal-dominant disorder characterized by extracellular amyloid deposition in nerves (sensorimotor and autonomic polyneuropathy), solid organs, and the eyes. It is caused by a single amino acid substitution of methionine for valine at position 30 of transthyretin (TTR), an abundant transport protein. Interestingly, liver transplantation potentially cures patients with TTR-related FAP because TTR is mainly produced in the liver. In the eye, production of amyloid from RPE causes its deposition in the vitreous cavity. Opacification of vitreous is a known clinical manifestation of FAP caused by amyloid deposition in the vitreous, leading to progressive decrease in VA. The incidence of vitreous opacities in FAP varies from 5.4% to 35%, and the amount and density of these opacities determine the VA and symptoms. Vitreoretinal amyloidosis manifests as 'lacy', 'cobweb-like', 'sheet-like' or 'stringy' veils of gray or yellowish-white material in the vitreous. Pseudopodia lentis, punctate dots on the posterior capsule resembling amoeboid foot processes, are considered pathognomonic of vitreoretinal amyloidosis. Amyloid deposits may appear to arise from the perivascular retina, although the retinal vessels themselves appear normal clinically and angiographically.

Management of vitreous amyloidosis requires small-gauge vitrectomy. Various reports have described vitrectomy as a safe treatment modality for vitreous amyloidosis. While visual recovery is substantial, chances of relapse persist. The challenges during vitrectomy in amyloidosis include stronger vitreoretinal adhesions along the blood vessels, equator, and periphery. Intraoperatively, we have found that PVD can be induced relatively easily but only up to the equator and not beyond

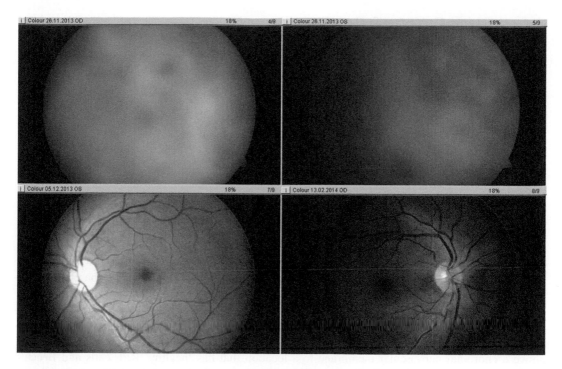

FIGURE 11.10 Fundus images of both eyes of patient with laboratory-confirmed intraocular amyloidosis, before [upper panel] and after surgery [lower panel].

[Figure 11.10]. It has been hypothesized that amyloid fibrils might weaken the vitreopapillary adhesions, leading to easier separation. Owing to possible attachments along the retinal blood vessels, there is a tendency for small, petechial haemorrhages to show up during vitrectomy. These quickly resolve in the early postoperative period without sequelae. Recurrence of vitreous opacities is a known phenomenon and can occur due to dispersion of residual vitreous opacities or continued intraocular production of amyloid fibrils from RPE. Reports indicate that almost 70% of patients who underwent incomplete vitrectomy developed recurrence and needed resurgery, while none of the patients who had undergone complete vitrectomy developed recurrence. Hence, to avoid early recurrence, vitrectomy should be as complete as is safely possible. It is believed that with complete vitrectomy, amyloid monomers are unable to polymerize and do not aggregate, thus reducing the risk of complications.

11.19 INTRALESIONAL DRUG INJECTION IN SUBRETINAL ABSCESS

Endogenous endophthalmitis involves suppurative inflammation of the inner ocular coats by an infective focus arising from a systemic source and accounts for 2%–6% of all endophthalmitis cases. Subretinal abscess is an uncommon presentation, accounts for approximately 5% of cases, and represents a more severe form of the disease. Appropriate systemic and local treatment may be helpful, but no standard management guidelines exist. A significant number of patients may need vitrectomy to control the infection and salvage the eye. We believe that subretinal abscess may respond better with intralesional antibiotic injection using a 41G cannula and have observed satisfactory response to this approach. In one such patient, we noted a large subretinal abscess after core vitrectomy. An elevated and relatively less vascular area was identified over the abscess and using a 41G needle [DORC International] vancomycin [0.05 mg/0.05 ml] was directly injected into the abscess [Video 11.4]. After air-fluid exchange, silicone oil [1000 cs] was injected to provide internal tamponade. Minimal subretinal bleed and fluid were noted in the initial postoperative period. By day 10, however, the abscess had shrunk significantly, and there was no evidence of any subretinal fluid. PPV with intravitreal antibiotics has been described as a treatment modality in the management of endogenous endophthalmitis. If the size of the subretinal abscess is smaller than four disc areas, PPV with intravitreal injection of antibiotics could be successful. However, in the presence of a larger abscess, the risk of failure is higher with PPV and intravitreal antibiotics alone. In such cases, internal drainage of the contents of subretinal abscess using conventional retinotomy has been reported. However, there is increased incidence of proliferative vitreoretinopathy and retinal detachment in these cases. Use of a 41G macular translocation needle allows for a minimally invasive means to deliver drugs into the intralesional or subretinal space and may be a useful intervention in patients with subretinal abscess.

11.20 MACULAR TRANSLOCATION

Foveal translocation was an exciting new surgical approach to managing subfoveal neovascular membranes in the era prior to anti-VEGF era. The idea of foveal translocation was based on anecdotal observations that macular heterotopia can be compatible with good visual recovery, especially in cases of operated GRT and in ROP. The technique had first been explored in experimental animals since the 1980s, attempts in humans were extremely limited. The objective in foveal translocation surgery is to physically shift the foveal neurosensory retina away from the 'unhealthy' location above a choroidal neovascular membrane to a location that has 'healthy' RPE cells and Bruch's membrane. The foveal shift achieved in various reports has varied from 300 to 1000 μm. To achieve satisfactory results, it has been recommended that the surgery should be carried out when the neurosensory retina is relatively less damaged.

Two approaches have been tried to obtain foveal translocation; one uses a large retinectomy to induce retinal redundancy, and the other uses scleral shortening. A more recent approach has been to use a scleral buckle in the periphery to induce redundancy and then steamroll the retina, and hence the fovea, to a position away from the subfoveal neovascular membrane.

The method of scleral shortening is claimed to have the advantage of being less invasive as it does not require a large retinectomy. In one report, scleral shortening for foveal translocation has been combined with simultaneous excision of a neovascular membrane. This report also demonstrated anatomic and functional recovery of the fovea following surgery using optical coherence tomography and scanning laser ophthalmoscope microperimetry. The approach in foveal translocation is to surgically induce a redundancy of the retina by retinal separation following either a giant retinotomy [Machemer approach] or by scleral shortening and limited retinotomy [de Juan Jr. approach]. Actual separation of the neurosensory retina from the RPE is obtained by a trans-scleral [external] or trans-retinal [internal] subretinal hydrodissection. This allows the retina to shift physically away from the choroidal neovascularization. In de Juan's approach, the direction of foveal shift is determined by the location and extent of the scleral shortening. After retinal separation, complete vitrectomy is performed followed by pneumo-hydraulic reattachment of the retina and injection of sulphur hexafluoride [SF6] gas. The redundant retina takes the form of a fold running beneath the area of scleral resection and can be seen postoperatively.

Foveal translocation has been performed for subfoveal choroidal neovascularization secondary to myopia, presumed ocular histoplasmosis syndrome, and ARMD. Although clinical reports on foveal translocation are few, the results showed promise. These procedures have a high risk of developing proliferative vitreoretinopathy and a torsional, binocular diplopia [when the angle of retinal rotation is large]. Owing to the success of anti-VEGF therapy in patients with neovascular AMD, this procedure is no longer considered as a necessary intervention.

11.21 SUBMACULAR SURGERY

Technical advances in vitreoretinal surgery enabled the evolution of submacular surgery for choroidal neovascular membranes. The success of submacular surgery in treating cases of presumed ocular histoplasmosis was first reported in the literature in 1991. De Juan and Machemer in 1988 had reported that their attempts at removing submacular scar by vitreoretinal surgery in patients with exudative ARMD was associated with a high incidence of proliferative vitreoretinopathy and disappointing visual results. These differences were attributed to the fact that in the latter study, a large retinotomy and less refined instrumentation were used compared with the small retinotomy and specially designed 31–36G instruments used by Thomas and colleagues. In addition, there was a difference in the aetiology and the location of the subfoveal membranes.

Histopathological studies by Gass have revealed that the nature of the choroidal neovascular membrane in ARMD is different from that secondary to other conditions. He has reported that subfoveal CNV secondary to ARMD is more commonly situated posterior to the RPE (type 1), while in other conditions, it is predominantly anterior to it (type 2). This classification is important to know because of its clinico-pathologic significance and its bearing on the visual outcome following submacular surgery as discussed earlier. It is obvious that attempts at removing a subfoveal neovascular membrane lying posterior to the RPE is technically more demanding and likely to cause greater trauma to the RPE. Experimentally, it has also been found that senescent RPE cells have a lesser capacity to regenerate, and this factor also contributes to the poorer outcome in patients with subfoveal choroidal neovascularization secondary to age-related macular degeneration. Other reports have also shown that the results of submacular surgery in age-related degeneration is less satisfactory than in presumed ocular histoplasmosis and myopia.

Submacular surgery at its inception was stated to have the advantages of being able to treat eyes with not only classic subfoveal neovascular membranes but also those with occult neovascularization and ill-defined margins and the potential to minimize damage to adjacent structures and to limit central visual loss. As for macular translocation, submacular surgery, too, has lost its relevance following the success of anti-VEGF treatment in patients with choroidal neovascularization.

11.22 RETINAL PIGMENT EPITHELIUM TRANSPLANTATION

The role of RPE in the pathogenesis of ARMD remains a matter of continued exploration. Although the molecular defect in ARMD remains unknown, histopathological evidence has revealed that the RPE is an early target of the disease. RPE cells are considered to have a bi-directional effect on the growth of endothelial cells owing to conflicting findings from various studies. One report has shown that these cells can promote endothelial cell proliferation by the production of VEGF under hypoxic conditions. However, there are other studies revealing the ability of RPE cells to prevent proliferation of endothelial cells in newly formed choroidal capillaries and in promoting maturation of aberrant new vessels. It is now established that RPE secretes both VEGF and pigment-derived growth factor.

In AMD, pathological studies have shown progressive changes in the Bruch's membrane, retinal pigment epithelial cells, and overlying photoreceptors. Experimental work undertaken on the Royal College of Surgeons [RCS] rats revealed that photoreceptor atrophy may be prevented for as long as 1 year by transplantation of RPE cells (both homografts and xenografts) into the subretinal space. Hence, efforts have been made to repair the damaged RPE cells by RPE transplantation in both exudative and atrophic forms of ARMD. Results in the exudative form of the disease were not as encouraging as in the atrophic form. Algvese and associates reported 'none of our patients have shown any visual improvement from the surgery and it is difficult to assess whether progression of the disease has been altered'. They also stated that their cases were of advanced disease, and hence if undertaken at earlier stages, the procedure may have been beneficial. Injection of RPE cell suspensions into the subretinal space through 50μ retinotomies rather than 200μ to 500-μ retinotomies [needed for patch transplants] was considered safer. In non-exudative ARMD, they concluded that it was technically feasible to transplant human RPE cells into the submacular space without adversely affecting visual function. RPE graft survival or rejection is dependent on the status of the blood–retinal barrier at the time of transplantation. The risk of rejection has been shown to be higher when the transplant is introduced into the subretinal space after removal of the neovascular membranes than when introduced into an avascular space [when the blood–retinal barrier is intact, as in atrophic form of ARMD]. Studies have shown that graft rejection is likely to occur because RPE cells express major histocompatibility antigens [particularly class I]. Currently, however, RPE transplantation is not a considered option in both neovascular and non-neovascular AMD. With better understanding of the reasons for developing dry AMD [e.g., hypoangiogenesis from RPE dysfunction] and advancements in cell culture techniques, RPE transplantation or its injection into the subretinal space may see a resurgence in the future.

11.23   RADIAL OPTIC NEUROTOMY

Central retinal vein occlusion [CRVO] is the most common RVO associated with severe visual compromise. Central retinal vein occlusion [CVO] study showed that 20% of all CRVO are ischemic, and around 45% of ischemic CRVO develop iris neovascularization [NVI] and neovascular glaucoma [NVG]. The study showed that there is no effective treatment for these eyes and that panretinal photocoagulation can only reduce occurrence of NVI and NVG. Radial optic neurotomy (RON) was introduced by Opremcak (2008) as a surgical modality for eyes with CRVO, with the hypothesis that in the majority of CRVO eyes, the vascular occlusion occurs at the level of lamina cribrosa, which acts as a tightly closed compartment. RON was believed to help decompress this compartment by transecting the lamina cribrosa at the level of scleral outlet, thus taking care of the hypothesized compartment syndrome. The approach to RON is a standard three port, pars-plana vitrectomy with PVD induction followed by radial incision of the nasal margin of the scleral ring. Care must be taken to avoid the major retinal vessels. A 20G micro-vitreoretinal blade is inserted up to its widest portion posteriorly into the optic disc. A radial incision of this manner is expected to transect the lamina cribrosa. Mild peripapillary and vitreous haemorrhage are likely, and this risk can be reduced by elevating the IOP before making the incision [Figure 11.11]. The earlier enthusiasm for this approach has waned owing to inconsistent results and advent of anti-VEGF–based pharmacotherapy.

11.24   NANOPHTHALMOS-RELATED RETINAL DETACHMENT

Nanophthalmos ['pure microphthalmos] is a disorder characterized by a small eye with good visual function, in the absence of amblyopia. The disorder may be sporadic or have a familial tendency with reports of both autosomal-dominant and recessive inheritance. Nanophthalmos tends to be bilateral and highly hyperopic with refractive errors as high as +20 D. There is no universally accepted value for the axial length at which to designate an eye as being nanophthalmic, but any eye with axial length less than 21 mm should be suspected to have the condition. In addition to exudative retinal detachment, these patients are prone to pupillary block and attacks of angle-closure glaucoma even at a younger age, owing to normal dimensions of the crystalline lens. The sine-qua-non feature of nanophthalmos is sclerochoroidal thickening. The thick sclera is hypothesized to prevent extravasated protein from escaping across the suprachoroidal space. Thick sclera also leads to vortex vein compression, further increasing the risk of outflow obstruction. Both these factors lead to the development of an exudative retinal detachment. Rarely, there is isolated or concurrent choroidal detachment. Scleral thickening is related to a genetic defect that promotes abnormal deposition of glycosaminoglycans within the sclera.

Resolution of the detachment following deroofing of the vortex vein and sclerotomy was first reported by Brockhurst. Subsequently, it was noted that partial-thickness sclerectomy alone

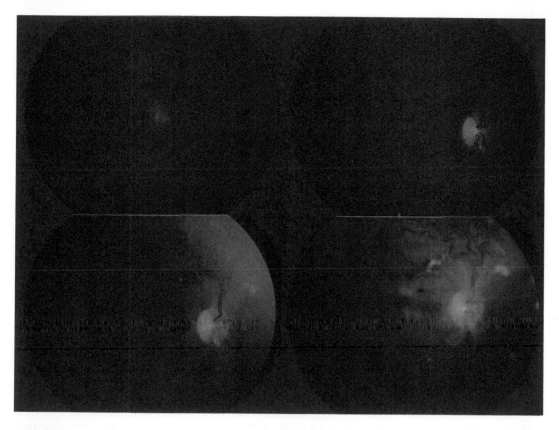

FIGURE 11.11   Sequential changes in the retinal vasculature after radial optic neurotomy over a period of 3 months.

at the equator brings about a steady resorption. The operative procedure starts with peritomy and bridle of the recti muscles. An area measuring 5 mm × 4 mm is marked over the region of the equator [with the anterior margin about 3 mm from the spiral of Tillaux] in two or more quadrants. Scleral flap is cautiously raised in the demarked area using a surgical blade braker or crescent blade. As the sclera is thickened, sclerectomy may have to be completed in layers so as to ensure an adequate dissection. The end point of dissection is indicated by the appearance of a violaceous hue at the sclera bed [due to the underlying choroidal vasculature]. Care must be taken to avoid penetration into the suprachoroidal or subretinal space. Local application of mitomycin C 0.02% solution [2 minutes using Merocel sponge] on the bed of the dissected sclera [followed by copious irrigation with normal saline] may improve the long-term results. [The scleral flap may be sent for pathological or microscopic studies.] The conjunctiva and tenon are then secured using Vicryl sutures. Resolution of retinal detachment occurs gradually over several weeks to months.

SUGGESTED READING

1. Teoh SC, Mayer EJ, Haynes RJ, Grey RH, Dick AD, Markham RH [2008]. Vitreoretinal surgery for retinal detachment in retinochoroidal colobomata. *Eur J Ophthalmol.* 18(2): 304–308.
2. Hocaoglu M, Karacorlu M, Ersoz MG, Sayman Muslubas I, Arf S [2019]. Outcomes of vitrectomy with silicone oil tamponade for management of retinal detachment in eyes with chorioretinal coloboma. *Retina.* 39(4): 736–742.
3. Gopal L, Badrinath SS, Sharma T, Parikh SN, Shanmugam MS et al [1998]. Surgical management of retinal detachments related to coloboma of the choroid. *Ophthalmol.* 105(5): 804–809.

4. Wu W, Lai C, Lin R et al [2011]. Modified 23-gauge vitrectomy system for stage 4 retinopathy of prema-
    turity. *Arch Ophthalmol.* 129(10): 1326–1331.
5. Klufas MA, Patel SN, Chan RVP [2014]. Surgical management of retinopathy of prematurity. In: Oh
    H, Oshima Y (Eds) *Microincision Vitrectomy Surgery.* Emerging Techniques and Technology, Dev
    Ophthalmol, Basel, Karger, vol. 54, 223–233.
6. Clarke B, Williamson TH, Gini G, Gupta B [2018]. Management of bacterial postoperative endophthal-
    mitis and the role of vitrectomy. *Surv Ophthalmol.* 63(5): 677–693.
7. Dib B, Morris RE, Oltmanns MH, Sapp MR, Glover JP, Kuhn F [2020]. Complete and early vitrectomy
    for endophthalmitis after cataract surgery: An alternative treatment paradigm. *Clin Ophthalmol.* 14:
    1945–1954.
8. Venkateswaran N, Cernichiaro-Espinosa LA, Negron C, Fallas B, Zhou XY et al [2018]. Subretinal cys-
    ticercosis extraction with bimanual, 3-D, heads-up-assisted pars plana vitrectomy: Clinicopathological
    correlation and surgical technique. *Ophthalmic Surg Lasers Imaging Retina.* 49(9): 708–711.
9. Sharma T, Sinha S, Shah N, Gopal L, Shanmugam MP et al [2003]. Intraocular cysticercosis: clinical
    characteristics and visual outcome after vitreoretinal surgery. *Ophthalmol.* 110(5): 996–1004.
10. Sen P, Singh N, Rishi E, Bhende P, Rao C et al [2020]. Outcomes of surgery in eyes with familial exuda-
    tive vitreoretinopathy associated retinal detachment. *Can J Ophthalmol.* 55(3): 253–262.
11. Huang L, Liang T, Lyu J, Jin H, Zhao P [2021]. Clinical features and surgical outcomes of encircling
    scleral buckling with cryotherapy in familial exudative vitreoretinopathy-associated rhegmatogenous
    retinal detachment encircling buckling for FEVR-RRD. *Retina.* PMID: 34393211.
12. Avci R, Yilmaz S, Inan UU, Kaderli B, Cevik SG [2017]. Vitreoretinal surgery for patients with severe
    exudative and proliferative manifestations of retinal capillary hemangioblastoma because of von Hippel-
    Lindau disease. *Retina.* 37(4): 782–788.
13. Gaudric A, Krivosic V, Duguid G, Massin P, Giraud S, Richard S [2011]. Vitreoretinal surgery for severe
    retinal capillary hemangiomas in von Hippel-Lindau disease. *Ophthalmol.* 118(1): 142–149.
14. Venkatesh P, Takkar B [2019]. Proposed classification system for retinal capillary angiomatosis.
    Ophthalmic Res. 61(2): 115–119.
15. Pastor-Idoate S, García-Arumí Fusté C, García-Onrubia L, Copete S, García-Arumí J [2020]. Surgical
    options for optic disc pit maculopathy: Perspectives and controversies. *Clin Ophthalmol.* 16(14): 1601–1608.
16. Pastor-Idoate S, Gómez-Resa M, Karam S, Copete S, Kyriakou D et al [2019]. Efficacy of internal limit-
    ing membrane flap techniques with vitrectomy for macular detachment associated with an optic disc pit.
    Ophthalmologica. 242(1): 38–48.
17. Babu N, Kohli P, Ramasamy K [2020]. Comparison of various surgical techniques for optic disc pit
    maculopathy: Vitrectomy with internal limiting membrane (ILM) peeling alone versus inverted ILM
    flap 'plug' versus autologous scleral 'plug'. *Br J Ophthalmol.* 104(11): 1567–1573.
18. Yuksel K, Celik U, Alagoz C, Dundar H, Celik B, Yazıcı AT [2015]. 23 gauge pars plana vitrectomy for
    the removal of retained intraocular foreign bodies. *BMC Ophthalmol.* 16(15): 75.
19. Venkatesh P, Keshavamurthy R, Verma L, Tewari HK [2003]. Removal of metallic intraocular for-
    eign body impacted in the retina by magnetizing the MVR blade using an external magnet. *Clin Exp
    Ophthalmol.* 31(5): 451–452.
20. Bata BM, Chiu HH, Mireskandari K, Ali A, Lam WC, Wan MJ [2019]. Long-term visual and anatomic
    outcomes following early surgery for persistent fetal vasculature: A single-centre, 20-year review. *J
    AAPOS.* 23(6): 327.e1.
21. Zahavi A, Weinberger D, Snir M, Ron Y [2019]. Management of severe persistent fetal vasculature: Case
    series and review of the literature. *Int Ophthalmol.* 39(3): 579–587.
22. Cabrera FJ, Wang DC, Reddy K, Acharya G, Shin CS [2019]. Challenges and opportunities for drug
    delivery to the posterior of the eye. *Drug Discov Today.* 24(8): 1679–1684.
23. Kang-Mieler JJ, Osswald CR, Mieler WF [2014]. Advances in ocular drug delivery: Emphasis on the
    posterior segment. *Expert Opin Drug Deliv.* 11(10): 1647–1660.
24. Giuliari GP, Chang PY, Thakuria P, Hinkle DM, Foster CS [2010]. Pars plana vitrectomy in the man-
    agement of paediatric uveitis: The Massachusetts eye research and surgery institution experience. *Eye.*
    24(1): 7–13.
25. Shin YU, Shin JY, Ma DJ, Cho H, Yu HG [2017]. Preoperative inflammatory control and surgical out-
    come of vitrectomy in intermediate uveitis. *J Ophthalmol.* 5946240.
26. Branson SV, McClafferty BR, Kurup SK [2017]. Vitrectomy for epiretinal membranes and macular
    holes in uveitis patients. *J Ocul Pharmacol Ther.* 33(4): 298–303.
27. Liu S, Wang D, Zhang X [2018]. The necessity and optimal time for performing pars plana vitrectomy
    in acute retinal necrosis patients. *BMC Ophthalmol.* 18: 15.

28. Li AL, Fine HF, Shantha JG, Yeh S [2019]. Update on the management of acute retinal necrosis. *Ophthalmic Surg Lasers Imaging Retina*. 50(12): 748–751.

29. Risseeuw S, de Boer JH, Ten Dam-van Loon NH, van Leeuwen R [2019]. Risk of rhegmatogenous retinal detachment in acute retinal necrosis with and without prophylactic intervention. *Am J Ophthalmol*. 206: 140–148.

30. Nasemann JE, Mutsch A, Wiltfang R, Klauss V [1995]. Early pars plana vitrectomy without buckling procedure in cytomegalovirus retinitis-induced retinal detachment. *Retina*. 15(2): 111–116.

31. García RF, Flores-Aguilar M, Quiceno JI, Capparelli EV, Munguia D et al [1995]. Results of rhegmatogenous retinal detachment repair in cytomegalovirus retinitis with and without scleral buckling. *Ophthalmol*. 102(2): 236–245.

32. Moharana B, Dogra M, Tigari B, Singh SR, Katoch D et al [2021]. Outcomes of 25-gauge pars plana vitrectomy for cytomegalovirus retinitis-related retinal detachment. *Indian J Ophthalmol*. Sept. 69(9): 2361–2366.

33. Sen S, Venkatesh P, Chand M [2003]. Primary intraocular hydatid cyst with glaucoma. *J Pediatr Ophthalmol Strabismus*. 40(5): 312–313.

34. de Souza EC, Nakashima Y [1995]. Diffuse unilateral subacute neuroretinitis: Report of transvitreal surgical removal of a subretinal nematode. *Ophthalmol*. 102(8): 1183–1186.

35. Rojanaporn D, Tipsuriyaporn B, Chulalaksiriboon P, Virankabutra T, Morakul S, Damato B [2021]. Fatal air embolism after choroidal melanoma endoresection without air infusion: A case report. *Ocul Oncol Pathol*. 7(5): 321–325.

36. Venkatesh P, Gogia V, Gupta S, Shah BM [2016]. 25 gauge endoresection for moderate to large choroidal melanoma. *Indian J Surg Oncol*. 7(3): 365–367.

37. Vidoris AAC, Maia A, Lowen M, Morales M, Isenberg J et al [2017]. Outcomes of primary endoresection for choroidal melanoma. *Int J Retina Vitreous*. 6(3): 42.

38. Venkatesh P, Kashyap S, Temkar S, Gogia V, Garg G, Bafna RK [2018]. Endoillumination (chandelier) and wide-angle viewing-assisted fine-needle aspiration biopsy of intraocular mass lesions. *Ind J Ophthalmol*. 66(6): 845–847.

39. van der Sommen CM, van Romunde SHM, van Overdam K [2021]. Surgery for combined hamartoma of the retina and retinal pigment epithelium. *Case Rep Ophthalmol*. 12(3): 778–783.

40. Venkatesh P, Gogia V, Khanduja S, Gupta S, Kumar L, Garg S [2015]. Therapeutic vitrectomy for vitreal recurrence of intraocular lymphoma resistant to intravitreal methotrexate post systemic chemotherapy. *J Cancer Res Ther*. 11(3): 668.

41. Venkatesh P, Keshavamurthy R, Bhaskar V, Garg SP, Tewari HK [2009]. Spontaneous resolution of macular exudation with good visual recovery in idiopathic retinal vasculitis, aneurysms, and neuroretinitis (IRVAN): A case report. *Neuro-Ophthalmol*. 29: 33–37.

42. Venkatesh P, Selvan H, Singh SB, Gupta D, Kashyap S et al [2017]. Vitreous amyloidosis: Ocular, systemic, and genetic insights. *Ophthalmol*. 124(7): 1014–1022.

43. Kakihara S, Hirano T, Imai A, Miyahara T, Murata T [2020]. Small gauge vitrectomy for vitreous amyloidosis and subsequent management of secondary glaucoma in patients with hereditary transthyretin amyloidosis. *Sci Rep*. 10(1): 5574.

44. Venkatesh P, Temkar S, Tripathy K, Chawla R [2016]. Intralesional antibiotic injection using 41G needle for the management of subretinal abscess in endogenous endophthalmitis. *Int J Retina Vitreous*. 2: 17.

45. van Romunde SHM, Polito A, Peroglio Deiro A, Bertazzi L, Guerriero M, Pertile G [2019]. Morphological changes in the diseased retina on a healthy choroid-retinal pigment epithelial complex after full macular translocation for exudative age-related macular degeneration. *Acta Ophthalmol*. 97(2): e283–e289.

46. van Romunde SH, Polito A, Bertazzi L, Guerriero M, Pertile G [2015]. Long-term results of full macular translocation for choroidal neovascularization in age-related macular degeneration. *Ophthalmol*. 122(7): 1366–1374.

47. Skaf AR, Mahmoud T [2011]. Surgical treatment of age-related macular degeneration. *Semin Ophthalmol*. 26(3): 181–191.

48. Romano MR, Valldeperas X, Vinciguerra P, Wong D [2011]. Sub-macular surgery: is still an option for age-related macular degeneration? *Curr Drug Targets*. 12(2): 190–198.

49. Caramoy A, Liakopoulos S, Kirchhof B [2011]. Recurrence of choroidal neovascular membrane after autologous transplantation of RPE and choroid for neovascular AMD. *Acta Ophthalmol*. 89(8): e666–e668.

50. Tsuboi K, Sasajima H, Kamei M [2018]. Chorioretinal shunt vessel in eyes with central retinal vein occlusion after radial optic neurotomy. *Ophthalmol*. 125(9): 1409.

51. Beck AP, Ryan EA, Lou PL, Kroll AJ [2005]. Controversies regarding radial optic neurotomy for central retinal vein occlusion. *Int Ophthalmol Clin.* 45(4): 153–161.

52. Venkatesh P, Majumdar SS, Kakkar A, Singh S, Gogia V, Garg S [2013]. Resolution of serous retinal detachment following partial sclerectomy with mitomycin C in nanophthalmos. *Ophthalmic Surg Lasers Imaging Retina.* 44(3): 287–289.

53. Mansour A, Stewart MW, Shields CL, Hamam R, Abdul Fattah M et al [2019]. Extensive circumferential partial-thickness sclerectomy in eyes with extreme nanophthalmos and spontaneous uveal effusion. *Br J Ophthalmol.* 103(12): 1862–1867.

54. Morris R, Witherspoon CD [1996]. *5th Vail vitreoretinal symposium.* Colorado.

55. Greenwald MJ, Wohl LG, Sell CH [1986 Sep–Oct]. Metastatic bacterial endophthalmitis: A contemporary reappraisal. *Surv Ophthalmol.* 31(2): 81–101.

56. Criswick VG, Schepens CL [1969 Oct]. Familial exudative vitreoretinopathy. *Am J Ophthalmol.* 68(4): 578–594.

57. Opremcak EM [2008 Sep]. Radial optic neurotomy. *Ophthalmology.* 115(9): 1638–1639.

12 Complications in Vitreoretinal Surgery

Similar to pharmacological interventions, every surgical intervention is associated with the risk of adverse events. These adverse events or complications could vary from mild events to severe adverse events [SAEs]. It is the responsibility of the surgeon to discuss the probability of all these risks [particularly of known SAEs] with the patient or guardians and obtain an informed written consent before the surgery. Some of the complications may not be entirely avoidable, but the risk can be lowered by taking adequate precautions before, during, and after the surgery. It is also a good habit to discuss probable complications that we could encounter with our peers or surgical team and get their perspective on how these could be avoided or reduced. This form of proactive discussion of anticipated complications with your seniors would help to minimize the risk by initiating preemptive steps and measures and taking additional precautions. There are several reasons for a complication to occur, and these range from preoperative to intraoperative to postoperative reasons. Preoperative reasons include incomplete history taking, inadequate clinical evaluation, failure to carry out appropriate investigations, wrong interpretation, and lack of discussion [in complex or unusual situations]. Intraoperative reasons include lack of prior mental planning and preparation for possible complications; inadequate comprehension of machine parameters, functioning, and implementation; machine and instrument failure; non-recognition of an incorrect prior step and continuation of the surgery; poor implementation of recommended or standard guidelines; extremely complex and tightly adherent normal-abnormal tissue relationship; assistant related missteps; and loss of patient cooperation during the surgery. Early recognition of a misstep helps prevent a complication altogether or at least prevents it from becoming an SAE. Postoperative complications may relate to lack of patient compliance with the medication, positioning, or other specific instructions; trauma to the eye; and vigorous rubbing of the eye [particularly in children]. Rapid advancements in technology, in particular over the past two decades, have greatly altered the panorama of vitreoretinal surgery by enabling true closed globe surgery. Reduction in port size, one-step entry with a trocar and cannula, and precise control of machine parameters, and their responsiveness in real time have not only improved the safety of surgical interventions but have also led to a significant reduction in the learning curve for vitreoretinal trainees. The latter in turn has further contributed to improved outcomes. A host of complications may occur; the majority are minor and resolve over a few days. Some complications are of greater concern but tend to resolve over weeks to months. However, there are a few complications that are of serious nature because they have the potential to progress and lead to complete loss of vision. These complications include scleral perforation, choroidal haemorrhage, intraoperative retinal tear, retinal detachment, and endophthalmitis.

Discussion regarding complications in vitreoretinal surgery can be approached in multiple ways such as time at which the event occurs (preoperative, intraoperative, or postoperative), the precise surgical step leading to the complication, the reason behind the surgical complication, or by simply listing the complications from the most severe to the minor side effects. Here, a region- or tissue-based approach is adopted for allowing a more complete and systematic coverage of possible complications that may result during or following vitreoretinal surgery. A complete list of complications would include vision and refractive complications [temporary reduction of vision with gaseous vitreous substitutes]; induced myopia, hyperopia, or astigmatism; ocular adnexal complications [ptosis, lid edema]; ocular motility complications [muscle rupture, muscle loss, restricted motility]; conjunctival or episcleral complications [tear, granuloma, retraction, haemorrhage, ingrowth]; corneal complications [epithelial defect, ulcer, band-shaped keratopathy, keratopathy, edema, decompensation];

DOI: 10.1201/9781003179320-13

scleral complications [scleral ectasia, scleritis, scleral abscess, scleral laceration, rupture]; anterior chamber complications [shallow chamber, hyphaema, hypopyon, gas migration, silicone oil migration, perfluorocarbon liquid (PFCL) migration]; pupil complications [inflammatory membrane, synechiae, dilated pupil, large inferior iridotomy]; iris complications [retraction, neovascularization, silicone oil deposition]; IOP complications [hypotony, ocular hypertension, glaucoma]; lens-related complications [lens touch, cataract, lens drop, lens subluxation, zonular dehiscence]; IOL-related complications [IOL subluxation or tilting, IOL drop, IOL–silicone oil adhesion, condensation of vapour, corneal touch]; vitreous-related complications [vitreous incarceration, residual vitreous contraction, endophthalmitis]; retina-related complications [retinal tear, retinal detachment, retinal incarceration, subretinal haemorrhage]; choroid-related complications [serous or haemorrhagic detachment, suprachoroidal air, suprachoroidal oil]; optic nerve–related complications [silicone oil neuropathy, disc pallor, glaucomatous atrophy]; orbital complications [retrobulbar haemorrhage, ecchymosis]; systemic complications [tetany, seizures, subcutaneous dissection of air, CNS migration of silicone oil]; and miscellaneous complications such as compression of ulnar nerve from prolonged postoperative positioning.

Some of these complications are unavoidable [e.g., reduction of vision when gaseous vitreous substitute is used] but must be explained to the patient prior to surgery. This reassures the patient and instills confidence in the surgical team. Complications related to the local anaesthetic injection can be addressed by noting high-risk features during history taking and clinical evaluation [these include anticoagulant use, recent intraocular surgery or trauma repair, cataract surgery, filtering surgery, prior vitrectomy or scleral buckling, high myopia, deep-set eye, one eyed] and taking extra precautions. Ocular adnexal and motility complications can be reduced by using the correct instruments [e.g., holding the conjunctiva with non-serrated forceps], dissecting only the necessary amount of tissue in a gentle manner [e.g., avoid 'rubbing' the muscle and scleral surface needlessly using a cotton swab, shearing the intermuscular septa more than necessary], avoiding abrupt and excessive traction on the extraocular muscles and the Whitnall ligament, recognizing and preventing splitting of the muscle or bridle of the superior oblique fibres, and proper closure of the peritomy at the end of surgery. Corneal complications like epithelial defect can be prevented by cautiously incising the eye drape at the beginning of surgery; maintaining a layer of viscoelastic on the corneal surface; avoiding a focused and high-intensity microscope light for long periods; maintaining tangential pull on the bridle sutures while gaining exposure to the equatorial sclera; resisting steps to debride the corneal epithelium and, if unavoidable, preventing damage to the Bowman's membrane and peripheral epithelium; avoiding high intraoperative IOP for a prolonged time; prophylactically using a dispersive viscoelastic in the anterior chamber when specular counts indicate high risk of corneal decompensation; and using viscoelastic instead of irrigating fluid under the contact lens and placing a bandage contact lens at the end of surgery in case a significant defect is noted at the end of surgery. In patients with diabetes, addition of dextrose to the irrigating fluid is said to lower the risk of corneal edema [and cataract], but this is not routinely practised.

Scleral complications can be avoided by preventing the tenotomy scissors from resting on the scleral surface while gaining exposure to the four intermuscular regions; carefully examining the exposed sclera for thinning, ectasia, and staphylomatous changes before performing indentation to locate and mark the retinal tear or undertaking cryotherapy, recognizing the appearance of any grey-black discoloration of the sclera [due to desiccation from intense light of the surgical microscope]; and immediately hydrating the region and passing the scleral sutures at the correct depth and width with a meticulous approach. In addition, if scleral incision has been extended for any reason [e.g., removal of RIOFB], the port needs to be closed tightly to avoid subsequent pigmented ectasia at the site. Crystalline lens–related complications can be minimized by paying attention to the distance and direction of entry of the scleral ports as well as introduction of intravitreal instruments [particularly curved instruments like scissors or endoilluminators], avoiding vitreous removal and tissue dissection with the instrument crossing the lens equator [safer to swap the instruments in the two superior ports], ensuring that the infusion cannula tip is not partially within the Petit's canal [would enhance the risk of zonular dehiscence], and minimizing anterior vitreous base dissection [preoperatively, if this is found to be absolutely necessary, combined or sequential surgery with phacoemulsification would be a better alternative]. In pseudophakic patients, it is important to note the type of IOL [if made of silicone, vitreous substitute would be limited to the use of gases], integrity of the posterior capsule, degree of capsular opacification, and stability of the capsular bag and IOL during the preoperative workup. Any high-risk instability must be explained to the patient beforehand, including the surgical options available to address this additional surgical challenge. Iatrogenic IOL complications can be minimized by avoidance of making a posterior capsular opening when the visualization is not very compromised, not undertaking excessive anterior dissection with scleral indentation, and avoiding use of high suction close to the capsular bag [in particular, during silicone oil removal].

Intraocular inflammatory and infectious complications like granuloma, abscess [Figure 12.1], buckle infection, intraocular inflammation, and endophthalmitis can be reduced by adhering to stringent protocols of asepsis and sterilization; use of betadine paint and wash; proper use of the surgical drape to keep the eyelashes away from the surgical field; meticulous and atraumatic tissue dissection; avoiding needless disturbance of the anterior chamber, iris, and lens capsule; soaking the buckle material in an antibiotic solution before placing it on the sclera; handling the sutures, buckle, and band using only forceps [avoid handling these directly using fingers]; avoiding excessive cryopexy, laser photocoagulation, and diathermy; preventing hypotony during surgery; minimizing intraocular haemorrhage; and never resorting to mixing of silicone oils. Combining cataract surgery with a vitreous procedure also has an increased risk of postoperative inflammation. The utility of routinely leaving behind or injecting triamcinolone into the vitreous cavity at the surgery to reduce the incidence of postoperative inflammation and proliferation remains contentious.

Other steps important in reducing the risk of surgery-related infections include preventing a direct tract across the conjunctiva into the scleral port and reducing the risk of posterior vitreous wick syndrome [by ensuring conjunctival displacement before placement of the trocar and cannula]; not hesitating to use a suture to close the scleral port whenever there is a suspicion of leak, when silicone oil is used [oil trapped within the track may impede would healing], and in high-risk patients [one eyed, poor lid hygiene and ocular surface, immunosuppressed and patient with diabetes]; meticulous closure of the episcleral tissue and conjunctiva [sometimes in two layers, particularly in the young]; and then irrigating the periocular space in all quadrants with an antibiotic solution.

During retinal detachment surgery, serious complications usually occur during or following external drainage of subretinal fluid. So, one must weigh these risks against the possibility of achieving successful reattachment with a non-drainage procedure. All three approaches to external drainage [scleral cut-down, needle drainage, and modified needle drainage] have the risk of inducing choroidal haemorrhage, subretinal haemorrhage, vitreous haemorrhage, vitreous incarceration,

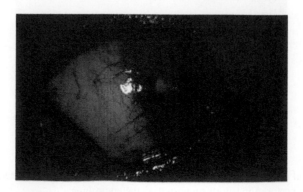

FIGURE 12.1   Scleral abscess in a patient following scleral buckling surgery for retinal detachment.

FIGURE 12.2A   Perforation of the retina by the needle during passage of scleral sutures at retinal detachment surgery.

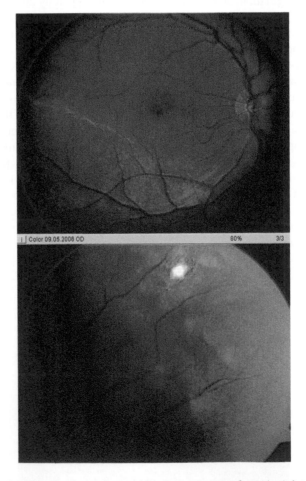

FIGURE 12.2B   Scleral perforation in another patient during surgery for retinal detachment. Unlike that in the previous figure, this perforation is well supported on the encirclage.

retinal incarceration, and retinal perforation. Similar complications may arise due to inadvertent perforation while passing the scleral sutures [Figure 12.2]. Another rare but potential cause of scleral rupture or intraocular haemorrhage is abrupt and sudden withdrawal of the cryotherapy probe [before waiting for it to thaw]. Choroidal haemorrhage may occur as a result of direct trauma with the needle or secondary to sudden hypotony and ocular decompression. The risk of these complications can be minimized by avoiding external drainage whenever possible, choosing the most optimal and safe site for drainage, and maintaining the IOP, both before [on the lower side during drainage by scleral cut down and slightly higher side for needle drainage] and after drainage.

The severity of complications induced is not always evident immediately and may only become manifest in the early days after surgery. So, these patients need a closer follow-up to decide on the subsequent course of action. For limited haemorrhage, no intervention is necessary, but for patients who develop massive submacular haemorrhage, it may become necessary to convert to a vitreoretinal procedure and drain the blood. Non-resolving and massive haemorrhagic choroidal detachments also have to be drained externally or in a combined approach, based on the status of the retina and presence of concurrent vitreous haemorrhage. If vitreous or retinal incarceration is well supported on the buckle and the retina remains attached, nothing further may have to be undertaken, or vitreoretinal surgery will need to be undertaken at the earliest. Retinal perforation alone can be treated with cryopexy, and the site supported by a band or buckle.

Choroidal detachment is the most common complication during the first 2 weeks after conventional retinal detachment surgery with drainage of subretinal fluid, the reported incidence varying form 22% to 44%. Although risk factors are known, the exact mechanism of its occurrence in human eyes is uncertain. Some of the known risk factors include advancing age, myopia, uncontrolled hypertension, head-down positioning of the patient, sudden hypotony, rapid withdrawal of the cryo probe before thawing, compression of the vortex veins, and direct injury to the choroidal vessels while passing scleral sutures or during drainage of subretinal fluid. The risk of choroidal detachment has been shown to increase with an increase in the extent of explant used for buckling. When the extent is less than 90 degrees, the reported incidence is 8%, and when more than 270 degrees, it is about 50%. There is also a definite but ill-defined relationship between the occurrence of choroidal detachment and venous outflow from the choroid. As the number of contributory factors increase, there seems to a corresponding increase in the risk of developing choroidal detachment after retinal detachment surgery. To reduce the risk of contribution by vortex vein compression, we have earlier proposed redesigning of the buckle intraoperatively by creating a notch in the region overlying the vortex vein.

During vitreous surgery, intraoperative complications can result at any stage of the surgery, from making of the scleral ports to closure of the scleral ports. So, the surgeon must be vigilant until the last step of the procedure. Most complications remain minor if recognized early and do not influence the final outcome; failure to recognize missteps and abnormal tissue response [e.g., hypotony and evolving choroidal mounds, due to faulty flow in the infusion line] in a prompt manner may, however, lead to a catastrophic situation. Some of these risks may be related to faulty manufacture [very rare], suboptimal design [e.g., non-beveled end on cannula, opaque shaft of the cannula], recycling of products meant for single use [including trocar and cannula, cutter], faulty application [excessive diathermy or laser], faulty technique and undetected or unanticipated systemic [e.g., anticoagulant use, sickle cell anaemia, spike in blood pressure, sudden coughing or movement], or intraocular pathology [nanophthalmos, pathological myopia, impacted and encapsulated foreign body and intraocular tumour (very rare)].

Complications related to passage of the trocar and cannula include injury to the crystalline lens, peripheral retina, bleeding from the pars plicata, placement of the cannula beneath the epithelium of the ciliary body or subretinal space or within the choroid, and jamming of the instruments [due to a manufacturing flaw–distal opening being marginally narrower than normal diameter, herniation and trapping of dense vitreous haemorrhage into the gap between the shaft of the cannula and the instrument]. The most frequent of these complications is location of the distal opening of the cannula within the ciliary epithelium or subretinal space. Risk factors for this complication include the presence of cilioretinochoroidal detachment, preoperative hypotony, repaired globe perforation, anterior proliferative vitreoretinopathy [PVR] with or without iris retraction, previous buckling surgery [particularly with high indent], endophthalmitis, and dense vitreous haemorrhage [when it may be difficult to visualize the location of the tip]. To avert this complication, it is most important to visualize not only the shining shaft of the cannula but also its distal opening within the vitreous cavity before switching on the infusion valve. Visualization of the tip is normally achieved by indenting the cannula into the vitreous cavity with one hand and simultaneously using an endoilluminator in the other hand to visualize the cannula and its opening, looking from outside the microscope field in a nasal to temporal manner with the surgeon's head tilted to an optimal angle. Sometimes the visualization can also be undertaken seeing through the microscope. If uncertainty still persists, it is very helpful to place the endoilluminator through one of the superior ports [keeping the infusion off] and try to obtain visualization of the infusion tip under a wide-angle lens. Infusion must be switched on only after this is doubly confirmed. Improvements in the configuration of the cannula from an end-on to a beveled design and availability of 6-mm small-gauge infusion tips would also help reduce these complications. Two other important risks related to the technique of making the scleral ports include endophthalmitis [by making the trocar entry without conjunctival displacement] and leakage from the port site at the conclusion of surgery.

After switching on the infusion at the commencement of surgery, air bubble(s) within the tubing [frequently encountered, despite priming of the machine] may flow into the vitreous cavity and get trapped within the fibrils near the periphery. Sometimes attempts to remove these bubbles can endanger the crystalline lens or result in traction on the vitreous base/retina. In the presence of a subluxated crystalline lens, lens notch [in eyes with coloboma], or capsular defect, the air can travel quickly even into the anterior chamber. In this instance, the surgeon would have to make an entry into the anterior chamber to remove the air bubble with the additional risk of its collapse, momentary hypotony, pupillary constriction, and loss of visualization. In addition, viscoelastic may have to be injected into the anterior chamber, a step that can increase the risk of postoperative IOP elevation. Hence, it is best to avoid getting air bubbles from the infusion line at the beginning of surgery. This situation can be avoided, first by physically looking for and removing any trapped air within the tubing. Second, once there is free flow of fluid, the tubing must be pinched at its distal end. The infusion is then stopped, and with the tubing still pinched, the steel tip is inserted into the port assigned for placement of the infusion cannula. Pinching of the tubing in this manner prevents air from reentering [even a small amount] into the tubing [due to negative pressure so generated] when the infusion is stopped. Entry of air into the vitreous cavity can also be prevented by placing the tip into the port with the fluid flowing. However, with this approach, there is risk of subretinal or choroidal infusion as the intravitreal location of the cannula is usually confirmed only after placement of the infusion tubing. Complications related to the infusion line also include hypotony by an inability of the machine to adequately compensate for high outflow of fluid during vitrectomy [if the lower end of the aspiration cassette and tubing are placed significantly higher than the patient's eye level] or by inadvertent pulling out of the tubing [e.g., by assistant during removal of instruments]. Until better designs become available, risk from the latter can be reduced by taping the tubing to the surgical drape.

Rarely, it is found that one or both of the superior ports have also not penetrated into the vitreous cavity and are lying beneath the ciliary epithelium [risk factors are the same as those mentioned earlier]. If this possibility is not recognized and instruments are rapidly introduced, serious damage to the peripheral retina or significant intraocular haemorrhage could result. To avoid this, the surgeon must introduce the endoilluminator and vitrector cautiously during their initial pass into the vitreous cavity under the observation of a wide-field lens. If the cannula is found to be in this location, a new one should be placed [however, there is no certainty that this would definitely go into the vitreous cavity]. Sometimes it may become necessary to perforate the tissue [not retina], which is preventing the instruments from passing into the vitreous cavity using the trocar itself or small-gauge microvitreoretinal [MVR] [23G or 25G if available] or the sharp tip of the diathermy probe. In a pseudophakic eye [and rarely phakic eye], ciliary tissue covering the infusion tip can be carefully teased away using an MVR blade introduced from the opposite port. Vitrectomy is only started once the scleral ports are secured and any possible complications related to them have been ruled out [as mentioned earlier].

The actual process of vitreous removal is very challenging as each surgery shows its own inherent variability. Being a very dynamic process and having multiple components, this step can be associated with some serious complications like creation of a retinal tear or dialysis and intraocular haemorrhage. These complications can occur at multiple times during the procedure, such as induction of PVD, shaving of the vitreous base, and removal of vitreous over detached retina. The risk is higher in paediatric patients, combined traction–rhegmatogenous detachment, tightly adherent hyaloid in the presence of a retinal detachment, posterior migration of the vitreous base [in older adult patients], presence of predisposing lesions like lattice degeneration, thin [e.g., pathological myopia], and atrophic retina and when there is machine [e.g., sudden hypotony] or instrument failure [e.g., inefficient cutting of the vitreous and resultant traction on the retina]. Rarely, these may result from an inappropriate or risky surgical approach. The risk of creating an iatrogenic break can be reduced by following the safest sequence of vitreous removal [port, posterior, posterior vitreous detachment, and then peripheral vitreous], using triamcinolone suspension to improve vitreous visualization, maintaining immaculate visualization of the vitreoretinal relationship at each time point [by appropriate use of the endoilluminator and visualization lenses], recognizing regions of increased vitreous adherence [vitreous base, lattice degeneration, posterior migration] and avoiding excessive use of suction, maintaining an eye on the margin and extent of induced posterior hyaloid separation, using PFCL in the presence of a firmly adherent hyaloid and retinal detachment, and performing fluid–fluid exchange at the earliest opportunity to convert a bullous detachment to a shallower detachment, before proceeding with further vitreous removal. Another measure that could help to reduce the risk of creating an iatrogenic retinal tear is to keep the opening on the vitreous cutter facing 90–180 degree away from the detached retina while performing vitrectomy [this is contrary to the recommendation in 20G surgery that the port should be facing towards the retina]. Control over the foot pedal, too, is an extremely useful way of reducing retinal tear formation. The surgeon should note [by asking the assistant or nurse] the minimal suction at which the vitreous is seen to travel into the opening of the vitreous cutter. With this is mind, an attempt must be made to remove or shave the vitreous away from a detached retina at this minimal necessary suction. [Sometimes this minimal force could be as low as 15 mmHg, while at other times it could be above 100 mmHg, based on a lot of variables.] An approach of this kind would certainly add to the surgical time but also add significantly to reduce the chances of creating an iatrogenic retinal tear. Inadvertent formation of a retinal tear is more likely while dealing with tractional retinal detachments and combined traction–rhegmatogenous detachments. In this situation, bimanual surgery using chandelier illumination through a fourth port may improve the safety of tissue dissection. However, the need for bimanual surgery is said to arise in only about 15%–20% of patients.

Intraocular haemorrhage during vitreoretinal surgery is a serious complication and may result in accumulation of blood in the anterior chamber, vitreous cavity, subretinal space, or choroidal layers [haemorrhagic choroidal detachment] and as a tenacious layering over the retinal surface. The incidence of haemorrhage within the eye during vitreoretinal surgery varies depending on the primary pathology for which the surgery is being performed. While it is relatively very infrequent during surgery for retinal detachment, the same is not true if the indication for surgery is proliferative vascular retinopathies, like diabetic retinopathy. The severity of intraocular haemorrhage may vary from mild to very severe. In addition to immediately compromising the visibility of the anatomical structures and impeding the surgical steps from being carried forward safely, intraocular haemorrhage may also impact the postoperative course and visual outcome. Even if the haemorrhage has been successfully controlled intraoperatively, these patients tend to have a higher incidence of postsurgical inflammation, microscopic to clearly visible hyphaema, corneal staining, fresh bleeding, and early development of PVR or silicone oil emulsification in the postoperative period. The location of intraocular haemorrhage may be the anterior chamber, the root of the iris and anterior chamber angle, layered over the lens or intraocular lens [IOL], between the IOL and the lens capsule, layered along the posterior capsule, confined to the vicinity of the port site, over or under the neurosensory retina, dispersed into the entire vitreous cavity, or within the choroid.

The cause of intraocular haemorrhage could be one or many, including sudden worsening of blood pressure, occult globe perforation during local anaesthesia, improper positioning of the patient [head end lowered], sudden hypotony, ingress through a limbal incision [e.g., explanting an IOL], ingress from the scleral port, pre-existing news vessels anteriorly [iris and trabecular meshwork], within the ciliary region [fibrovascular downgrowth], or posteriorly [at the disc or elsewhere], iatrogenic injury to the pars plicata, retinal blood vessels, vessels over the optic nerve head, or vascular stroma of the choroid, planned retinotomy or retinectomy, trimming of the retinal flap [large tear, giant retinal tear], retinal and retinochoroidal biopsy, or resection of intraocular tumours [e.g., choroidal melanoma]. External drainage of subretinal fluid and perforation of the sclera while placing sutures for a buckle or encirclage are additional sources of intraocular haemorrhage. Sudden removal of the cryoprobe before complete thawing could also be a source of intraocular haemorrhage. An infrequent cause could be avulsion or compression of the vortex vein during bridling of extraocular muscles and placement of the explant. Globe rupture and expulsive haemorrhage are very rare but grievous forms of intraocular haemorrhage. The risk of haemorrhage occurring intraoperatively can be reduced by taking certain precautions before and during surgery. Preoperatively, it is important to be aware of both the systemic risk factors [e.g., older adult patient with poorly controlled hypertension, those on anti-platelet medication] as well as ocular risk factors [high myopia, recent trauma or surgery, iris or angle neovascularization, diagnosed proliferative vitreoretinopathy, hypotony, anterior PVR, retracted iris]. Intraoperatively, all surgical steps must be carried out with utmost care. Sometimes it is useful to modify the surgical plan thought of in the preoperative period [e.g., may be safer to avoid indentation or passing scleral sutures for an explant if significant scleral thinning is noted]. In patients with active iris neovascularization or proliferative vessels over the disc or elsewhere (even if these are seemingly regressed clinically), intravitreal injection of bevacizumab 12–72 hours before surgery significantly reduces the risk of intraocular haemorrhage.

Intraocular haemorrhage from surgical maneuvers themselves can be minimized by anticipating the possibility and instituting measures to lower the risk before performing the surgical step. These measures include laser or diathermizing retinal vessels before excision of neovascular tissue, trimming of retinal flap, undertaking retinotomy or retinectomy, and creating a retinal free flap for transplantation. A useful method to achieve better 'constriction' of news vessels within proliferative tissues [e.g., in diabetic vitreous surgery] is to place the diathermy tip beneath the membrane [i.e., on the undersurface] rather than over the membrane. This is more efficient because it causes contraction of not only the distal but also the proximal, usually patent part of the feeding vessel. However, during this approach, it is important to ensure that there is a safe cleavage plain between the retinal surface and neovascular tissue. In addition, it is also prudent to increase the IOP before excising any neovascular tissue or undertaking a surgical step that is known to be fraught with high risk of inducing intraoperative haemorrhage. Preventive increase of intraoperative IOP is more useful and simpler than increasing the IOP after the onset of haemorrhage. Risk of intraocular haemorrhage is also lowered by sharp dissection [with scissors or small-gauge vitreous cutter] of tissues to be excised than by using blunt dissection [with forceps].

Complications could also be noted in the early or late postoperative period. These include rebleed into the vitreous cavity, hyphaema, migration of the vitreous substitute [air, gas, silicone oil, PFCL] into the anterior chamber, hypotony, elevated intraocular pressure, choroidal detachment [Figure 12.3], retinal tear formation and detachment [Figure 12.4], redetachment, subretinal gas or silicone oil, retained PFCL bubble, corneal epithelial defect, corneal edema, fibrinoid anterior

FIGURE 12.3 Localized choroidal detachment and early vitreous haemorrhage following pars plana vitrectomy and endolaser in a patient with proliferative diabetic retinopathy.

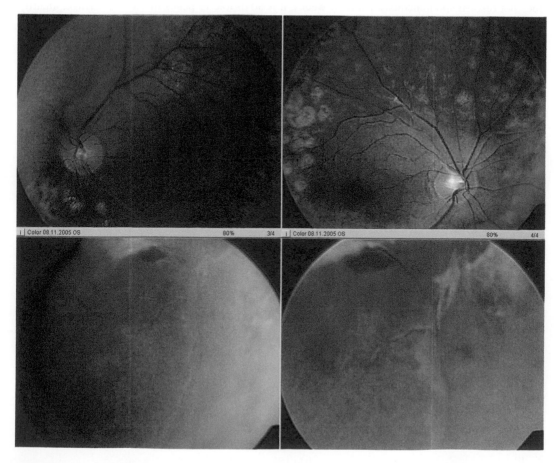

FIGURE 12.4 Peripheral retinal tear with detachment of the retina after pars plana vitrectomy.

chamber reaction, inflammatory pupillary membrane, severe intraocular inflammation, anterior hyaloidal fibrovascular proliferation [Figure 12.5], recurrent epiretinal proliferation [Figure 12.6], proliferation from the retinotomy site [Figure 12.7], and endophthalmitis. Ways of reducing the occurrence of these complications have been mentioned earlier. If, however, they develop despite taking all precautions, management decisions must be individualized. Redetachment occurring a few days after surgery may also be related to poor compliance with positioning. Re-emphasis about the same and prompt laser augmentation may sometimes resolve the complication [Figure 12.8]. Vitreous rebleed in the early postoperative period is usually minimal and transient and may need no intervention other than to keep the patient in a propped-up position [and avoiding prone position] for a day or two. Early rebleed is usually a manifestation of dissolution of residual blood that was left behind [because it was layered to the anterior hyaloid in a phakic patient, was trapped in the vitreous base and extreme periphery of the retina, or was tenaciously adherent to the retinal surface or masked near the port site] at the conclusion of surgery. If these reasons are ruled out, then it could be indicative of ooze from dissected ends of neovascular tissue and retinotomy or retinectomy sites. This could result from elevated blood pressure during the postoperative period or may be precipitated from prone positioning. Early rebleed in the vitreous sometimes tends to be associated with variable degree of blood in the anterior chamber, from microscopic hyphaema to frank hyphaema. Most of these resolve spontaneously with a conservative approach. When the view of the retina is significantly obscured by the rebleed, it is prudent to undertake USG at 7- to 10-day intervals for early detection of potential retinal detachment. If vitreous rebleed in the early postoperative period does not resolve spontaneously within 4 weeks, it is advisable to perform vitreous lavage, identify and treat any possible risk factor, and consider tamponade with a long-acting vitreous substitute.

Vitreous haemorrhage that shows up a few weeks after the surgery is usually an ominous feature and may be indicative of anterior hyaloidal proliferation. Anterior hyaloidal fibrovascular proliferation occurs as a result of vascular ingrowth from the scleral port site onto the anterior hyaloidal

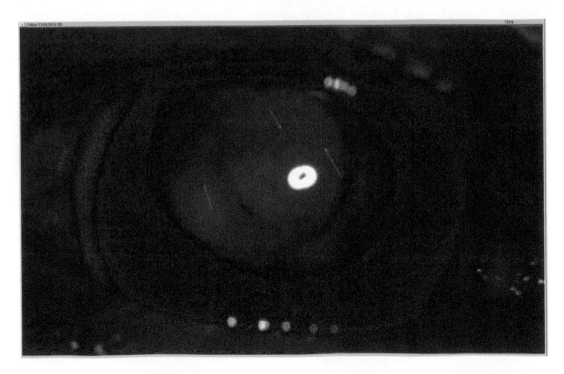

FIGURE 12.5   Anterior hyaloidal fibrovascular proliferation in a young woman after surgery for proliferative diabetic retinopathy.

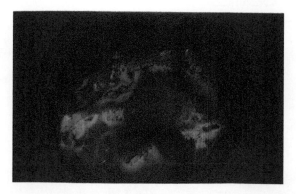

FIGURE 12.6A Focal epiretinal membrane formation [in the temporal macula] after vitreoretinal surgery with silicone oil tamponade in a patient with retinal detachment and proliferative vitreoretinopathy.

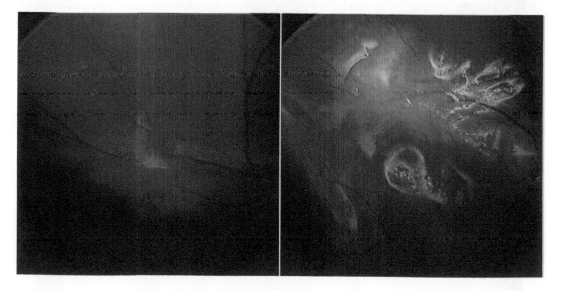

FIGURE 12.6B Preoperative and postoperative images following removal of an epiretinal membrane under silicone oil [2007] in a patient with operated vitreoretinal surgery.

phase. It is usually seen following surgery for complications of diabetic retinopathy and in the presence of a severely ischemic and unlasered retina. It may rarely be a complication of surgery for vitreous haemorrhage in young patients with retinal vasculitis. With the widespread availability of endolaser, wide-angle visualization, and peripheral vitreous debulking, this complication is now infrequently encountered. Early recognition of anterior hyaloidal proliferation is important because it tends to progress rapidly to a vascularized cyclitic membrane followed by ciliary body traction, hypotony, and phthisis. In its early stages, it may be possible to arrest the condition by immediately performing vitreous lavage with cryoablation of neovascular tissue at the scleral port site, debulking the peripheral vitreous, applying additional endolaser, intravitreal injection of anti–vascular endothelial growth factor [anti-VEGF], and long-term tamponade with silicone oil. In established cases, it may be possible to prevent phthisis by undertaking complete [including lens capsule] removal of the crystalline lens or IOL as well as the anterior hyaloidal phase in addition to these steps. More frequent and better manageable cause of late vitreous haemorrhage is progression of the original proliferative disease or from rupture of the initial but undetected and active neovascular tissue. The

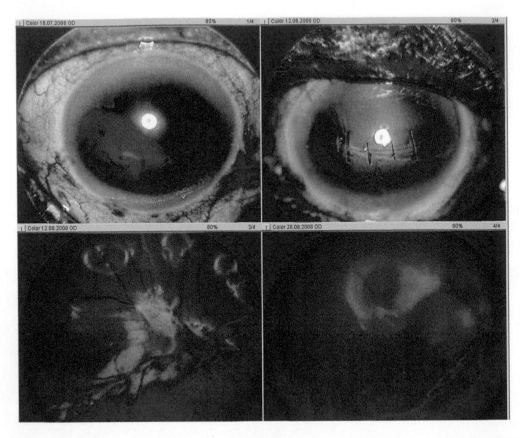

FIGURE 12.6C Removal of epimacular membrane under oil in a patient with repaired corneal perforation and prior vitreoretinal surgery.

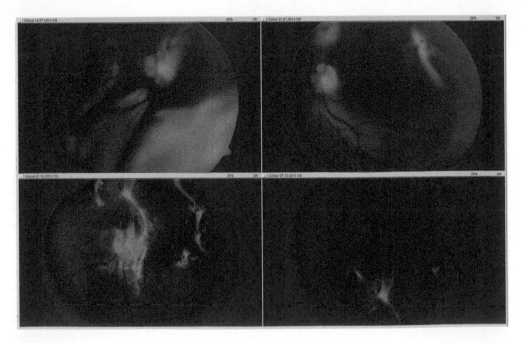

FIGURE 12.7 Preoperative and postoperative image showing proliferation of tractional membrane from the site of internal drainage retinotomy after vitreoretinal surgery.

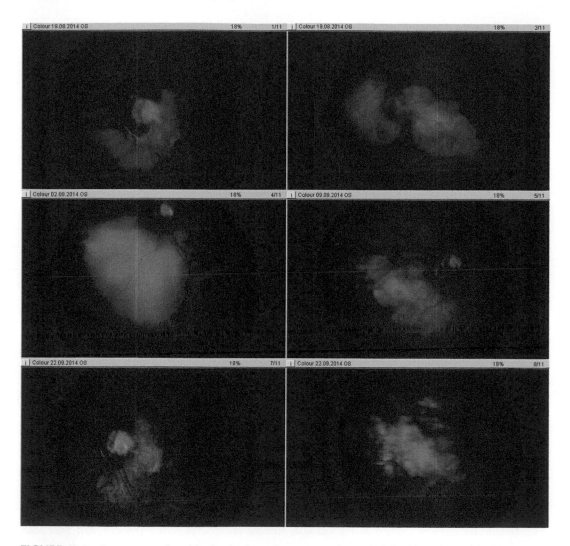

FIGURE 12.8 Importance of positioning in the early postoperative period. In this patient with high myopia, localized accumulation of subretinal fluid was noted around the retinotomy site in the early postoperative period [middle panel, left column]. Prompt counselling about the need for strict prone positioning led to resorption of subretinal fluid [following which laser around the retinotomy site was augmented].

latter situation can be avoided by making it a habit to undertake fluorescein angiographic assessment of the operated eye within the first 4–6 weeks of surgery for patients with diagnosed proliferative vascular disease. This helps identify active neovascular tissue, which can then be controlled by additional laser photocoagulation. If anterior hyaloidal proliferation can be ruled out with reasonable certainty, then non-resolving late onset vitreous haemorrhage can be managed by vitreous lavage after waiting about 4 weeks for spontaneous resolution. It may also be useful to treat these eyes with intravitreal anti-VEGF injection as some patients are known to have benefited from this intervention alone. Most proliferative conditions are bilateral, so it is important to continue meticulous monitoring of the fellow eye and not focus all the efforts on managing the situation in the operated eye alone.

Fibrinoid anterior chamber reaction is another serious complication that is commonly seen after diabetic vitreous surgery. It is seen in the early postoperative period and may mimic endophthalmitis. Eyes without prior laser, nephropathy, excessive tissue manipulation, and combined phacoemulsification surgery are some risk factors for its occurrence. The condition can be treated by increasing the frequency of topical steroids, intravitreal steroid injection, and systemic steroids. Some patients in whom silicone oil has been used as vitreous substitute tend to develop appreciable anterior chamber inflammation on day 2 or 3 after the surgery. This could be accompanied by the development a translucent pupillary membrane. Prompt treatment with frequent corticosteroid drops, cycloplegics, and a short course of oral corticosteroids usually results in retraction of the pupillary membrane and resolution of the complication.

SUGGESTED READING

1. Chandra A, Xing W, Kadhim MR, Williamson TH [2014]. Suprachoroidal hemorrhage in pars plana vitrectomy. *Ophthalmol.* 121(1): 311–317.
2. Covert DJ [2012]. Intraoperative retinal tear formation and postoperative rhegmatogenous retinal detachment in transconjunctival cannulated vitrectomy systems compared with the standard 20-gauge system. *Arch Ophthalmol.* 130(2): 186.
3. McLoone E [2001]. Silicone oil-intraocular lens interaction: Which lens to use? *Br J Ophthalmol.* 85(5): 543–545.
4. Park JC, Ramasamy B, Ling RH, Prasad S [2011]. Endophthalmitis following vitrectomy. *Eye.* 26(3): 482–482.
5. Chronopoulos A [2015]. Complications of encircling bands-prevention and management. *J Clin Exp Ophthalmol.* 6(3).
6. Toyokawa N, Kimura H, Matsumura M, Kuroda S [2015]. Incidence of late-onset ocular hypertension following uncomplicated pars plana vitrectomy in pseudophakic eyes. *Am J Ophthalmol.* 159(4): 727–732.
7. Apple DJ, Federman JL, Krolicki TJ, Sims JCR et al [1996]. Irreversible silicone oil adhesion to silicone intraocular lenses. *Ophthalmol.* 103(10): 1555–1562.
8. Mimouni M, Abualhasan H, Derman L, Feldman A, Mazzawi F, Barak Y [2020]. Incidence and risk factors for hypotony after 25-gauge pars plana vitrectomy with nonexpansile endotamponade. *Retina.* 40(1): 41–46.
9. Mariotti C, Nicolai M, Saitta A [2015]. Management of intraoperative and postoperative complications during vitrectomy for retinal detachment. In: Patelli F, Rizzo S (Eds) *Management of complicated vitreoretinal diseases.* Springer, Cham.
10. Verma L, Venkatesh P, Chawla R, Tewari HK [2004]. Choroidal detachment following retinal detachment surgery: An analysis and a new hypothesis to minimize its occurrence in high-risk cases. *Eur J Ophthalmol.* Jul–Aug. 14(4): 325–329.
11. Branisteanu D, Moraru A, Maranduca M, Branisteanu D, Stoleriu G, Branisteanu C, Balta F [2020]. Intraocular pressure changes during and after silicone oil endotamponade (review). *Exp Ther Med.* 20(6): 1.
12. Venkatesh P, Verma L, Tewari H [2002]. Posterior vitreous wick syndrome: A potential cause of endophthalmitis following vitreo-retinal surgery. *Med Hypotheses.* 58(6): 513–515.

13 Important Studies in Vitreoretinal Surgery

13.1 SILICONE OIL STUDY

This was a multicentric, randomized comparative study to determine the efficacy and safety of vitreous tamponade with silicone oil or long-acting intraocular gas [sulphur hexafluoride, SF6 or perfluorocyclopraprane, C3F8]. The study was conducted over a 6-year period between 1985 and 1991. Patients with proliferative retinopathy of proliferative vitreoretinopathy [PVR] C3 and PVR D [Retina Society classification] were enrolled into the study. Two groups of patients were evaluated, those undergoing surgery for the first time [group 1] and those for redetachment [first surgery having been performed outside of the study]. Random allocation to the type of tamponade was undertaken after the surgery was performed using a set of standard steps, and intraoperative attachment was confirmed following air-fluid exchange. Patients were followed up for 3 years. Resurgery was allowed in case of failures noted during follow-up. Outcome measures were visual acuity more than 5/200 and macular attachment for 6 months after the final surgical procedure. A total of 555 patients were recruited of whom 113 received SF6 [all in group 1], 232 received C3F8 [all in group 2], and 210 received silicone oil [38 in group 1 and 172 in group 2]. The study team developed a new system for classification of PVR based on changes at and anterior to the vitreous base [broadly categorized as anterior PVR and posterior PVR]. Some of the observations were, chronically elevated intraocular pressure [IOP] in 5% [silicone oil, more than gas], and chronic hypotony in 24% [gas more than oil, anterior diffuse contraction of the retina was a risk factor]; macular pucker developed in 15% [unrelated to type of tamponade] and relaxing retinectomy was more often necessary in group 2. Patients with anterior PVR fared better with silicone oil, but their overall outcomes were poorer. An extension study [6 years of follow-up] found that beneficial results noted at 3 years were maintained in the long run, and those who had successful reattachment of the retina following a single surgery had better visual acuity outcomes.

As an outcome of this study, silicone oil is now routinely used as long-term tamponade in the management of complex retinal detachment [RD]. If silicone oil is retained beyond 3 to 6 months, emulsification of silicone oil can be very significant, resulting in hyperoleon formation. Hyperoleon can be removed at surgery using one of two methods: injecting jets of fluid into the anterior chamber or simultaneous irrigation and aspiration using cannulas meant for extracapsular cataract surgery [e.g., Simcoe cannula; Video 13.1]. As described by the Oxford centre for evidence based medicine [Figure 13.1] randomized studies and systematic reviews are considered as having the highest level of scientific value. Some of the studies that have been undertaken in vitreoretinal surgery generating high levels of evidence through randomized studies and unbiased systematic reviews are described here.

13.2 DIABETIC RETINOPATHY VITRECTOMY STUDY

The main objectives of the Diabetic Retinopathy Vitrectomy Study [DVRS] were to determine the natural course of eyes with severe proliferative diabetic retinopathy [PDR], determine the effect of vitreous surgery on eyes with severe PDR, and identify surgical complications. Another key objective was to determine when to perform vitrectomy in patients with severe proliferative disease. Patients were randomized into three groups—the natural history study group [to determine the outcome of conventional management, group N], merits of surgical intervention in eyes with severe PDR and without severe visual loss [SVL] group [group NR], and comparison of early vitreous surgery versus conventional management [deferral of surgery for 1 year] in eyes with vitreous haemorrhage [group

DOI: 10.1201/9781003179320-14

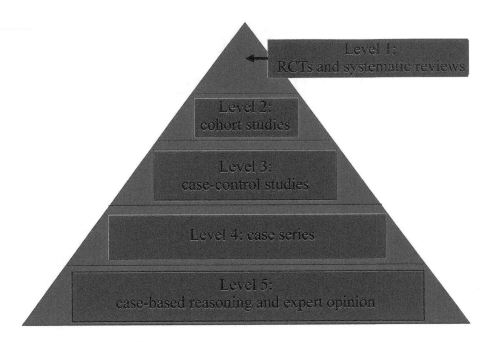

FIGURE 13.1   Oxford Centre for Evidence Based Medicine: Levels of Evidence

H]. Group N patients were further sub-grouped as NN [new vessels only], ND [detachment], and NH [haemorrhage] subgroup. Group NR subgroups were NVC-1 [least severe new vessels], NVC-2 [moderately severe new vessels], NVC-3 [severe new vessels], and NVC-4 [very severe new vessels]. Group H subgroups were early vitrectomy group [operated within a few days of randomization] and deferral group [offered surgery 1 year after randomization if SVL and vitreous haemorrhage persisted]. The study enrolled 616 eyes with severe vitreous haemorrhage of recent onset [less than 1 month duration] and 370 eyes with active and advanced PDR with useful baseline vision [more than 10/200]. Major observations of the study were as follows: In the early vitrectomy group [insulin-dependent diabetes mellitus patients], at 2 years after treatment, three times more patients had recovery of good vision [defined as vision better than 10/20] than in the conventional group [36% vs. 12%]; 4 years after treatment, five times more patients had maintained good vision than in the conventional group [50% vs. 10%]. However, in the first 18 months of follow-up, a greater number of eyes undergoing vitrectomy had no light perception [this needs to be specifically informed and discussed with the patient] than the conventional group. After 18 months, however, this difference was negligible. Final recommendations of the study were to advocate early vitrectomy in three categories of patients: patients with type 1 diabetes mellitus with severe vitreous haemorrhage of more than 1 month duration, monocular patients [any group of diabetes], and patients with active and advanced PDR [even with useful baseline vision] in whom laser photocoagulation has not caused adequate regression of new vessels or in whom vitreous haemorrhage prevents laser photocoagulation. Endolaser was not widely available, and there was no knowledge about anti–vascular endothelial growth factor during the conduct of this study. The routine use of these two beneficial procedures for managing patients with features similar to those enrolled in DRVS may have significantly improved the outcomes further and may have also reduced the risk of losing light perception vision in the postoperative course.

13.3   ENDOPHTHALMITIS VITRECTOMY STUDY

This study was primarily undertaken to determine the role of initial pars plana vitrectomy versus intravitreal injection [vancomycin and amikacin] in patients with acute [within 6 weeks of surgery] bacterial postoperative [mainly after cataract surgery and secondary IOL] endophthalmitis. Other objectives were to assess the role of intravenous antibiotics [ceftazidime and amikacin] and to identify any other prognostic factors [other than the type of treatment]. The study was conducted over a 5-year period between 1990 and 1995 as an interventional, multicentric, randomized study. Visual acuity for enrolment was between 20/50 and light perception or better. Reasonable corneal clarity to allow vitreous surgery was a prerequisite for enrolment. Follow-up was for 9 months, reinjection was allowed for patients did poorly after vitrectomy [within 36–60 hours], and vitrectomy was allowed for patients who did poorly with primary tap and injection. A total of 420 patients were enrolled, and the main outcome measures were improvement in visual acuity and improvement in media clarity at the end of 3 to 9-month follow-up. Patients with a history of other intraocular surgeries, presentation after 6 weeks, fungal endophthalmitis, trauma, or age younger than 18 years were not included in the study. Patients with history of previous intraocular antibiotic administration, other causes of poor vision, presence of retinal or choroidal detachment, and drug sensitivity to lactams were also excluded from the study. The patients were randomly categorized into four groups: pars plana vitrectomy [PPV] with systemic antibiotics, PPV without systemic antibiotics, TAP vitreous biopsy with intravitreal antibiotic injection with systemic antibiotics, and TAP without systemic antibiotics. The mean interval between surgery and onset of symptoms was 4 days and visit to a vitreous surgeon, 6 days. Treatment was initiated in all patients within 6 hours of presentation. The intravitreal drugs used in this study were vancomycin [1000 µg in 0.1 ml] and amikacin [400 µg in 0.1 ml]. No intravitreal corticosteroids were given. For systemic [parenteral] administration, the chosen drugs were ceftazidime [2 gm, 8 hourly] and amikacin [7.5 mg/kg initially and then 6 mg/kg every 12 hours]. In those allergic to lactams, ciprofloxacillin 750 mg orally twice daily was used as an alternative. Systemic medication was given for a period of 5–10 days. The surgical interventions performed were vitreous tap and intravitreal injection, vitreous biopsy and intravitreal injection, or PPV and intravitreal injection. The goal of vitrectomy in eyes with no obvious vitreous separation was to remove at least 50% of the vitreous gel. Additional surgery [re-vitrectomy, re-vitreous tap, or vitrectomy] was undertaken in eyes doing poorly 36–60 hours after the first intervention. Signs of worsening were an absent red reflex or increasing opacification, a 1-mm increase in the height of hypopyon, development of a corneal ring infiltrate, and worsening pain. The study concluded that there is no difference in outcome between immediate vitrectomy or intravitreal antibiotics when visual acuity was hand movements or better. If initial vision was only light perception, then final visual acuity and media clarity were substantially better in patients undergoing vitrectomy and intravitreal injection. Intravenous antibiotics had no impact on the results.

13.4 SCLERAL BUCKLING VERSUS PRIMARY VITRECTOMY STUDY

Scleral buckling versus primary vitrectomy study in rhegmatogenous RD [SPR] was a prospective randomized, multicentric study evaluating the safety and efficacy of RD surgery versus primary vitrectomy in phakic and pseudophakic patients having RD of medium severity. The study was conducted over a 5-year period from 1998 to 2003 [25 centres and 45 surgeons]. The numbers of phakic and pseudophakic patients recruited were 416 and 265, respectively. Of 416 phakic patients, 209 underwent scleral buckling [SB], and 207 underwent primary vitrectomy. Corresponding figures for pseudophakic patients were 133 for SB and 132 for vitrectomy. In the phakic trial, the overall single surgery success rate was only 64% [133 of 209 in the SB group and 132 of 207 the PPV group]. Using a multivariate regression model, anatomical success was found to be related to number of breaks, extent of break, irregular margins of the break, subretinal fluid drainage, and use of cryotherapy. Similarly, overall primary anatomical success in the pseudophakic trial subgroup was 63% [71 of 133 in the SB group and 95 of 132 in the PPV group]. In this group, anatomical success was related to prior yttrium aluminum garnet capsulotomy, number of breaks, and intraoperative use of laser. The low primary anatomical outcome at 1-year follow-up was attributed by the authors to the restrictive definition of success used in the study, according to which primary success was defined as retinal attachment without secondary interventions like laser photocoagulation, cryotherapy, intraocular gas injection, buckle revision, and revision vitrectomy for removal of macular pucker. The final anatomical success at the end of 1 year with secondary interventions were, however, good [97% in the phakic group and 94% in the pseudophakic group]. Results of this study provided affirmation that scleral buckle surgery must be considered as the surgery of first choice in phakic patients with RD of medium severity. In pseudophakic patients, however, SB tended to be inferior to primary vitrectomy.

13.5   PNEUMATIC RETINOPEXY VERSUS SCLERAL BUCKLING

Unlike the SPR study, which was undertaken in patients with RD of medium severity, this trial was conducted on patients with simple RD. The study was conducted by the RD study group. A total of 198 patients were randomly assigned to either pneumatic retinopexy [PR] or SB surgery. The 6-month and 2-year outcomes were presented as two separate reports. At 6 months, the single operation success rate was 82% [SB] versus 73% [PR], 84% versus 81% with one additional procedure like laser or cryopexy and 98% versus 99% after further surgery. Final visual acuity of 20/50 or better [in patients who had RD for less than 2 weeks] was better in the PR group [56% vs. 50%]. Proliferative vitreoretinopathy was 3% and 5% in the SB and PR group, respectively, while new tear formation was significantly higher [13% vs. 23%] in PR group. Favorable results, comparable to SB, were noted at the 2-year follow-up as well.

13.6   VITREOMACULAR TRACTION STUDIES

Based on results of the Microplasmin IntraVitreal Injection [MIVI]-Trust study, Food and Drug Administration [FDA] approval was granted for the clinical use of ocriplasmin [for details on ocriplasmin, see section on enzymatic vitreolysis] in patients with symptomatic vitreomacular traction [VMT]. Following this, other randomized studies for management of patients with symptomatic VMT using ocriplasmin have been undertaken, some concluded and others ongoing. These studies include the Oasis study, Orbit study, and Inject study and those comparing the role of intraocular gas injection versus primary PPV.

MIVI-Trust study. In this study, 652 patients [464 in the ocriplasmin group and 188 in the placebo injection group] with focal symptomatic vitreomacular adhesion [VMA] were evaluated. Focal VMA was defined as attachment of the vitreous to the central 6-mm field of the macula with elevation of the posterior vitreous cortex. About 27% of patients achieved the primary end point of pharmacologic vitreolysis by day 28 [compared with 10% in the placebo group]. Secondary end points of total PVD [on ultrasonography] and closure of macular hole was achieved in 13% versus 4% and 41% versus 11%, respectively. In this study, patients with epimacular membrane had a significantly lower response. Vitrectomy rates were 18% and 27% in the ocriplasmin and placebo groups, respectively. Two patients in the treatment group developed retinal tear and detachment and were managed surgically.

Oasis study. This study included 220 patients with VMA, VMT, or full-thickness macular hole and randomized them to receive either ocriplasmin [0.125 mg] intravitreal injection [146 patients], or sham injection [74 patients] [2:1 enrolment ratio]. Patients with hole size more than 400 μ and those with epimacular membranes were ineligible for recruitment. All patients were followed for a period of 2 years. Primary outcome was relief from preoperative pathology at 28 days. Secondary outcome measures were assessed at month 24 and included change in visual acuity, macular hole closure without vitrectomy, vitrectomy rates, and visual function questionnaire responses. The primary end point was noted in 42% of patients receiving ocriplasmin compared with 6% in the sham group. At the secondary outcome point [24-month follow-up], visual acuity improvement of more than two lines was noted in 50% of those who received ocriplasmin [compared with 40% in the sham group], and nonsurgical closure of macular hole was seen in 30% [ocriplasmin group] versus 15% in sham group. Most side effects were mild to moderate. Phakic patients with focal VMA and prior hole seemed to fare better following ocriplasmin treatment.

Orbit study. This was a phase IV study to determine outcomes and safety of ocriplasmin in a real-world setting. Of 480 patients treated with ocriplasmin for VMA or VMT, resolution was seen in about 46% at 1 month and 60% at 1 year. About one in three patients had closure of macular hole at 1-month follow-up [and about the same at 1 year]. Rates of macular hole closure was highest for those with holes that were smaller than 250 μ. However, visual acuity gain was only modest, and those with visual acuity less than 20/50 before injection seemed to show better results. Mean time to vitrectomy in patients without macular hole closure was 63 days and was more common in those with hole sizes larger than 400 μ. Serious adverse events were noted in 5% of patients and included photopsia and floaters. Retinal tear, detachment, lens dislocation, zonular dehiscence, ellipsoid zone disruption, and endophthalmitis were not observed in any patient.

Inject study. This was also a was a phase IV study that analysed outcomes and safety of ocriplasmin [Jetrea] in patients [*n* = 395] treated outside of the United States [Europe and Canada]. VMT resolution was reported in 41% and closure of macular hole in 36%. Adverse events were similar to those observed in the Orbit study.

Ozone. This study was a post-hoc analysis of changes in the ellipsoid zone following ocriplasmin injection.

13.7   MACULAR HOLE STUDIES

Approaches to management of macular hole include observation, vitrectomy, intravitreal injection of gas [when associated with VMA or VMT], intravitreal injection of ocriplasmin [when associated with VMA or VMT], and no intervention. Factors that influence the decision are the patient's visual needs and motivation, status of the fellow eye, duration of the macular hole, size of the macular hole, and presence of concurrent pathology [e.g., choroidal rupture, resolved subfoveal haemorrhage, traumatic optic neuropathy, foveal schisis]. Although surgery is widely performed nowadays, only a few randomized controlled trials have been considered to be of high quality in terms of randomization, data concealment, and analysis. One study compared the safety and efficacy of vitrectomy versus observation in patients with stage 2 macular hole [see section on macular hole], and the remaining two studies compared the safety and efficacy of surgery in those with stage 3 and stage 4 macular hole. In the study on stage 2 macular hole, 36 patients [of the enrolled 40, having 12-month follow-up] were randomized [21 to observation and 15 to surgery] and were followed up for 12 months. Surgery was vitrectomy with PVD separation [and no internal limiting membrane (ILM) peeling]. About 71% of patients in the observation group were found to progress to stage 3 and 4 hole compared with 20% in the PPV group. Final hole size was smaller in those who underwent surgery. Although visual outcomes, in terms of word reading and potential acuity meter, were better in the interventional group, no significant difference was observed on Early Treatment of Diabetic Retinopathy Study [ETDRS] chart and contrast sensitivity. In a randomized controlled trial (RCT) for stage 3 and stage 4 hole published in 1997, 129 eyes [120 patients] were randomized into two groups, PPV [64 eyes] or observation [65 eyes]. This was part of Vitrectomy in Macular Hole Study [VMHS] vitrectomy for macular hole study. Surgical steps included meticulous removal of the vitreous and any membrane attached to the macular hole and drainage of subretinal fluid after air-fluid exchange [sometimes after a waiting time of 10–15 minutes] followed by 16% perfluorocycloprapane tamponade. Strict prone positioning was maintained for 2 weeks. No ILM peeling was undertaken. This study reported hole closure rate of 69% compared with 4% in the observation group. Visual acuity improved by two or more lines in 19% versus 5% [observation], while 34% of patients in the surgery group also lost one line of vision [largely from progression of nuclear sclerosis]. Posterior segment complications in this study were published separately. According to this report, complications were noted: 41%–33% had retinal pigment epithelial changes [on fundus imaging, optical coherence tomography [OCT] not being available], 11% had retinal detachment, 2% had reopening of the hole, and 2% had endophthalmitis and a few other complications. The applicability of these results may no longer be appropriate because several factors have added to the safety and efficacy of macular hole surgery, including preoperative OCT and advances in vitreous machine technology, chromovitrectomy, and ILM peeling. The high incidence of nuclear sclerosis is being overcome by performing combined phaco-macular hole surgery. However, there is a lack of high-evidence randomized, multicentric, prospective studies using a standardized approach and comparing it with various other approaches that have been described over the past decade.

13.8   DRUG DELIVERY SYSTEM STUDIES

Drug delivery for diseases of the posterior segment has always been challenging because of restricted availability of drugs administered systemically owing to the blood–ocular barrier, the chronicity of many of these conditions, and the risk of systemic complications from prolonged drug administration [e.g., corticosteroids]. To bypass these challenges, local delivery using intravitreal implants has been extensively explored, but only a few have received FDA approval. Twin challenges while using drug implants include risks related to the procedure such as endophthalmitis, vitreous haemorrhage, retinal detachment, extrusion, and dislocation and those related to the drug itself, like elevated IOP and progression of cataract. Some of the diseases that have been managed using intravitreal drug implants include cytomegalovirus retinitis [Vitrasert]; chronic, non-infectious uveitis [Retisert, Iluvien, Posurdex]; diabetic macular edema [Retisert, Iluvien, Posurdex]; and exudative age-related macular degeneration [port delivery system, Susmivo]. An entirely different route to deliver drugs into the posterior segment that is under active exploration is suprachoroidal delivery using microinjectors.

13.8.1 RETISERT STUDY

This was the first intravitreal implant to undergo extensive evaluation for the management of chronic, non-infectious posterior and intermediate uveitis. The active drug is fluocinolone acetonide. Each implant contains 0.59 µg of the drug, and the release rate varies between 0.6 and 0.3 µg/ day over a period of 24–36 months. The implant has a flattened plate-like platform with a tablet of the active drug affixed at one end and a strut with a suture hole at the opposite end. The tablet is encased in a silicone elastomer cup with a release orifice covered by polyvinyl alcohol membrane. The tablet itself is glued onto the polyvinyl plate using silicone glue. It has dimensions of 5 mm × 3 mm × 2 mm [increased thickness is due to the tablet] and has to be inserted at the pars plana through a 3.2-mm scleral section [see section of intravitreal drug implants]. A total of 227 patients were evaluated in two parallel RCTs, with the primary end point as the rate of recurrence for a 34-month period before and after implantation. The difference was found to be extremely significant, at 40%–54% versus 7%–14%. Alongside the decrease in recurrence of uveitis, serious adverse effects were also noted, with 60% needing IOP-lowering medication, 32% needing a filtering procedure, and almost all phakic patients needing cataract surgery. In addition, it was also associated with other adverse events like extrusion, dislocation, endophthalmitis, and retinal detachment. The device was one of its kind at the time of its development and was approved by FDA for clinical use despite these serious adverse events. It was, however, not released worldwide because of cost considerations. This macro-implant was soon also dominated by the introduction of micro-implants like Iluvien and Posurdex.

13.8.2 FLUCINOLONE ACETONIDE MACULAR EDEMA [FAME] STUDY

This was the first study to use a prefilled syringe for intravitreal delivery of an implant. The implant is non-biodegradable and contains 0.19 µg of fluocinolone acetonide [FAc]. It is cylindrical in shape with a length of 3.5 mm and diameter of 0.35 mm and is injected through a 25G needle. The release rate is 0.2 µg/day, and the release duration is 36 months. Following submission of results from two parallel studies [FAME A-in the United States and FAME B-in Canada, Europe, and India] with the same protocol but in different geographic locations of the world, it was approved by the FDA in 2013 for use as second-line therapy in patients with chronic or resistant diabetic macular edema. FAME studies were multicentric, randomized, and double masked with three study arms [low-dose 0.20-μg implant, high-dose 0.50-μg implant, and placebo]. The main inclusion criteria was persistent diabetic macular edema [mean duration, 3 years]. A total of 953 patients were randomized in the ratio 2:2:1; 375 with the low-dose implant, 393 with the high-dose implant, and 185 with placebo. Visual gain of 15 or more letters was seen in 28% of treatment eyes versus 16% in placebo eyes [both 2- and 3-year end points]. Treated patients also needed much lower secondary interventions like laser and/or other intravitreal injections. This implant is marketed as Iluvien and has been further evaluated with phase 4 studies like the ICE-UK study [Iluvien Clinical Evaluation, United Kingdom], RESPOND study [evaluation of safety and efficacy in patients with chronic diabetic macular edema and inconsistent response to other therapies], Medisoft audit study, and Retro-IDEAL study. Some ongoing studies include PALADIN study [primary outcome being the need for intraocular pressure lowering procedures] and NEW DAY study [to evaluate Iluvien as baseline therapy in diabetic macular edema].

13.8.3 PORT DELIVERY SYSTEM STUDIES

The **Ladder study** was a phase 2 evaluation to assess the safety and efficacy of ranibizumab delivered in escalating doses [10 mg/ml, 40 mg/ml, and 100 mg/ml] through a port delivery system in patients with neovascular age-related macular degeneration [ARMD] and compare this with monthly ranibizumab 0.5-mg injections. A total of 220 patients were randomized in a ratio of 3:3:3:2. Port delivery system [PDS] 100 mg/ml was found to have the same response as that of monthly intravitreal injection of bevacizumab. Over a 16-month period, 2.4 PDS refills with 100 mg/ml were needed compared with 16 ranibizumab injections. Vitreous haemorrhage was a serious adverse event and was seen in 4.5% of patients receiving PDS refillable implants.

The **Archway study** was a phase 3 study comparing ranibizumab PDS 100 mg/ml with monthly injections of ranibizumab 0.5 mg in patients with neovascular ARMD. The mean time to refill the implant was fixed at 24 weeks. The primary outcome measure was change in best corrected visual acuity [BCVA]. A total of 418 patients were randomly assigned to the two comparator arms; 248 received PDS, and 167 received monthly injections of ranibizumab. At week 40, change in BCVA in the two groups was found to be comparable [+0.2 in the implant group and +0.5 in the injection group], demonstrating the non-inferiority of PDS to monthly injections.

The **Pilot study** is an ongoing phase 3 extension study in which the systemic and ocular safety and tolerability of PDS with intermittent refilling are being assessed over a period of 144 weeks [see section on PDS for implant details].

13.9 COCHRANE REVIEWS

A recent systematic review [1307 participants] compared **SB versus primary PPV** in patients with simple rhegmatogenous retinal detachment. The results indicated comparable outcomes in terms of anatomical success and visual recovery. Redetachment rates between 3 and 36 months were 28 and 21%, in the SB and PPV group, respectively. Adverse events in the PPV group included a higher incidence of cataract and a relative risk of 9 for the occurrence of iatrogenic breaks in the PPV group [none in the SB group]. Patients undergoing SB had a 0.19 higher relative risk of choroidal detachment. It is important to emphasize, however, that the evidence level [see section on levels of evidence] gathered was stated as low to very low and that all the studies had high to unclear risk of bias. The role of **pneumatic retinopexy** in the management of simple retinal detachment continues to have two categories of surgeons, one convinced about its utility and the other totally lacking in belief about its efficacy. Another Cochrane review published in 2020, found only two RCTs [218 patients] with moderate level of evidence that SB may have a lower relative risk of recurrent detachment. At the same time, SB was also found to have a higher operative adverse event [including choroidal detachment]. Another review highlighted the absence of evidence for determining the utility of surgery with scleral buckle and encirclage and direct PPV in patients with various grades of **giant retinal tear**.

SUGGESTED READING

1. Vitrectomy with silicone oil or sulfur hexafluoride gas in eyes with severe proliferative vitreoretinopathy: Results of a randomized clinical trial [1992]. Silicone study report 1. *Arch Ophthalmol.* 110(6): 770–779.
2. McCuen BW, Azen SP, Stern W, Lai MY, Lean JS, Linton KL, Ryan SJ [1992]. Vitrectomy with silicone oil or perfluoropropane gas in eyes with severe proliferative vitreoretinopathy: Results of a randomized clinical trial: Silicone study report 2. *Arch Ophthalmol.* 110(6): 780–792.
3. McCuen BW, Azen SP, Stern W, Lai MY, Lean JS, Linton KL, Ryan SJ [1993]. Vitrectomy with silicone oil or perfluoropropane gas in eyes with severe proliferative vitreoretinopathy: Silicone study report 3. *Retina.* 13(4): 279–284.
4. Abrams GW, Azen SP, McCuen BW 2nd, Flynn HW Jr, Lai MY, Ryan SJ [1997]. Vitrectomy with silicone oil or long-acting gas in eyes with severe proliferative vitreoretinopathy: Results of additional and long-term follow-up. Silicone study report 11. *Arch Ophthalmol.* 115(3): 335–344.
5. Two-year course of visual acuity in severe proliferative diabetic retinopathy with conventional management [1985]. Diabetic retinopathy vitrectomy study (DRVS) report #1. *Ophthalmol.* 92(4): 492–502.
6. Results of the Endophthalmitis Vitrectomy Study [1995]. A randomized trial of immediate vitrectomy and of intravenous antibiotics for the treatment of postoperative bacterial endophthalmitis: Endophthalmitis vitrectomy study group. *Arch Ophthalmol.* 113(12): 1479–1496.
7. Flynn HW Jr, Scott IU [2008]. Legacy of the endophthalmitis vitrectomy study. *Arch Ophthalmol.* 126(4): 559–561.
8. Heimann H, Bartz-Schmidt KU, Bornfeld N, Weiss C, Hilgers RD, Foerster MH [2007]. Scleral buckling versus primary vitrectomy in rhegmatogenous retinal detachment study group: A prospective randomized multicenter clinical study. *Ophthalmol.* 114(12): 2142–2154.
9. Tornambe PE, Hilton GF [1989]. Pneumatic retinopexy: A multicenter randomized controlled clinical trial comparing pneumatic retinopexy with scleral buckling. The retinal detachment study group. *Ophthalmol.* 96(6): 772–783.
10. Hatef E, Sena DF, Fallano KA, Crews J, Do DV [2015]. Pneumatic retinopexy versus scleral buckle for repairing simple rhegmatogenous retinal detachments. *Cochrane Database Syst Rev.* 5(5): CD008350.
11. Stalmans P, Benz MS, Gandorfer A, Kampik A, Girach A et al [2012]. MIVI-TRUST study group: Enzymatic vitreolysis with ocriplasmin for vitreomacular traction and macular holes. *N Engl J Med.* 16(367(7)): 606–615.
12. Schneider EW, Jaffe GJ [2020]. Baseline characteristics of vitreomacular traction progressing to full-thickness macular or lamellar holes in the phase III trials of enzymatic vitreolysis. *Retina.* 40(8): 1579–1584.
13. Dugel PU, Tolentino M, Feiner L, Kozma P, Leroy A [2016]. Results of the 2-year ocriplasmin for treatment for symptomatic vitreomacular adhesion including macular hole (OASIS) randomized trial. *Ophthalmol.* 123(10): 2232–2247.
14. Drenser KA, Pieramici DJ, Gunn JM, Rosberger DF, Kozma P et al [2021]. Retrospective study of ellipsoid zone integrity following treatment with intravitreal ocriplasmin (OZONE study). *Clin Ophthalmol.* 16(15): 3109–3120.
15. Steel DHW, Patton N, Stappler T, Karia N, Hoerauf H, INJECT Study Investigators et al [2021]. Ocriplasmin for vitreomacular traction in clinical practice: The INJECT study. *Retina.* 41(2): 266–276.
16. Benson WE, Cruickshanks KC, Fong DS, Williams GA, Bloome MA et al [2001]. Surgical management of macular holes: a report by the American academy of ophthalmology. *Ophthalmol.* 108(7): 1328–1335.
17. Freeman WR, Azen SP, Kim JW, el-Haig W, Mishell DR 3rd Bailey I [1997]. Vitrectomy for the treatment of full-thickness stage 3 or 4 macular holes: Results of a multicentred randomized clinical trial. The vitrectomy for treatment of macular hole study group. *Arch Ophthalmol.* 115(1): 11–21.
18. Mester V, Kuhn F [2000]. Internal limiting membrane removal in the management of full-thickness macular holes. *Am J Ophthalmol.* 129(6): 769–777.
19. Spiteri Cornish K, Lois N, Scott N, Burr J, Cook J et al [2013]. Vitrectomy with internal limiting membrane (ILM) peeling versus vitrectomy with no peeling for idiopathic full-thickness macular hole (FTMH). *Cochrane Database Syst Rev.* 5(6): CD009306.

20. Yeh S, Khurana RN, Shah M, Henry CR, Wang RC, PEACHTREE Study Investigators et al [2020]. Efficacy and safety of suprachoroidal CLS-TA for macular edema secondary to non-infectious uveitis: Phase 3 randomized trial. *Ophthalmol.* 127(7): 948–955.

21. Merrill PT, Henry CR, Nguyen QD, Reddy A, Kapik B, Ciulla TA [2021]. Suprachoroidal CLS-TA with and without systemic corticosteroid and/or steroid-sparing therapy: A post-hoc analysis of the Phase 3 PEACHTREE clinical trial. *Ocul Immunol Inflamm.* 18: 1–8.

22. Conrady CD, Yeh S [2021]. A review of ocular drug delivery platforms and drugs for infectious and noninfectious uveitis: The past, present, and future. *Pharmaceutics.* 13(8): 1224.

23. Brady CJ, Villanti AC, Law HA, Rahimy E, Reddy R et al [2016]. Corticosteroid implants for chronic non-infectious uveitis. *Cochrane Database Syst Rev.* 2(2): CD010469.

24. Jaffe GJ, Martin D, Callanan D, Pearson PA, Levy B, Comstock T, Fluocinolone Acetonide Uveitis Study Group et al [2006]. Fluocinolone acetonide implant (Retisert) for noninfectious posterior uveitis: Thirty-four-week results of a multicenter randomized clinical study. *Ophthalmol.* 113(6): 1020–1027.

25. Mansour SE, Kiernan DF, Roth DB, Eichenbaum D, Holekamp NM et al [2021]. Two-year interim safety results of the 0.2 µg/day fluocinolone acetonide intravitreal implant for the treatment of diabetic macular oedema: the observational PALADIN study. *Br J Ophthalmol.* 105(3): 414–419.

26. Fallico M, Maugeri A, Lotery A, Longo A, Bonfiglio V et al [2021]. Fluocinolone acetonide vitreous insert for chronic diabetic macular oedema: A systematic review with meta-analysis of real-world experience. *Sci Rep.* 11(1): 4800.

27. Campochiaro PA, Marcus DM, Awh CC, Regillo C, Adamis AP et al [2019]. The port delivery system with ranibizumab for neovascular age-related macular degeneration: Results from the randomized phase 2 ladder clinical trial. *Ophthalmol.* 126(8): 1141–1154.

28. Holekamp NM, Campochiaro PA, Chang M, Miller D, Pieramici D, Archway Investigators et al [2021]. Archway randomized phase 3 trial of the port delivery system with ranibizumab for neovascular age-related macular degeneration. *Ophthalmol.* S0161–6420(21)00734.

29. Gutierrez M, Rodriguez JL, Zamora-de La Cruz D, Flores Pimentel MA, Jimenez-Corona A et al [2019]. Pars plana vitrectomy combined with scleral buckle versus pars plana vitrectomy for giant retinal tear. *Cochrane Database Syst Rev.* 12(12): CD012646.

14 Futuristic Approaches in Vitreoretinal Surgery

14.1 AUGMENTED REALITY–ASSISTED SURGERY

Technology is now able to significantly influence human experience, thinking, and senses by providing additional data about the current environment or digitally transporting into a remote, unreal, or simulated environment. Technology also enables the person to interact with the altered environment through digital means. An umbrella term for such technology is extended reality [XR]. It includes virtual reality [VR, wherein the experience is with a simulated or remote environment, e.g., Google Glass], augmented reality [AR, wherein the experience in the immediate surroundings is enhanced by superimposed digital cues or editing tools, e.g., the game Pokémon GO; Snapchat lenses], and mixed reality [MR, wherein objects in the real world and digital world interact, e.g., Microsoft HoloLens]. As the name suggests, AR is a state wherein the perspective of a real environment [e.g., the surgical field] is enhanced. This is achieved by digitally superimposing related and useful data as well as suggesting alternate pathways, solutions, and approaches. The superimposed data, for example, could be related to dimensions of a mass, depth at which it is located, or important structures adjacent to the mass; in addition, it could suggest which surgical approach is likely to provide the safest outcome. In the realm of vitreoretinal surgery, for example, it could project a thickness map of the patient's internal limiting membrane ILM, into the surgical field, during 3D surgery for macular hole. Based on this and the proximity of large blood vessels, it could suggest the best site at which to initiate ILM peel. It could also project dimensions and various indices of the macular hole, as well as indicate which approach would likely provide the best probability of achieving closure after surgery. It is true that preoperatively, every surgeon [and her or his team] analysis available data, variables, and results from prior studies and forms a plan that is likely to provide the best results. However, there is always a possibility of human fallibility and errors of the moment. AR attempts to provide, in real time, data and decision outcomes that are likely to be less biased and more objective. It is like performing surgery under the guidance of an omnipresent and knowledgeable mentor [digital, invisible], throughout the surgery. AR not only projects data points collected before surgery [e.g., optical coherence tomography (OCT) numeric or thickness map] but also collects and analyses data points in real time, as the surgery is being performed. Feedback is provided after a synthesis of all the available [prior and real time] data points and again an updated analysis and outcome probability is projected. Two types of AR can be used—with markers and without markers. In AR with marker, the image [e.g., computed tomography of the brain] is preprogramed into the device along with some reference points. These points act as indicators for the AR to determine the pose [position and orientation] of its camera when AR is being used during surgery. Markerless AR uses cues such as colour, pattern, and so on and an identification algorithm for recognition. One application of using digital markers in retinal surgery is said to be localization of retinal breaks that are sometimes 'lost' during air-fluid exchange. Another application is using AR as preoperative simulator to identify the best fit surgical settings for subretinal prosthesis implantation.

How is this achieved? For AR to work, the surgeon has to share the surgical field with a camera [special headset, smart phone, overhead camera], which routes this into a data processing unit [computer software, smartphone app]. These data, obtained in real time, are rapidly analysed and compared with preoperative data, as well as comparable data from literature datasets and the Internet of Things [IoT]. The combined data are synthesized, and the best-fit pathway possibilities are projected back digitally into the surgical field for the surgeon [and his team] to process and consider.

                                                  DOI: 10.1201/9781003179320-15

The surgeon is then able to modify the intervention [taking his or her own experience and expertise into consideration] to obtain the best outcome. AR is already in use in fields like neurosurgery wherein surgeons use an AR projection of the patient's brain in three dimension to gain a better perspective and aid them through the surgical steps. Robocop glasses, an AR-based device, is being evaluated to train vitreoretinal surgeons. The surgical field [real world] in this is augmented by magnification of the image virtually [about eight times, the same as microscope magnification] and by projecting guidelines [using, e.g., arrows] on how to proceed with removing a retinal membrane using an intravitreal forceps. Unlike virtual reality, in AR, the surgeon is also able to see real-world attributes like her or his hands and the position of the surgical instruments.

Surgery or its preoperative planning [using data available from colour, multimodal, and volume data] using AR is best accomplished using a head-mounted system [HMS]. Case series of vitreous procedures using HMS-3000MT, Clarity HMS, and Avegant Glyph retinal projection systems have been recently reported. In HMS systems, images from high-resolution 3D cameras mounted on the surgical microscope are projected separately [but rapidly] for the right and left eye using dual video input. Fusion of these images creates a high-resolution stereoscopic image. Some systems, such as Avegant, use mirrors and microarray to directly project images independently into the right and left eyes of the surgeon. None of these systems have currently undergone comparative clinical studies. In the future, AR is likely to become integrated with robotic-assisted surgery, and only then is its full potential likely to unravel.

14.2 ROBOTIC VITREORETINAL SURGERY

The word *robot* is derived from the Slavic *robota*, which translates to servant or slave and was first introduced in a play almost a century ago. With advancements in technology and computing, robotics has evolved into an area of specialization within the field of engineering. Robotics involves the conceptualization, design, and applications of machinery that can emulate and reproduce mechanical tasks that are performed by human beings. These machines have been in use for several decades in areas that are beyond human capability such as space exploration and repair and deep-sea exploration. More recently, they are being used to replace human labour in homes and workplaces. In combination with the exponential improvements in deep learning and machine learning, robot-assisted surgery is expected to achieve a quantum leap in terms of precision and clinical applicability. It is also expected to improve the quality and standardization of surgical training. Limitations of robotic surgery include the technical complexity, cost, and questions on responsibility assignment, consent, ethics, and liability. Although robotic platforms provide 3D visualization, access to tissues and better dexterity to the surgeon, surgical aspects like traction, applied force, suture tying strength, dissection, and tissue response are based largely on visual cues. To overcome some of these limitations, approaches like the haptic feedback systems and tactile feedback systems have been studied.

Robotic-assisted surgery has been in clinical use for many decades as well but is a relatively recent area of research in the field of vitreoretinal surgery. All robotic platforms adhere to the master–slave principle wherein the surgeon remotely controls the telemetry of the robotic movements through the intermediary of a complex control panel. All robotic platforms have a clearly defined working space [volume] centered on the handle position, force capability, and bandwidth. Although the first robotic-assisted ocular surgery was reported in 1989 by Guerrouad and Vidan using their stereotactic micromanipulator, to date, there are only a few centers worldwide pioneering in this area of research. Hence, it is likely to take a decade or more before it makes its way into the vitreoretinal surgical suite. Some of the centres involved in advanced level research on applications of robotics in vitreoretinal surgery include München, Germany; Johns Hopkins University, University of California, and Columbia University, United States; Lausanne, Switzerland; and Tokyo University. The first experimental robotic vitreoretinal surgery on human eye, peeling of a 10-μm membrane by Maclaren and his team, was at the Oxford University in 2016.

Although the anatomical success of most vitreoretinal surgeries has currently reached levels above 90%, there are situations like endovascular, subretinal, intraretinal, and choroidal interventions that are beyond routine possibility. In addition, there is a level of natural hand tremor during surgical procedures, and it is believed that eliminating the physiological tremor by the use of robotics would improve the precision and reduce the risk of collateral tissue damage and complications during vitreoretinal interventions.

Robotic platforms usually consist of a head fixation system, eye fixation ring, micromanipulator, and dual surgeon control panel. Four types of robotic platforms are recognized for vitreoretinal surgery: assistive hand-held devices, co-manipulation platforms, tele-manipulation platforms, and devices for special applications [Octomag and Microhand].

Following are some of the studies on robotic-assisted VR surgery that have been conducted experimentally.

1. Delicate peeling of membranes using an innovative micromanipulator called 'Micron'. Using active tremor cancelling, significant reduction in oscillations in the range of 2–20 Hz has been noted. In addition, the peeling forces were found to be below 7 mN. Unlike most robotic platforms, which are mounted on a table, Micron is a fully handheld system. In Micron, the position information is provided by optical sensors, and it operates by activating three piezoelectric actuators, each with a motion range of 400 μm.
2. Integration of intraoperative OCT into the robotic platform to improve target localization and assist with the delivery of pharmacologic agents, stem cells, and gene vectors into the subretinal space. Intuitive localization of the surgical tool with this approach is said to approach 5 μ.

In the coming years, surgery using robotic technology would have greater penetrance into the operation theatres. However, autonomous robotic surgeries are unlikely to gain acceptance any time in the future. This is because robots have no means of recognizing tissues by themselves. Experimentally, recognition of tissues by robots has been achieved on cadavers by using dyes and contrast agents and more recently by tool–tissue interaction. In addition, autonomous robotic surgery has a higher scale of all the other limitations indicated earlier.

14.3 RETINAL PROSTHESES

A prosthetic device is an artificial device that is used for rehabilitation when tissue rejuvenation or replacement is not possible. Unlike limb or cardiac prostheses in which the key effect of the device is mechanical function, retinal prostheses would need advanced neural functioning for image capture, transmission, interpretation, and feedback. In addition, they need to be miniature in size. Retinal prostheses are useful only when the native retinal tissue still has some residual functioning elements such as photoceptors and first- and second-order neurons. In the absence of functioning retinal elements, studies using optic nerve prosthesis are underway. Optic nerve prosthesis like AV-DONE [artificial vision by direct optic nerve electrode] uses three to seven 0.05-mm wire electrodes embedded into the optic nerve [after vitrectomy]. Owing to complex requirements, safety concerns, challenging surgical approach, and negligible possibility of achieving even form vision [most experiments have been able to generate phosphenes], advances in the field of retinal prosthesis has been slow but steady. As testimonial to the perseverance and ingenuity of pioneers in this field [who were able to consistently achieve some form vision], the FDA approved clinical use of the Argus II device a few years ago. The basic construct of retinal prostheses includes integration of stimulus perceived using an electronic receiver, transmission of the signal, and secondary feedbacks. The components of the prostheses are embedded into biologically inert substances like polyimide or silicone. Visual signals are usually received by a camera, chip, microarray, or wire electrode. Received images are then either processed digitally and relayed back to the chip, from where it is hoped that these signals would get picked up and be further transmitted along the bipolar and ganglion cells to the lateral geniculate body and visual cortex. The ideal scenario would be when the prosthesis takes over the role of the photoreceptors and the rest of the image processing and transmission happens through intact retinal and visual pathway. However, technology is many decades away from being able to invent an electronic array with the same resolving capability of the retinal photoreceptors. Even if this were to be achieved, its integration with the next cellular relay would remain an arduous task to achieve.

Devices being tested to function as an artificial retina can be classified, based on the location of implantation, into epiretinal prosthesis, subretinal prosthesis, and suprachoroidal prosthesis. Each of these has unique advantages and disadvantages in terms of safety, ease of implantation, and efficacy. **In a suprachoroidal approach**, a 49-electrode array is placed within a scleral pocket and another reference electrode into the vitreous cavity. There is a secondary coil and image processing chip that is surgically implanted sub-dermally over the temporal scalp. This device aims at suprachoroidal–transretinal stimulation. A suprachoroidal prosthesis seems the safest because it does not carry the risk of damaging residual retinal tissue elements. However, being located away from the neurosensory retina, higher energy is necessary to drive the device, and there is significant degradation of the signals and loss of resolution during transmission. **Subretinal prostheses** uses a chip made of micro-photodiode array [MPDA] for capture of light and images passing through normal ocular media. This image is then expected to relay forward through intact bipolar and ganglion cells. Implantation of the array into the subretinal space has been achieved through an internal approach [pars plana vitrectomy], external approach [scleral window followed by choroidal entry and placement of the implant], or a combined approach. Creation of submacular detachment by injecting balanced salt solution into the subretinal space using a 41G cannula helps in implantation of the microarray. Some of these implants may have two types of microarrays, a light-dependent [with 1500 elements] and a light-independent electrode array of 16 electrodes. MPDA, in addition to detecting light signals, amplifies and connects the signal through fine electrodes into the neurosensory retina. The battery and other operations of the device are controlled remotely through a cable connected to the microarray. The cable extends beneath the lateral rectus subcutaneously over the auricle and then connects to the control device on a neck band. The MPDA array is about $1000\,\mu \times 1000\,\mu$ in overall size, and each electrode is $50\,\mu \times 50\,\mu$. The number of electrodes may vary from 1500 to 5000 depending on the model. Subretinal protheses have several advantages, including stabile location without the need for fixation, stimulation by lesser current [as they lie in close association with the neurosensory retina], and lack of dependency on external cameras and image processors. These implants are also thought to provide neurotrophic and neuroprotective effect as they enhance survival of the remaining photoreceptors. A contrary opinion is that subretinal prostheses may actually increase the risk of thermal damage [due to current flow] to the surviving photoreceptors. Other disadvantages are the need for a more surgically challenging procedure, risk of implant corrosion, and degradation. A third approach to artificial retina is the epiretinal prosthesis. The intraocular 'chip' is affixed onto the retinal surface using tacks after vitrectomy. It is connected through a cable to an external camera, image processing chip, and battery. The external component of the device is carried on a spectacle. So, it can be noticed that the epiretinal component, unlike the subretinal protheses, does not receive or capture light or image directly. It only receives images captured and processed outside the eye and helps in transmitting this processed image directly into the ganglion cells [through fine microelectrodes]. In the Argus II prostheses, which has been FDA approved [second sight retinal prostheses], the electronic stimulator and processor are sutured onto the sclera itself using a silicone encircling band. With this device, patients had better localization and motion detection capability. This device has enabled some patients to achieve visual acuity of 20/1260. Serious adverse events from the surgical procedure include retinal detachment and endophthalmitis. **Epiret** is a recent approach in which the image receiver is implanted into the capsular bag [similar to a standard intraocular lens]. A microcable connects the capsular bag receiver to an epiretinal image receiver [fixed to the retinal surface with tacks] that transmits images through microelectrodes into the inner retina. In this device, image capture and processing are through spectacle mounted camera. Despite FDA approval, the evolution of retinal prostheses is still in its nascent stages, and routine usage is likely to take another decade. Until this time, conventional low vision rehabilitation measures remain cost effective and superior to available retinal prostheses in enabling patients to navigate.

14.4   LASER, FUGO BLADE, AND PULSED ELECTRON KNIFE VITREOUS SURGERY

Until a decade ago, the maximum cut rate possible with mechanical vitreous cutters was about 2500 c/m. To cut the vitreous fibrils, mechanical cutters have to first draw in the fibrils into the port using vacuum. In the absence of posterior vitreous detachment, the vacuum force could get transmitted to the retina via the vitreous fibrils. Hence, mechanical cutters were considered as suboptimal tools for vitrectomy with a higher risk for producing iatrogenic breaks due to the force of aspiration. So, there were continued efforts at identifying a safer method for performing vitrectomy. Some of these methods included laser vitreolysis, Fugo blade, and pulsed electron avalanche knife [PEAK] surgery. Experiments with holmium: yttrium aluminum garnet [YAG] laser were not successful as the results were not reproducible, and the depth of laser effect was very variable. Subsequently, erbium (Er): YAG laser was found to be a suitable candidate for **laser-assisted vitreous surgery.** While Erbium is a rare earth element, Er: YAG is a solid-state laser with YAG ($Y_3Al_5O_{12}$) serving as a dopant [substance added in minute amounts to another pure substance to alter its conductivity]. It emits light in the infrared range at a wavelength of 2940 nm, and the emission is strongly absorbed by water. For vitreous surgery, the emitted laser is coupled with a zirconium–fluoride (ZrF) optical fibre. This fibre terminates into a cavity located within a quartz tip of 320 μ, of the handpiece. At 200-ms duration, Er: YAG laser has a cutting threshold between 2 and 8 mJ. Probes with graduated output between 0.2 and 5mJ/pulse and repetition rate of 2–30 Hz have been used in patients for maneuvers like transection, incision, vitreous liquefaction, ablation of membranes, retinotomy, and coagulation of retinal vessels. It has been found to produce fewer tissue vibrations and movements and to be able to liquefy vitreous in the same amount of time [average, 4.5 minutes of laser time for basic vitrectomy] but with lower vacuum. Reduced traction on the vitreous fibrils is thought to decrease the risk of suction-induced retinal tears during surgery. Lateral thermal damage during ablation was also found to be restricted to 50 μ. Hence, the Er: YAG vitrectomy probe was considered safer than mechanical vitreous cutters. However, a major limitation noted was the extreme caution needed [and hence the slow pace of surgery] while working close to the retinal surface [e.g., dissection of epiretinal membrane]. In addition, the device is costly and large. These disadvantages have prevented the acceptance of laser assisted vitreous surgery into routine practice. Most recently, the diode-pumped Q switched Nd: YAG laser has been evaluated in porcine eye for vitreous surgery. **Fugo blade** [after the inventor, Richard Fugo] is a handheld surgical tool devised for high-precision, resistance-free making of incisions and molecular dissolution of tissues. The handpiece consists of a tiny filament that on activation produces a cloud of plasma [also called the fourth state of matter], a conglomeration of highly energized thermal, or non-thermal ionized gases. The plasma appears as a yellow light when the handpiece is switched on and is created by focused electromagnetic waves generated by four C cell battery– [standard size of dry cell battery] powered sources. The Fugo blade comes in multiple tip sizes and is chosen based the task at hand. Each tip produces a track slightly larger than the tip itself [e.g., a 300-μ tip is known to result in a 450-μ track]. The energy within the plasma cloud is able to break molecular bonds within tissues through a process of resonance. This ability is confined only to tissues with which it is in contact, and there is no collateral spread, charring, or burning. As a result, the incision and tissue ablation are very precise [said to be sharper than an incision made with a diamond blade]. In addition, it has the ability to cut through thick, avascular, and fibrotic membranes, as well as vascularized membranes, without producing any bleeding. This property has been used to manage patients with retinal hemangioblastomas and complex retinal detachments. This blade has been approved by the FDA for capsulotomy and iridotomy but not for vitreous surgery due to safety concerns about the effect of plasma on the retina while carrying out ablation of membranes lying in close proximity. Routine use of the Fugo blade is also impractical owing to the prohibitive cost [in 2007] of the handpiece [$20,000] and each disposable tip [$20]. The handpiece is also bulky and non-ergonomic.

PEAK is a type of plasma blade introduced after the Fugo blade for performing surgical dissection with precision and relatively avascular manner. It allows coagulation of bleeders and traction free tissue dissection depending on the mode of operation [hot or cold respectively]. The modes can be switched without having to remove the probe from the vitreous cavity. The probe has an integrated light source, and the tip has a 50-μ wire protruding about 0.3–0.6 mm. Power and pulse adjustment is possible based on the type of tissue to be dissected. Tissue dissection produced with PEAK is precise and reproducible, but collateral damage could result depending on the voltage, probe length, and distance of the tip from the retina. It has been successfully used to dissect epiretinal membranes and other avascular and vascular membranes, as well as make drainage and relaxing retinotomy. In the absence of a safe plane and distance of separation between the retina and the abnormal tissue, bimanual dissection may be helpful. Formation of air bubbles could obscure visualization of the surgical field. Unlike the Er: YAG laser developed for vitreous surgery, the Fugo blade and PEAK do not have the ability for aspiration and irrigation. This could be an advantage as it can be easily integrated with standard multiport vitreous surgery. Currently, advances in technology of mechanical cutters with the ability to achieve ultrahigh cuts rates [5000–16,000 cpm] have reduced the risk of traction-induced retinal breaks during surgery. Hence, it is unlikely that laser-assisted and plasma blade–assisted surgery would find acceptance in the near future unless they become more ergonomic and cost-effective. It is also possible that there may be a revival of these tools with advances in robotic vitreoretinal surgery and 3D surgery.

14.5 PHARMACOTHERAPY OF PROLIFERATIVE VITREORETINOPATHY

Improvements in instrumentation and technological advancements in vitreous machines, illumination, and viewing systems have helped to improve the success rate of vitreoretinal surgery for PVR from about 75% to about 90%. However, recurrent proliferation still occurs in a significant number of patients and remains the number one cause of redetachment. Since PVR is a dynamic cellular process with recognizable risk factors, efforts at reducing the same through pharmacological measures have been made. Depending on the time of the cell cycle at which a drug acts, two categories have been identified. They are cycle-specific and phase-specific drugs. The former is effective only when the cells are in the growth phase, while the latter is effective at a specific phase of the cell cycle [e.g., the S phase (synthesis phase)]. The synthesis phase is the most critical step when cells are amenable to pharmacological modulation. Inhibitors of PVR can be broadly grouped into anti-inflammatory agents, inhibitors of cellular proliferation, and modulators of extracellular matrix [ECM].

Several of the agents that have been evaluated in the past include 5-flurouracil [a fluoropyrimidine that acts by inhibiting thymidylate synthetase and 'corrupts' ribosomal RNA, thereby inhibiting cellular proliferation and reducing contractility], daunorubicin [an anthracycline antibiotic that inhibits cellular proliferation independent of the cell cycle by DNA binding, ion chelation, and free radical formation], colchicine [an alkaloid that suppress cellular proliferation by inhibiting sol-gel transformation in mitotic spindle and hence motility], Taxol [inhibits cellular proliferation by retarding contraction of the collagen gel], Cis hydroxyproline [modulates ECM by inhibiting synthesis of hydroxyproline and destabilizing collagen fibres], penicillamine [chelates copper and hence inhibits the enzyme lysyl oxidase, thereby affecting ECM formation], Arginyl-Glycyl, Aspertyl-Serine [RGDS] tetrapeptide [blocks fibronectin attachment to cells], and heparin [inhibits fibroblast adhesion to fibronectin, blocks Go-phase transition and inhibits polymerization of collagen]. Currently, the only interventions under clinical evaluation as inhibitors of recurrent PVR after vitreoretinal surgery are intravitreal triamcinolone and dexamethasone sustained-release implants.

14.6   ENZYMATIC VITREOLYSIS

Separation of the posterior hyaloid from the retinal surface occurs naturally during the senile process of PVD. In a majority of patients, PVD does not result in any untoward serious sequelae. Patients who have had safe PVD are said to be protected from retinal pathologies such as vitreomacular traction, epiretinal membrane, macular hole, and proliferative vascular retinopathies. In addition, it is well recognized that the presence of complete preoperative PVD significantly improves the safety of vitreoretinal surgeries. Also, features of evolving PVD may be seen on OCT in some patients with early stages of macular hole and vitreomacular traction. While it is now common practice to induce PVD during vitreoretinal surgery, this entails a major surgical intervention and is hence fraught with significant risks. Surgical induction of PVD is particularly challenging during paediatric vitreoretinal surgery and diabetic vitreoretinal surgery and in patients with familial vitreoretinopathies. Owing to all of these observations on the advantage conferred by PVD and the risks associated with its surgical induction, efforts continue to be made to find an intravitreal agent that can safely induce separation of the posterior hyaloid from the retinal surface. Since the hyaloidoretinal interface is maintained largely by laminin, fibronectin, and chondroitin sulphate, the majority of the agents for that have been evaluated for inducing chemical vitreolysis have been enzymes [hence, enzymatic vitreolysis]. These enzymes include hyaluronidase, urokinase, dispase, plasmin, chondroitinase, and tissue plasminogen activator [tPA].

Hyaluronidase is routinely used as an adjunct during periocular anaesthesia to improve diffusion and uptake of the anaesthetic. On intravitreal injection, it acts on hyaluron, the major macro molecule within the vitreous, and destabilizes its structure. This results in liquefaction of the vitreous but does not produce PVD. Earlier reports indicated that following intravitreal administration in low concentration [1 IU/0.1mL] along with 0.2 ml of C3F8, PVD could be induced in vitro. However, more recent experimental studies using hyaluronidase alone have failed to detect signs of PVD on electron microscopic evaluation. Human trials with 55 IU of highly purified ovine hyaluronidase [Vitrase] have found the injection to be safe and able to hasten the clearing of vitreous haemorrhage secondary to diabetic retinopathy. This could be secondary to liquefaction of the vitreous rather than PVD induction. Chondroitinase is a nonspecific enzyme that has a potential to induce PVD as chondroitin sulphate is an important component of the hyaloid–ILM interface. However, chondroitin sulphate is also an important component of the interphotoreceptor matrix, so there is a risk of photoreceptor toxicity. One clinical study found quicker induction of PVD following injection of chondroitinase at the beginning of vitreous surgery. However, it remains poorly explored. Dispase is a protease enzyme isolated from *Bacillus polymyxa* and having a selective effect on collagen type 4 [basement collagen] and fibronectin. Due to its action on fibronectin, it has been explored for experimental induction of PVD. Studies, however, found that while PVD does result, there is also significant damage to the ILM. The latter effect is now exploited to induce experimental proliferative vitreoretinopathy [Dispase model of PVR].

Plasmin is a naturally occurring protease enzyme within the serum and is primarily responsible for fibrinolysis. However, it has also been found to have a broad range of action on coagulation factors, ECM proteins [including laminin and fibronectin]. Plasmin has a very short half-life and is almost immediately neutralized by alpha-2 antiplasmin. It is generated [when its action is deemed necessary within the body] by the cleavage of circulating plasminogen under the effect of tPA. Plasmin has been found to be the most effective agent in creating PVD in both experimental and clinical studies. However, it is very labile and difficult to synthesize and maintain. Hence, its practical utility is limited. It can be separated from the patient's own autologous blood, but the process is tedious and takes over 2 days [starting with withdrawal of blood and further steps] to procure.

Using recombinant technology, a truncated fraction of plasmin [called microplasmin] containing its catalytic domain was synthesized. Following multiple clinical studies, this agent [ocriplasmin] was approved by the FDA for the management of symptomatic patients with vitreomacular traction. It was commercially available as Jetrea, and the recommended dose for intravitreal injection was 1.25 µg in 0.1 ml. Though effective in inducing PVD in a significant number of patients with vitreomacular traction [VMT], it failed to gain widespread usage owing to the high cost [almost $4000], absence of clear guidelines for real-world management of VMT, and rapidly improving ease and safety of vitreoretinal surgery. The production and sale of Jetrea were halted in 2020 due to business reasons, and it is no longer available commercially.

As an in vivo surrogate for plasmin, studies have been undertaken to induce PVD using tPA [converts plasminogen to plasmin]. In addition, it is commercially available and affordable and can be procured without difficulty. Being synthesized using recombinant technology, it is devoid of contaminants. However, several aspects of its usage remain unexplored, including the dose and time frame when it is most effective [a few minutes or/ hours before surgery], so it is not routinely being used. In the future, sequential injection of autologous serum into the vitreous followed by tPA injection may be found effective. Experimental induction of PVD has also been obtained by intravitreal injection of lysine plasminogen and recombinant urokinase.

Research into enzymatic vitreolysis is again likely to gain pace if the natural history, risk factors for progression, severity grades and high-risk features for developing complications in patients with vitreomacular traction is unequivocally defined. In addition to the beneficial effects of PVD in VMT, enzymatic vitreolysis would have a potential role during vitreoretinal surgery in young children, familial vitreoretinopathies, and other complex detachments [e.g., coloboma, pathological myopia]. As the protective effect of PVD in patient with diabetes is well documented, enzymatic vitreolysis may also have a role in preventing progression of severe non-proliferative diabetic retinopathy to proliferative diabetic retinopathy.

14.7   ENDOSCOPIC VITRECTOMY

Visualization of structures internalized within the human body using narrow, rigid, or flexible viewing systems, passed through small surface openings, has been in routine use for many decades in fields like orthopaedics, gastroenterology, urology, and pulmonary medicine. In some of these fields, simultaneous surgical interventions like collecting biopsy specimens or resecting polyps are also performed. [Use of endoscopes is also common in the field of engineering to study defects in machine components.] The basic components and design of an endoscope depend on its purpose, to simply be able to visualize hidden structures or to be able to perform additional functions like taking a tissue specimen. Endoscopes designed for the sole purpose of visualization consist of a system of lenses [that can be focused to a limited extent] and a means [usually fiberoptic] for transmitting the images to a viewing monitor. Extended purpose endoscopes, in addition, may have integrated channels to aspirate and irrigate tissue and collect specimens. All these functions are controlled remotely. Endoscopes for the purpose of vitreous surgery need more miniaturization, sophistication, precision, and additional functions [cutting, laser]. Optical clarity of the human eye generally allows good visualization of structures within the posterior segment, both for evaluation as well as surgical intervention. Despite a clear media, there remain structures like the ciliary body [often involved in severe pathologies like cyclitic membrane, anterior loop traction, impacted foreign body] that are difficult to visualize. A more common difficulty faced in the clinic is assessment of posterior segment structures due to severe abnormalities in the anterior segment [e.g., opaque cornea, dense pupillary membrane with flat anterior chamber]. In these situations, one can indirectly determine the anatomical status and functional capacity of the posterior segment using clinical tests like assessing for inverse relative afferent pupillary defect, ultrasonography, ultrasound biomicroscopy, and electrophysiological tests. The endoscope, by allowing direct visualization and assessment of posterior segment structures is claimed to allow better decision making and prognostication. The exact role and impact of vitreous surgery under an endoscope remain less certain as postoperative evaluation remains impossible, and the visual disability persists at the conclusion of surgery. Thus, the use of endoscopic procedures remains limited, although clinical studies on vitreous surgery using an endoscope began about three decades ago. Endoscopes for vitreous surgery when introduced were 20G, but more recently, 23G and 25G devices have become available. Similar to the vitreous infusion suction cutter, these probes have multifunction capability. In its early clinical use, it was found to be extremely useful in furthering our understanding about reasons for failure of retinal detachment surgery and in deciphering the pathogenesis and complexity of anterior PVR in clinical situations.

The typical endoscope has an objective lens [Hopkins-rod lenses or gradient index (GRIN) lenses] located along the central axis at the tip of the fiberoptic cable and multiple fibres for imaging, for illumination, and for laser. Imaging fibres run coherently along the core of the cable, while fibres for illumination lie at the periphery. The fibre for laser is solitary and runs within the peripheral fibres. Endoscope allows 360-degree visualization of the peripheral structures without needing scleral indentation. Based on the angulation, structures in front [frontal view] as well as those adjacent [tangential view] can be visualized. The field of view [FOV] and magnification depends on the distance of the endoscope tip. FOV is panoramic when the endoscope is at the site of insertion and becomes increasingly focal as it is taken closer to the area of interest. Magnification can vary from 5× to 20× depending on the distance between the probe and tissue [retinal capillaries could also be visualized]. Recent endoscopes have relatively higher resolution [17,000 pixels]. The device can be used safely in phakic eyes but only after going past an initial learning phase [about tens of cases] in pseudophakic eyes. Becoming accustomed to the orientation [side-on view compared with top-bottom view of the microscope; a rotational axis, in addition to the x and y axes], dynamic tissue magnification, judging distance of the probe from the tissue [due to lack of stereopsis], higher glare [as illumination and light capture is coaxial], and locating the intraocular instruments [due to narrow FOV, as the endoscope is taken closer to the tissue] remain challenges during endoscopic surgery. Recently, surgical manoeuvres using the endoscope [to visualize ciliary sulcus and anterior PVR] have been carried out using 3D visualization [Ngenuity]. This is said to be possible due to split-screen option, data fusion software, and digital image enhancement [reduces glare]. As 3D surgery gains greater acceptance, it is likely that combined surgery using endoscopic viewing would become common practice during procedures like scleral fixation and management of severe anterior PVR. The latter, in particular, is likely to prevent chronic hypotony and improve long-term outcomes. In addition, it may be found useful [in combination with 3D surgery] in performing paediatric surgeries in advanced retinopathy of prematurity with significant involvement of the retro-iridial structures.

14.8   GENE THERAPY

In disease processes, cell death may occur by either apoptosis or necrosis, while in degenerative process, it is largely by apoptosis. Apoptosis is also known as programmed cell death or induced cell death and is initiated by endogenous cellular processes triggered by a gene or set of genes. Programmed cell death is an energy-requiring process of self-elimination of cells without production of cellular debris to attract macrophages. Programmed cell death is normally known to occur during embryogenesis and morphogenesis to regulate the size and shape of organs by deletion of selective cells. It is also known to occur physiologically in the normal turnover of intestinal epithelial cells, prostate epithelium, hormone-mediated regression of uterine epithelium, deletion of lymphocyte clones, regression of lactating mammalian gland, and atresia of ovarian follicles. Necrosis, in contrast, is inflicted by noxious stimulus in which macrophages are attracted and cell death occurs in clusters.

Degenerative diseases of the retina, involving the retinal pigment epithelium and photoreceptors, like retinitis pigmentosa, Leber's congenital amaurosis [LCA], and Stargardt's disease contribute significantly to the burden of low vision globally. Until a few decades ago, the mechanism of cell death in photoreceptors and retinal pigment epithelium was not known. However, studies on Royal College of Surgeons [RCS] rats have now shown that apoptosis is a predominant method. It has also been found that photoreceptor cell death often occurs secondary to a genetic defect in the neighbouring retinal pigment epithelial cells. It has been demonstrated that in transfected cell cultures and transgenic mouse lines, expression of certain genes can prevent apoptosis. Hence, for gene-mediated disease, advances in gene therapy may play a significant role in preventing, reversing, or retarding the degenerative process. Studies have also tried to precisely determine the nature of cell death in age-related macular degeneration [ARMD].

Genes have been experimentally introduced to rescue photoreceptor cells from degeneration, and corrective genes have also been introduced into cultured retinal pigment epithelial cells using retrovirus as a vector. As this requires dividing cells for the gene transfer to occur, it cannot be used in the adult retina wherein the cells are not replicating. However, methods have now also been devised to transfer exogenous genes into differentiated living animals with procedures such as injection of naked DNA or DNA mixed with a highly polar lipid vehicle. Replication deficient adenoviruses used as vectors for gene transfer in post-mitotic cells have not been found to cause any severe tissue damage. Adenovirus has also been tried to transfect post-mitotic photoreceptors and retinal pigment epithelial cells in vivo. Whether they can control gene expression in these cells remains poorly understood. Attempts at gene modification of retinal pigment epithelial cells to inhibit programmed cell death by injecting therapeutically modified adenovirus E1 and E4 vectors into the subretinal space have also been made for several decades.

Based on the results in the canine model, three independent clinical pilot studies were initiated in 2008 on RPE65 deficient patients with LCA. No untoward systemic immunological response and serious ocular adverse events were noted in these three studies. One of these trials was conducted at the Children's Hospital of Philadelphia [CHOP] and its collaborating partners. Sub retinal injection of AAV-RPE65 was delivered in three patients aged 19–26 years. Visual improvement was noted on pupillometry, nystagmus charting, visual acuity, visual fields, and mobility charting after 15 days. Macular hole was noted as a complication in one patient. In a dose escalation phase 1 trial, the number of patients was increased to 12 by the same study group, and encouraging results were seen. It was noted that earlier treatment had better chances of visual gain. In contrast, a pilot study undertaken on three young adults at the University College of London and Moorfield's Eye Hospital using sub-retinal injections of recombinant AAV2-RPE65 complementary DNA found no statistical improvement in the visual parameters. Some positive change on dark adaptometry and microperimetry was observed in one subject. While studying 12 additional participants in an open-label trial, improvements were seen in retinal sensitivity in six patients for up to 3 years. This improvement was noted to peak at 6–12 months and then gradually decline. Although efficacy remained doubtful, safety was established. In the third trial carried out at University of Florida and University of Pennsylvania on three patients ages 21–24 years, the procedure was again reported to be same and some increment in photoreceptor sensitivity was observed. Currently, CHOP and University of Iowa have launched a collaborative phase 3 study on patients with LCA. Primary outcome measure is mobility testing at 1 year. Thirty-one patients older than 3 years of age have been enrolled, and the study is estimated to be completed in 2029. Preliminary reports suggest satisfactory improvement in mobility and visual sensitivity but not visual acuity. While introducing genes into the intraocular space or tissues seems to have a potential in managing some degenerative disorders of the retina, there is still a long road that basic scientists and clinicians have to travel, before precise guidelines on patient selection, outcome expectations, and follow-up can be made. Administering the therapeutic gene vector will likely become less invasive and safer with advances in 3D vitrectomy and robotic vitreoretinal surgery.

14.9 PORT DELIVERY SYSTEM

Intravitreal pharmacotherapy has become the mainstay for management of complications secondary to ARMD, diabetic retinopathy, and retinal vascular occlusions. Owing to the universal short half-life of all currently available anti–vascular endothelial growth factor agents and their inability to eradicate the basic pathology, they have to be administered into the vitreous cavity every 4–8 weeks. Almost 8–12 injections are needed in the first year, followed by continued monitoring and reinjection in the following years over an indefinite time frame. This approach is not time efficient for both the surgeon and the patient. In addition, there is a theoretical cumulative increase of the associated risks, following each additional injection. Alternate drug delivery systems [DDS], which minimize the need for repeated intravitreal injections, are being explored to enable sustained drug delivery. Some of these approaches include sustained-release intravitreal implants, refillable implants, injectable particulate systems, encapsulated cell delivery, iontophoresis, and nanotechnology. Alternate delivery routes like transscleral and suprachoroidal delivery have also been suggested. Of these, the most studied device clinically and currently undergoing phase 3 evaluation is the port delivery system (PDS). This is a refillable device for long-term delivery of drugs into the posterior segment and has to be placed surgically through a 3.2-mm scleral incision. A large incision is necessary to accommodate the diameter of the rigid drug reservoir. Insertion of this device requires prior surgical training to minimize complication rates. [Initial rates of complications were found to be very high, as more than 50% cases developed vitreous haemorrhage]. To reduce the risks, the procedure was then modified. Modification of the procedure involves partial dissection followed by laser and cauterization of the pars plana. Despite the modification, risk of serious adverse events, though diminished, continues to persist. Following recent results of phase 3 studies, the FDA has approved the PDS device [which is being marketed as **Susvimo**]. It is said to have the ability to maintain the stability of patients with wet ARMD with just two treatments annually. However, a major concern remains a nearly threefold higher risk of endophthalmitis [2%] in the Archway trial. The long-term safety and efficacy of Susvimo in wet ARMD are being further evaluated in the PORTAL study. Other ongoing trials with this device include VELODROME [to study efficacy with 9 month refill in wet ARMD], PAGODA [in diabetic macular edema], and PAVILION [in diabetic retinopathy without macular edema].

It is a general observation that larger the scleral incision, the greater the likelihood short- and long-term complications related to the procedure. A DDS that can be inserted without a scleral incision would make the procedure more safe and simpler. Towards this objective, we recently introduced the concept of PDS with an inflatable reservoir. The proposed DDS would have three parts; extrascleral, intrascleral, and intravitreal, with protective septae. The extrascleral and scleral parts of the DDS may be made of non-compliant materials, whereas the intravitreal part may be made of a more compliant material that allows inflation or expansion. The extrascleral part should be an easily identifiable solid non-transparent port with a safe septum through which the reservoir can be refilled. The diameter of the extrascleral part should be slightly more than the conjoining scleral part to prevent internal prolapse of the device. The scleral part may be around 0.5–0.7 mm in diameter, which is the size of a 23G–25G vitreous surgery cannula. Its length should be more than 1.5 mm, so that the internal opening of the device is safely within the intravitreal cavity, and not the suprachoroidal space [SCS]. The scleral and the extra-scleral parts should be separated by septum that permits passage of a refilling needle and acts as barrier. [This kind of septum has also been employed in the PDS being evaluated in clinical studies.] The distal-most 'inflatable' part of the DDS should be made of a semipermeable material, which will allow continuous but controlled release of the drug. At the outset of its implantation, the intravitreal part of the DDS can be kept folded inside the scleral conduit. Following a trans scleral stab incision with a 23G–25G microvitreoretinal knife in the pars plana region under aseptic precautions, the DDS can be gently inserted inside the incision manually or even with an injector. The extra-scleral part of the DDS, being larger in diameter than the incision, will stay flush on the scleral surface. As the length of the scleral part is designed to be more than the thickness of the outer coat of the eyeball, the distal end of the device would lie within the intravitreal space.

A fine needle can now be used to inject the drug into the reservoir system by penetrating the valvular septum using a pre-filled drug injector. Due to the compliant nature of the inflatable reservoir, it expands to accommodate a pre-designated volume of the injected drug. The inflated reservoir and retinal periphery could be evaluated using indirect ophthalmoscopy. Subsequently, following a pre-determined period or on the basis of clinical signs, refilling of the reservoir can be planned. The refilling procedure shall involve a simple injection of the drug as in the primary procedure. If therapy is deemed completed and the drug is no longer required, the implant can be easily removed [ensuring that the reservoir is completely deflated] by simply hinging the external part of the DDS and gentle externalization. If required, limited conjunctival dissection may be done. The chief difference between the DDS proposed by us and the ones existing or under evaluation is the 'expandable' reservoir. This reservoir shall be advantageous in bringing down the incision size needed from about 3 mm to 0.5 mm, thus six times less. This decrease shall obviate the need for surgical training and make the procedure much easier to learn. Even the refilling and the removal procedures would be simple. However, the chief advantage of using an inflatable reservoir would be in decreasing the complication rates by negating the necessity for a large scleral incision.

14.10 SUPRACHOROIDAL DRUG DELIVERY

The suprachoroidal approach is a newer method of drug delivery under investigation, providing higher levels of the drug to the posterior ocular tissues with minimal systemic adverse effects. Because of its proximity to the choroid, Bruch's membrane, and retinal pigment epithelium [RPE], drugs delivered into the SCS may reach these tissues at higher levels than intravitreal or transscleral routes. In addition, suprachoroidal injections do not disturb the vitreous body and are less likely to cause significant disturbances in visual acuity and changes in vitreous. Injection into SCS may also increase the duration of a drug effect [e.g., animal studies of triamcinolone acetonide injected into SCS of monkey and pig eyes have demonstrated a tissue resident time of about 120 days]. Currently, clinical trials on suprachoroidal injection of triamcinolone using microneedles are ongoing in patients with non-infectious chronic uveitis. The control arm in this study is given a sham injection. The drug comes in a prefilled syringe, and there are two needle lengths available for injection, one 900 µm and the other 1100 µm. The latter is chosen if the sclera is presumed to be thicker or if resistance to free drug delivery is noted while using the 900-µm needle. The injection is given at the pars plana, 3.5 to 4 mm away from the limbus. It is important to penetrate the sclera perpendicular to its surface. Pressure is then applied at the penetration site so that the hub is flush with the sclera and some dimpling is noted [Video 14.1]. The drug is only then injected. There is a small learning curve while using this method, so it would be useful to first practice using dummy eyes. One unusual observation noted by the author while using this device as part of a multicentric study has been the significant hardening of the eyeball and elevation of the IOP immediately after the injection. Hence, it would be necessary to monitor the IOP for about 15–30 minutes post-injection. Suprachoroidal delivery of triamcinolone using **Xipere** [formerly CLS-TA] has been recently given approval by FDA [based on the results of Peachtree trial and its extension, the Magnolia trial] for use in patients with uveitis.

14.11. TELESCOPIC INTRAOCULAR IMPLANTS

There are several chronic disorders of the retina in which central vision is significantly impaired. These include hereditary macular dystrophies and degenerations in the young and ARMD in adults. Until some decades ago, the only form of rehabilitation available was the prescription of low-vision aids in the form of optical and digital magnifiers. These devices have well-established limitations, so user acceptance is less than desirable. Implantation of an IOL that could function like a telescope and be able to deflect the image to a healthier part of the macula is a concept that is gaining ground in the management of patients with non-progressive, relatively stable central vision loss. The majority of these implants are currently used only in patients with geographic atrophy. There are several implant designs available, but their optical design is based on one of four principles: Galilean telescope [with one convex and one concave lens e.g., implantable miniature telescope [IMT], intraocular lens for visually impaired patients [IOL-VIP] system, intraocular lens in age-related macular degeneration [iolAMD]], Cassegrain approach [uses mirrors instead of lenses, Lipschitz implant], Fresnel prisms, and simple magnification at the centre of the IOL using a high plus lens [Scharioth macula lens].

IMT is a fixed-focus device measuring 4.5 mm in thickness, 3.2 mm in lens aperture, and 13.5 mm in diameter. It has to be implanted into the capsular bag after removal of the crystalline lens through a 12-mm incision. It is made of quartz and carries two lenses separated in air [hence achieving higher magnification]. The device is carried on a PMMA [polymethyl methacrylate] base with modified haptics. In combination with the cornea, it provides 3× magnification and 24-degree field of view projected over 55 degrees of the retina. Following the success of clinical trials [with a significant number of patients showing improvement in central vision of greater than two lines], the device was approved by FDA for use in patients older than 65 years of age with moderate and advanced dry ARMD. Only uniocular implantation is recommended as the device severely restricts the peripheral field. Hence, the patient has to go through proper counselling and a period of training so as to be able to use the implanted eye for central vision and unimplanted eye for peripheral vision. Although the device is bulky, endothelial cell loss is said to be comparable to conventional IOLs.

The **IOL-VIP** telescopic system is surgically created by the implantation of two high-powered PMMA, ultraviolet-filtering lenses, one biconcave [-66D, serves as eyepiece] into the capsular bag and another, biconvex [+55D, serves as objective], into the anterior chamber. Intense training of the patient, both before and after surgery, to determine an ideal retinal locus is considered important for success of the procedure. The lenses are implanted through a 7-mm incision after standard phacoemulsification. The capsulorrhexis has to be large to accommodate the high-power biconcave lens. Since shallowing of the anterior chamber is inevitable, there is a high risk of pupillary block. Hence, preoperative laser iridotomy is recommended. Unlike IMT, this procedure does not result in constriction of the visual field, so binocular activities are not impaired.

The **iolAMD** is similar to IOL-VIP in using two lenses to create a Galilean system, but the lenses are foldable and can be inserted through 3-mm incisions. The lenses are made of hydrophobic acrylic. The capsular bag implanted IOL is -49D and has 4-mm optic and a 11.0 overall diameter. The sulcus fixated IOL is +63D, 5-mm optic, and 12-mm diameter. The IOLs are decentred by 0.85 mm, and this allows an image shift of 3 degrees on the retina. These lenses are available only in the powers mentioned and so can be used only in eyes with 21—23 mm. There is a potential for pupillary block and higher endothelial cell loss with this lens.

The **Scharioth macula lens** is an add on intraocular implant for improving near visual acuity in patients with ARMD. It is a foldable PMMA lens [can be inserted through a 2.2-mm incision], with an overall diameter of 13 mm and has to be placed in the ciliary sulcus. It has a 1.5-mm optic zone with +10D power, the remaining lens component being neutral. It can be inserted during primary phacoemulsification over the standard IOL or as a secondary procedure in patients with uncomplicated pseudophakia and devoid of posterior capsular opacification. It must be reiterated to the patient that the macula add-on lens only enhances near vision and not intermediate or distance vision. The lens does not impede peripheral vision and binocularity.

The **Lipschitz macular implant** [LMI] is based on the Cassegrain telescopic system. It uses small mirrors in such a manner that the reflected image gets magnified 2.5 times on the retina. It is similar to a conventional IOL in its dimensions, 13 mm in overall diameter with 6.5-mm optic. It is implanted into the capsular bag through a 6.5-mm incision. Within the optic, there are two mirrors [1–2 mm in thickness], anterior [measuring 1.4 mm] and posterior [measuring 2.8 mm]. There is a

1.4-mm central opening in the posterior mirror. The mirrors are coated on their reflecting surface with titanium oxide and silicone dioxide. To improve biocompatibility, the entire lens is coated with poly-paraxylene. The outer zone of the optic allows normal peripheral vision. The newer LMI-SI is a non-foldable IOL that needs to be placed over a regular IOL implanted into the capsular bag.

The **Fresnel prism intraocular implant** does not provide any optical magnification but is capable of displacing the image to a region where the macula is healthy. It was introduced as a simpler alternate to the complex surgery of macular translocation. It has fixed central optical power of +20D with the Fresnel prism IOL designed on its posterior surface. The prism produces 6 degrees of deviation, corresponding to 1.8-mm displacement of the image on the retinal surface. However, this image shift would lead to fusional and hence oculomotor difficulties.

Telescopic IOLs have a certain degree of advantage over conventional low vision aids; however, they also have limitations that impede their routine use in practice. In addition, there seems to be less impetus for refining and customizing telescopic IOLs because highly potent pharmacotherapy currently available for macular disorders may have significantly delayed the onset and prevalence of disabling blindness in ARMD.

SUGGESTED READING

1. Güneş A, Koray K, Afsun S, Pablo A, Hakan U [2021]. Applications of augmented reality in ophthalmology [invited]. *Biomed Opt Express*. 12: 511–538.
2. Ong CW, Tan MCJ, Lam M, Koh VTC [2021]. Applications of extended reality in ophthalmology: Systematic review. *J Med Internet Res*. 23(8): e24152.
3. Forslund JM, Konge L, Alberti M, la Cour M, Park YS et al [2020]. Robot-assisted vitreoretinal surgery improves surgical accuracy compared with manual surgery. *Retina*. 40(11): 2091–2098.
4. Roizenblatt M, Edwards TL, Gehlbach PL [2018]. Robot-assisted vitreoretinal surgery: Current perspectives. *Robot Surg*. 5: 1–11.
5. Bloch E, Luo Y, da Cruz L [2019]. Advances in retinal prosthesis systems. *Ther Adv Ophthalmol*. 11: 25.
6. Weiland JD, Humayun MS [2014]. Retinal prosthesis. *IEEE Trans Biomed Eng*. 61(5): 1412–1424.
7. Uthoff D, Oravecz R, Kuehnl R et al [2020]. A promising approach in laser vitrectomy executed by plasma-mediated removal of vitreous body via a diode-pumped Q-switched Nd: YAG laser. *Sci Rep*. 10: 21710.
8. Berger JW, D'Amico J [1997]. Modelling of erbium: YAG laser mediated explosive photovapourization. *Impli Vitreoretl Surg*. 28(2): 133–139.
9. Priglinger SG, Haritoglou C, Mueller A, Grueterich M, Strauss RW et al [2005]. Pulsed electron avalanche knife in vitreoretinal surgery. *Retina*. 25(7): 889–896.
10. Priglinger SG, Haritoglou C, Palanker DV, Alge CS, Gandorfer A, Kampik A [2005]. Pulsed electron avalanche knife (PEAK-fc) for dissection of retinal tissue. *Arch Ophthalmol*. 123(10): 1412–1418.
11. Moysidis SN, Thanos A, Vavvas DG [2012]. Mechanisms of inflammation in proliferative vitreoretinopathy: From bench to bedside. *Mediators Inflamm*. 815937.
12. Schaub F, Hoerster R, Schiller P, Felsch M, Kraus D, et al [2018]. Prophylactic intravitreal 5-fluorouracil and heparin to prevent proliferative vitreoretinopathy in high-risk patients with retinal detachment: study protocol for a randomized controlled trial. *Trials*. 384.
13. Lopez-Lopez F, Rodriguez-Blanco M, Gómez-Ulla F, Marticorena J [2009]. Enzymatic vitreolysis. *Curr Diabetes Rev*. 5(1): 57–62.
14. Raczyńska D, Lipowski P, Zorena K, Skorek A, Glasner P [2015]. Enzymatic vitreolysis with recombinant tissue plasminogen activator for vitreomacular traction. *Drug Des Devel Ther*. 9: 6259–6268.
15. Ajlan RS, Desai AA, Mainster MA [2019]. Endoscopic vitreoretinal surgery: principles, applications and new directions. *Int J Retin Vitr*. 5: 15.
16. Lai FHP, Wong EWN, Lam WC, Lee TC, Wong SC et al [2021]. Endoscopic vitreoretinal surgery: Review of current applications and future trends. *Surv Ophthalmol*. 66(2): 198–212.
17. Campa C, Gallenga CE, Bolletta E, Perri P [2017]. The role of gene therapy in the treatment of retinal diseases: A review. *Curr Gene Ther*. 17(3): 194–213.
18. DiCarlo JE, Mahajan VB, Tsang SH [2018]. Gene therapy and genome surgery in the retina. *J Clin Invest*. 128(6): 2177–2188.
19. Khanani AM, Aziz AA, Weng CY, Lin WV, Vannavong J et al [2021]. Port delivery system: a novel drug delivery platform to treat retinal diseases. *Expert Opin Drug Deliv*. 18(11): 1571–1576.

20. Campochiaro PA, Marcus DM, Awh CC, Regillo C, Adamis AP et al [2019]. The port delivery system with ranibizumab for neovascular age-related macular degeneration: Results from the randomized phase 2 ladder clinical trial. *Ophthalmol.* 126(8): 1141–1154.

21. Jung JH, Chae JJ, Prausnitz MR [2019]. Targeting drug delivery within the suprachoroidal space. *Drug Discov Today.* 24(8): 1654–1659.

22. Yeh S, Khurana RN, Shah M, Henry CR, Wang RC, PEACHTREE Study Investigators et al [2020]. Efficacy and safety of suprachoroidal CLS-TA for macular edema secondary to non-infectious uveitis: Phase 3 randomized trial. *Ophthalmol.* 127(7): 948–955.

23. Dag MY, Afrashi F, Nalcaci S, Mentes J, Akkin C [2019]. The efficacy of "IOL-Vip revolution" telescopic intraocular lens in age-related macular degeneration cases with senile cataract. *Eur J Ophthalmol.* 29(6): 615–620.

24. Grzybowski A, Wang J, Mao F, Wang D, Wang N [2020]. Intraocular vision-improving devices in age-related macular degeneration. *Ann Transl Med.* 8(22): 1549.

Index

Note: Page number is *italics* indicate a figure and page numbers in **bold** indicate a table.

Printed and bound by CPI Group (UK) Ltd, Croydon, CR0 4YY

17/10/2024

01775698-0007